Health Promotion Evaluation Practices
in the Americas

Louise Potvin · David V. McQueen
Editors

With
Mary Hall · Ligia de Salazar
Laurie M. Anderson · Zulmira M. A. Hartz

Health Promotion Evaluation Practices in the Americas

Values and Research

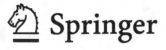
Springer

Editors
Louise Potvin
University of Montreal
Montreal
QC, Canada
louise.potvin@umontreal.ca

David McQueen
National Center for Chronic Disease
Atlanta
GA, USA
dvmcqueen@cdc.gov

ISBN: 978-1-4419-2726-2   e-ISBN: 978-0-387-79733-5
DOI: 10.1007/978-0-387-79733-5

Printed on acid-free paper

springer.com

Contributors

Denis Allard

Denis Allard holds a PhD in sociology from Université du Québec à Montréal. He is a researcher at the Montréal Public Health Department and with GRAVE-ARDEC, a research group on child welfare and development in the community, at Université de Montréal. His research interests include public planning, monitoring and program evaluation, methodologies of participation and figurative thinking.

Laurie M. Anderson

Laurie Anderson, PhD, MPH, conducts systematic reviews for evidence synthesis to inform public health practice and policy recommendations of the U.S. Task Force on Community Preventive Services. Content areas include public health nutrition, obesity prevention and control, and sociocultural determinants of health inequalities. Dr. Anderson serves on the Advisory Group to the Cochrane Collaboration Health Promotion & Public Health Field. She is a scientist with the U.S. Centers for Disease Control & Prevention and an affiliate professor in the Department of Epidemiology, School of Public Health, University of Washington, Seattle.

Juan Carlos Aneiros Fernandez

Juan Carlos Aneiros Fernandez is the coordinator of the Permanent Education nucleus of the Center of Studies Research and Documentation on Healthy Cities – (CEPEDOC Cidades Saudáveis) and researcher in the evaluation area, since 2003. The Center is in the process of being recognized as a Collaborating Center of the World Health Organization. He has a degree in Social Sciences from the School of Philosophy of the University of Sao Paulo (USP), Brazil and is now a doctoral student in Public Health – Health Promotion area – at the School of Public Health, University of Sao Paulo.

Angèle Bilodeau

Angèle Bilodeau holds a PhD in applied human sciences from Université de Montréal. She is a researcher at the Montréal Public Health Department and professor in the Department of Social and Preventive Medicine at Université de Montréal. She is also a researcher with the Centre de recherche Léa-Roback sur les inégalités sociales de la santé de Montréal, with the Chair in Community Approaches and Health Inequalities and with GRAVE-ARDEC, a research group on child welfare and development in the community, at Université de Montréal. Her research interests include public and participatory planning, action in partnership and social innovation, inter-organisation collaborations, intersectoral action and public/community collaborations in public program.

Sherri Bisset
Sherri Bisset just completed her PhD in Public Health (Health promotion option) at the Université de Montréal. Her thesis presents a study of the implementation of a nutrition education program in the school setting using the sociology of translation as a theoretical framework to understand how the nutrition interventionists negotiate their own health promotion goals with education actors. She is continuing her research training with a post doctorate fellowship in Education where she will study the social context of the school as a health determinant. Health promotion and education in schools is an area of research which she aims to develop.

Regina Bodstein
Regina Bodstein is Professor of Social Science and Health in the Department of Social Science at the National School of Public Health (ENSP), Fundação Oswaldo Cruz, Rio de Janeiro, Brazil. She trained as a Post-Doctoral research fellow in health promotion evaluation at the University of Montreal, Canada, 2005. She has been coordinator of the evaluation project of Sustainable and Integrated Local Development – Manguinhos in collaboration with Health Promotion in Action Project (Canada/Brazil, 2003). She is currently the ENSP coordination of Brazil-Canada project "Intersectoral Action for Health: Health Promotion as Strategy for Sustainable Local Development". Her main areas of interest include health promotion practices, and Health Family Program in Brazil and the theory and qualitative methodology in health promotion practice and evaluation.

Margaret Cargo
Margaret Cargo is senior lecturer in the School of Health Sciences, University of South Australia in Adelaide, with adjunct appointments in the Department of Psychiatry, McGill University and the McGill affiliated, Douglas Mental Health University Institute in Montréal. For the last 15 years, she has applied the principles of participatory research to the process evaluation of health promotion and disease prevention interventions in marginalized populations. She seeks to integrate this practical experience with social theory and method to advance the understanding of change processes and "best processes" in complex participatory interventions.

Jean-Louis Denis
Jean-Louis Denis, PhD, is Director of the Interdisciplinary Health Research Group, Professor at the Health Administration Department. He holds a CHSRF/CIHR Chair/Professorship on the transformation and governance of health care organizations at the Université de Montréal. He has taught for more than twenty years, the transformation of health organizations and systems to health managers and researchers. Author of many scientific publications on strategic change, leadership and regulation of health organizations, he pursues research on the regionalization and integration of health care, primary care strategy and the role of scientific

evidence in the adoption of clinical and managerial innovations. He is a member of the Royal Society of Canada and member of the advisory committee of CIHR's Institute of Health Services and Policy Research. He was the academic coordinator of the FORCES/EXTRA initiative from 2003 to 2007, a training program which aims at developing Canada's health managers' competencies in research use.

Ana Cláudia Figueiró

Ana Cláudia Figueiró is a nutritionist-hygienist, with an MSc in Public Health Nutrition from the Federal University of Pernambuco. She is a researcher and coordinator of the Group of Studies of Evaluation in Health (GEAS) of the Infantile Maternal Institute of Pernambuco (IMIP) in Recife, Brazil. She has also been the executive director of Education and Communication in Health of the State General Office of Health in Pernambuco; manager of the Coordination of Evaluation of the Alimentary Safety's and Combat the Hunger of the Extraordinary Ministry of Federal Government and technical consultant of the Coordination of Monitoring and Evaluation of the Department of Basic Attention in Brazilian Ministry of Health. She is also active in and, co-author of publications in other areas on Public Health: health promotion; popular education; evaluation capacity building and in evaluation of institutionalized programs and policies.

Maria Cristina Franceschini

Maria Cristina Franceschini is a consultant with the Sustainable Development and Environmental Health Unit of the Pan American Health Organization (PAHO) in Washington, DC. She has been working with PAHO's Healthy Municipalities, Cities and Communities Initiative since May, 2003. Prior to this position, she worked as a consultant for the World Bank, Social Development Unit/HIV/AIDS program, and for the World Bank Institute, Health, Nutrition and Population team. She has also worked with World Food Program in Cape Verde, and the Johns Hopkins School of Public Health. She holds a degree in anthropology and a master's degree in public health and social and behavioral interventions.

Nicholas Freudenberg

Nicholas Freudenberg is Distinguished Professor of Public Health and Social Psychology at Hunter College and the Graduate Center of City University of New York and Director of the City University of New York's Doctoral Program in Public Health. Freudenberg's research focuses on the social determinants of the health of urban populations. For the past 15 years, he has implemented and evaluated interventions to reduce drug use, HIV risk and recidivism among young people leaving New York City jails. He is also lead editor of *Cities and the Health of the Public* (Vanderbilt Press, 2006), a synthesis of recent scholarship on how city living affects health. More recently, Freudenberg has investigated how the alcohol, automobile, tobacco, firearms, food and pharmaceutical industries contribute to socioeconomic and racial/ethnic disparities in health and the role of public health advocacy in modifying health damaging corporate practices.

Katherine Frohlich

Katherine Frohlich is trained in Political Science and Public Health. She is Assistant Professor with the Département de médecine sociale et préventive, Université de Montréal, Research Associate with the Manitoba Centre for Health Policy, the Groupe de recherche interdisciplinaire en santé (GRIS), as well as the Centre de recherche Léa Roback sur les inégalités sociales de santé. Her research interests include social inequalities in health-related practices, social theory in social epidemiology and health promotion and the sociology of smoking. She currently holds CIHR funding to undertake a comparative Montreal/Vancouver study of the social context of smoking among youth and the need for reflexivity among tobacco control practitioners. She also holds pilot funding for a large-scale longitudinal survey that she and colleagues at the Centre Léa Roback are developing to examine social inequalities in smoking in neighbourhoods across Montreal.

Sylvie Gendron

Sylvie Gendron is Associate Professor in the Faculty of Nursing at Université de Montréal, Canada. Her current research focuses on the evaluation of a multi-system health promotion initiative for young parents in Québec and on nurses' health promotion practices in primary health care. Through her research, she collaborates in the creation of participatory spaces to engage with diverse actors (health professionals, community workers, decision-makers and representatives of program users) in order to ensure that her work is consistent with practice and program development issues. Her ongoing interest is to contribute to the methodology of participatory tools and approaches that are conducive to knowledge development and practice for the health of socially vulnerable groups.

Mita Giacomini

Mita Giacomini is a Professor in the Department of Clinical Epidemiology and Biostatistics, Director of the PhD Program in Health Policy, and a member of the Centre for Health Economics and Policy Analysis at McMaster University, Hamilton, Canada. Her research interests include ethical and political reasoning in health technology assessment, healthcare rationing, and the role of values and ethics in Canadian policy making. She has provided consultation and service to several local, provincial, national and international health agencies in areas related to technology assessment, resource allocation, and health policy.

Carmelle Goldberg

Carmelle Goldberg is a candidate in the PhD in Public Health program (Health Promotion option) at Université de Montréal. She is interested in meta evaluation and the role of evaluation in the improvement of community development programs.

Mary Hall

Mary Hall is a Program Analyst at the National Center for Chronic Disease Prevention and Health Promotion, U.S. Centers for Disease Control and Prevention, Atlanta, Georgia. Her interest areas are mainly capacity-building in health promotion evaluation at the community level, and strengthening organizational capacity in evaluation. She holds a master's degree in public health in behavioral sciences and health education.

Zulmira Hartz

Zulmira Hartz, MD, MSc and PhD in Public Health from Université de Montréal, is a researcher (retired) at Epidemiology Department at the National School of Public Health (ENSP/Fiocruz) in Rio de Janeirao, Brazil. Major posts held include Director of the Department of Epidemiology of Rio de Janeiro State, Vice-Director and Teaching Coordinator of ENSP, and Dean for Graduated Studies at Fiocruz. Guest professor at the Department of Social and Preventive Medicine, Université de Montréal (2004–2006), she is an associate researcher of the Interdisciplinary Health Research Group (Montreal University), and in the Group for Studies on Health Evaluation (GEAS), of the Maternal and Infant Institute of Pernambuco. As evaluation advisor, she has been giving advice to several national health programs and policies. She is an active member of the American, Canadian and European Evaluation Associations, as well as of the Brazilian Association of Collective Health (Abrasco).

Alvaro Hideyoshi Matida

Alvaro Hideyoshi Matida MD, PhD in Public Health/Epidemiology from the Escola National de Saúde Pública FIOCRUZ, ENSP, Brazil; Director of HIV/AIDS Control Unit from the Health Department of the State of Rio de Janeiro (1985–1997); Deputy Executive Director of the Brazilian Association on Collective Health (ABRASCO_1997–2003). Currently, he is (1) Executive Director of the Brazilian Association on Collective Health; (2) Associated researcher in the project "Intersectoral Action for Health: Health Promotion as an strategy for local development" (Canadian International Development Agency/Brazilian Cooperation Agency); (3) *Co-editor of the Electronic Journal of Communication Information and Innovation in Health – RECIIS*; (4) Member of the Ethical Committee of the Technical Public Health School/ Fiocruz. He is active in the areas on Public Health; International Health; HIV/Aids program development and Health program evaluation. Over the past years he has published articles in these areas.

Felicia Schanche Hodge

Felicia Hodge (Dr. P.H.) a member of the Wailaki tribe in Northern California, holds a joint position as Professor of Health Services in the School of Public Health and Professor in the School of Nursing. She teaches courses in Nursing Health-Related Theories, Research Methods, and Qualitative Research Methods for Indigenous Populations. Dr. Hodge received her MPH and DrPH from the University of California at Berkeley. Dr. Hodge's research is in the area of chronic health conditions among American Indian and indigenous populations. Current studies examine the cultural constructs of cancer symptoms among Southwest American Indians and test an intervention to alleviate barriers to self-management of cancer symptoms, environmental management, and illness beliefs. Past projects tested diabetes, cervical cancer, breast, nutrition and smoking cessation interventions among tribes in the Northern Plains, Minnesota, and California regions. Dr. Hodge is a member of the

National Institute of Nursing Research National Advisory Council, UCLA Graduate Council, is the director of the Center for American Indian/Indigenous Research and Education, and is Chair of the UCLA American Indian Studies Interdepartmental Program.

Jeremiah Hurley

Jeremiah Hurley is a Professor in the Departments of Economics and Clinical Epidemiology and Biostatistics, and Associate Director of the Centre for Health Economics and Policy Analysis at McMaster University, Hamilton, Canada. He received his PhD in Economics from the University of Wisconsin at Madison. He has worked extensively on issues of resource allocation in health care, particularly needs-based funding methods and the effects of alternative health care financing arrangements. He is currently engaged in research empirically investigating the public's understanding of equity in resource allocation and in assessing equity in the utilization of health care services in Canada.

Marjorie MacDonald

Marjorie MacDonald has a background in nursing, public health and health education. She is currently an Associate Professor in the School of Nursing at the University of Victoria, in Victoria, British Columbia. Her research interests include the implementation and evaluation of health promotion and public health initiatives, school and adolescent health, adolescent health literacy, and the integration of public health and primary health care. All of her research is collaborative, with some projects more participatory than others. A common theme in her research is theorizing practice and processes inherent in the phenomena of interest.

David McQueen

David McQueen is a Senior Biomedical Research Scientist at CDC in Atlanta, Georgia. For ten years he has been the Associate Director for Global Health Promotion in the Office of the Director at the National Center for Chronic Disease Prevention and Health Promotion (NCCDPHP); prior to1998 Director of the Division of Adult and Community Health at NCCDPHP, as well as Chief of the nationwide Behavioral Risk Factor Surveillance System. Prior to CDC he was Professor and Founding Director of the Research Unit in Health and Behavioral Change at the University of Edinburgh, Scotland (1983–1992), and prior to that Associate Professor of Behavioral Sciences at the Johns Hopkins University School of Hygiene and Public Health in Baltimore. His Doctoral training was in behavioral sciences at Johns Hopkins University. He has an extensive record of presentations and publications in health promotion and evaluation. In recent years he has led in the development of behavioral risk factor surveillance systems globally and in the assessment of evaluation and effectiveness in health promotion. Currently he is president of the International Union for Health Promotion and Education (IUHPE), as well as leader of the IUHPE Global Program on Health Promotion Effectiveness.

Geneviève Mercille

Geneviève Mercille is a student in the Health Promotion option of the PhD program in Public Health at Université de Montréal. Before enrolling in this program she has worked several years as a community nutritionist in Aboriginal communities in Québec, Canada before completing a masters in Community Health. Her interest for research synthesis focuses on how to make it more relevant and appropriate for health promotion practitioners.

Elizabeth Moreira dos Santos

Elizabeth Moreira dos Santos, MD (1974), MPh (1986), PhD in Community Health from University of Illinois – Urbana Champaign (1993) is a full researcher at the Department of Endemic Diseases at the National School of Public Health (ENSP/FIOCRUZ) in Rio de Janeiro, Brazil. Currently she teaches three graduate courses in program evaluation, and coordinates the first Professional Master Program in Health Evaluation in the country. This course has been adapted and it is currently implemented in Ethiopia in Collaboration with Tulane University and the CDC. She has coordinated and developed several national evaluation of endemic diseases control programs such as malaria, HIV, Tuberculosis, Leprosy. Her academic experience involves advising around 30 Master thesis and 10 PhD dissertations. She published nine book chapters, seven books as author and editor and 16 peer-reviewed journal articles. She is active in the areas of endemic disease program development and program evaluation with national and international experience especially in African countries such as Ethiopia, Guiné-Bissau and Angola.

Jennifer Mullett

Jennifer Mullett is a Community Psychologist and an Adjunct Assistant Professor in the faculty of Human and Social Development at the University of Victoria, Victoria, British Columbia. She works collaboratively with government and non-governmental agencies to implement and evaluate interventions at the community level. Her former positions include: Research Scholar in Community Based Research supported by the British Columbia Health Research Foundation and Director of Research and Evaluation for the Ministry of Health. Her current research projects include: the reorganization of mental health services for children, articulating an ecological approach to create healthy, literate communities, documenting the implementation of a multi-disciplinary program to build community competence in parenting skills and developing research methods appropriate for community action projects with the Queen Alexandra Foundation.

Blake Poland

Blake Poland is Associate Professor in the Department of Public Health Sciences at the University of Toronto. He is currently the Director of the Collaborative Program in Community Development at the University of Toronto, where he was the Director of the MHSc Program in Health Promotion from 1999 to 2007. Drawing on a combination of critical social theory and qualitative research methods, his recent and ongoing research foci include the settings approach (*Settings for Health Promotion*, Sage, 2000), hospital-community collaboration, environmental health promotion, and community development as an arena of practice for health professionals.

Louise Potvin

Louise Potvin completed her doctorate in Public Health from Université de Montréal and post doctoral training in program evaluation with one of the pioneer figures in the field, Donald T. Campbell. She is currently professor at the Department of Social and Preventive Medicine, Université de Montreal and Scientific director of the Centre de recherche Léa-Roback sur les inégalités sociales de santé de Montréal. She holds the CHSRF/CIHR Chair on Community Approaches and Health Inequalities. This Chair aims at documenting how public health interventions in support to local social development contribute to the reduction of health inequalities in urban settings. Her main research interests are the evaluation of community health promotion programs and how local social environments are conducive to health. She was a member of the WHO Working Group on the evaluation of health promotion. She is a Fellow of the Canadian Academy of Health Sciences.

Marilyn Rice

Marilyn Rice is the Regional Advisor in Healthy Municipalities and Urban Health for the Pan American Health Organization (PAHO), the Regional Office for the Americas of the World Health Organization (WHO). She has worked for PAHO for 15 years and the Global Office of WHO for 7 years. She has also held the position of Project Director of the National Resource Center for Prevention of Perinatal Abuse of Alcohol and Other Drugs and Branch Chief of the Perinatal Branch for the US Center for Substance Abuse Prevention (part of the U.S. Department of Health and Human Services). Ms. Rice is also the Vice President for the North American Regional Office of the International Union for Health Promotion and Education (IUHPE) and the Chair of the International and Cross-Cultural Health Special Interest Group of the Society for Public Health Education (SOPHE). She holds a degree in sociology and masters training in public health and health education.

Ligia de Salazar

Ligia de Salazar holds a doctorate in Epidemiology from McGill University, Montreal, Canada, a Masters degree in Community Health from Liverpool University, England; and in Health Administration from Universidad del Valle, Colombia. She is senior professor and researcher of the School of Public Health, Universidad del Valle, Cali, Colombia, and director of the Center for Evaluation of Public Health Policy and Technology, CEDETES, at the same University. She is Leader and Regional Coordinator of the Latin American Regional Project of Health Promotion Effectiveness, promoted by the International Union for Health Promotion, IUHPE. Dr. Salazar is Principal investigator and coordinator of national and international projects as well as consultant for several institutions, invited as temporary professor in several Latin American Universities. Dr. Salazar has been member of different committees and scientific associations as well as member of Advisory Committee on Health Research, CAIS, PAHO. She has authored six books, and several scientific articles about local development, surveillance, evaluation in public health and health promotion in line with her research and academic interests.

June Strickland

June Strickland is Cherokee and an Associate Professor in Psychosocial and Community Health in the School of Nursing at the University of Washington, Seattle. She is a member of the National Cancer Institute Native Research Network and has been conducting research with Native communities for over twenty years. Her research focus has been in advancing the understanding of transcultural issues in prevention. While she has conducted both qualitative and quantitative research, her major aim has been to lay the foundation for evidence based intervention for Indian people through her work with rural tribal communities in the Pacific Northwest using qualitative research methodologies. She is committed to tribal sovereignty and building community capacity through models that assure tribal empowerment such as community based participatory research.

Lillian Tom-Orme

Lillian Tom-Orme, PhD, MPH, RN, FAAN, a member of the Dine' or Navajo Nation, was born and raised on the Navajo Indian reservation in New Mexico. Dine' was her first language and she remains fluent in her native tongue. Dr. Tom-Orme is Research Assistant Professor in the Department of Internal Medicine, University of Utah School of Medicine and has adjunct appointments in the Departments of Oncological Science and Pediatrics. Dr. Tom-Orme holds graduate degrees in transcultural nursing and public health from the Nursing, University of Utah. Dr. Tom-Orme has been active in several local and national committees related to the health of American Indians. Consistent with her beliefs in increasing the number of ethnic students involved in research, she serves as mentor to many students throughout the country. Dr. Tom-Orme chaired the Cultural Diversity Committee for the University of Utah College of Nursing. She is a consultant and author in transcultural nursing and health. She also is active in the work of the local Indian Walk-in Center serving as consultant in its Special Diabetes Program for urban-based American Indians. Her current research includes patterns of cancer care and a national public health study of chronic conditions among a cohort of American Indian/Alaska Natives.

Marcia Faria Westphal

Marcia Faria Westphal was Vice- President for Latin America of the International Union for Health Promotion and Education from 1998 to 2007. She was also vice Dean of the School of Public Health of the University of Sao Paulo, from 1998 to 2001. She is currently Professor of the Department of Health Practices of the School of Public Health of the University of Sao Paulo, Brazil, and President of the Center of Studies Research and Documentation on Healthy Cities – (CEPEDOC CIDADES SAUDÁVEIS – The Center is in the process of being recognized as a Collaborating Center of World Health Organization). She has a degree in Political and Social Sciences from PUC (Pontifícia Universidade Católica) in Sao Paulo (Brazil) and master's degree and doctorate in Public Health from the University of Sao Paulo. She has been publishing and advising master and doctoral students in the Health Promotion area, since 1988.

Contents

Part III   Aligning Evaluation with Health Promotion Principles: Experiences from the Americas

Chapter 1
Introduction. Aligning Evaluation Research and Health Promotion Values: Practices from the Americas

Louise Potvin, David V. Mcqueen, and Mary Hall

A little more than 20 years after its birth, marked by the launching of its foundational document at an international WHO conference in Ottawa (World Health Organization, 1986), health promotion appears to be well and alive. Many western countries have now incorporated health promotion into mainstream public health practice. In Australia, for example, health promotion is defined as one of the core public health functions (National Public Health Partnership, 2000). The "Health on equal terms", Swedish national public health program (Swedish National Committee for Public Health, 2000), is clearly a deliberate attempt to operationalize and implement values such as equity and action principles such as intersectoral action, spelled out in the Ottawa Charter (World Health Organization, 1986). In addition to this institutionalization in western states where it was an essential element of the strategy to meet the Alma Ata declaration goal of "Health for All in the year 2000" (Kickbusch, 2003), health promotion is now spreading in developing countries where it is increasingly conceived as an appropriate response to the enormous task of addressing the challenges associated with the epidemiological transition from infectious to chronic disease (Reddy, 2002) and from rural to urban life (Neiman & Hall, 2007). A decade ago, a leading scholar from the field of epidemiology characterized health promotion as the third revolution of public health (Breslow, 1999). Recently, the Bangkok Charter (World Health Organization, 2005) reiterated the relevance and appropriateness of health promotion to face the challenges of a globalized world. Clearly, what started in 1986 as a regional reform for public health has become a strong global current that shapes and orients public health practice (Kickbusch, 2007).

In the Continuity of the Work by WHO-EURO Working Group on Health Promotion Evaluation

Associated with this mainstreaming and expansion of health promotion is an increasing demand for it to prove its worth. During the past 10 years various initiatives

L. Potvin
Department of Social and Preventive Medicine, Université de Montreal, Montreal, QC, Canada

L. Potvin, D. McQueen (eds.), *Health Promotion Evaluation Practices in the Americas*,
DOI: 10.1007/978-0-387-79733-5_1, © Springer Science+Business Media, LLC 2008

have been launched in western countries in order to demonstrate that interventions designed along the strategies of the Ottawa Charter can impact population health. From the Centers for Disease Control in the United States (Zaza, Briss, & Harris, 2005), to the International Union for Health Promotion and Education (McQueen, & Jones, 2007a), to the Cochrane collaboration (Waters et al., 2006), various groups and organizations have come to the conclusion that much more primary evaluation research should be undertaken in order for health promotion to show its actual value as a public health approach to population health intervention (McQueen & Jones, 2007b). To answer this call, however, researchers and evaluators have to take into account many of the specificities that define health promotion. Outlining many of those challenges, the WHO-EURO Working Group on Health Promotion Evaluation concluded that failing to consider the specificities of health promotion in the design and implementation of evaluation research may lead to inaccurate results and eventually to misguided policy decisions about population health interventions (Rootman et al., 2001). Finally, the recent debate about the nature of evidence that is needed to feed evidence-informed public health decision-making (McQueen, 2001; Rychetnik, Frommer, Hawe, & Shiell, 2002) as well as the best practice and evidence-based practice movements in health promotion (Ziglio, 1997) have reactivated the need for an in-depth reflection and discussion on whether or not health promotion evaluation should be approached any differently from any other evaluation endeavor and if yes, what and how pitfalls should be avoided (Potvin, Gendron, Bilodeau, & Chabot, 2005).

Early attempts at developing a perspective on health promotion evaluation were linked to health education and were synthesized in two books (Green & Lewis; 1986; Windsor, Baranowski, Clark & Cutter, 1984). These publications adopted a post-positivist Campbellian perspective on evaluation founded in a quasi-experimental approach to evaluation, in which random assignment of subjects into different study arms corresponding to being exposed or not to the program, or versions of it, is seen as the gold standard for establishing causal relationships between an intervention and an effect (Shadish, Cook, & Leviton, 1991). In line with the quasi-experimental paradigm, early evaluators in health promotion primarily defined evaluation as a methodological tool for establishing internally valid causal links between an intervention and its measured effects, advocating for strong investigator control over the parameters of the intervention that was to be conceived as a fixed package. Context was mainly conceptualized as a source of confounding to be controlled for. These pioneer works established a strong affiliation between health promotion evaluation and a methodologically oriented tradition of evaluation that emphasizes the importance of an objective appraisal of interventions and primacy of internal validity and causal reasoning as epistemological tools to achieve this goal. What was missing in this import of a Campbellian thinking into the field of health education/health promotion, however, was Campbell's critical discussion on the need for closure or quasi-closure for establishing causal relations in real-life situations (Cook & Campbell, 1979) and on the inherently fuzzy nature of the interventions to be evaluated, that is interventions are complex treatment packages, the components of which are acting in synergistic manner (Campbell, 1986). The failure of the first American community prevention projects to demonstrate positive effects, specifically in the domain of heart health, led several top epidemiologists to question the adequacy of the experimental/quasi-experimental paradigm for the evaluation of health promotion and prevention projects (Susser, 1995; Winkleby, 1994).

The first project clearly addressing evaluation issues specific to the field of health promotion was the work of the WHO-EURO Working Group on Health Promotion Evaluation that was active from 1995 to 1998 and which produced a policy statement (WHO European Working Group on Health Promotion Evaluation, 1998), a practical guide (Springett, 1998) and a book (Rootman et al., 2001). Formed by scholars from Europe and North America, this group developed a perspective for health promotion evaluation that (1) calls for policy makers to fund evaluation of health promotion projects, (2) is broader in concern and methods than the traditional quasi-experimental approach and (3) advocates for opening up the field to a variety of actors outside the scientific world. Despite these features that situate this work as more aligned to the principles underlying the Ottawa Charter than what had been previously published, the outcome of this working group nevertheless reiterates the primacy of methodological issues in defining the contour and articulating the content of health promotion evaluation. It also failed to develop a clear and coherent vision, as well as a critical appraisal of the role of evaluation with regard to the evolution of the field of health promotion. Further, because of a highly delayed publication schedule, much of the impact was reduced as the debate about evaluation and evidence had moved on.

In the meanwhile, more recent endeavors in health promotion evaluation were all concerned with the issue of effectiveness evaluation. Four projects, international in scope, need to be acknowledged: (1) the Cochrane collaboration group on health promotion; (2) the CDC Community preventive services synthesis; (3) the IUHPE European work on the effectiveness of health promotion; and (4) the IUHPE Global project on health promotion effectiveness.

Some of these projects are ongoing; however, most have pursued either or both of the following goals. The first was to estimate overall benefits, both in qualitative and in quantitative terms, of public investments in health promotion. This was the primary goal of the two IUHPE projects. In its first report to the European Commission, the IUHPE "provides a summary of the main evidence, and puts forward a case for ensuring that Health Promotion is properly resourced. This will enable Health Promotion to play its full part in the public health policy framework which is currently being shaped by the European Commission" (International Union for Health Promotion and Education, 1999, p. i). Later, in their first report on the IUHPE Global Program on Health Promotion Effectiveness, McQueen & Jones (2007b), taking stock of the field of health promotion evaluation, raised three issues that limit our capacity to estimate the overall value of investments in health promotion: there is a wide variety of methods used in health promotion evaluation; those evaluations are often conducted internally by people involved in program delivery; and there are not enough evaluation studies conducted as yet to produce any clear evidence. Such a goal clearly establishes evaluation as a management instrument to support decision-making about health promotion as a general item in the gigantic hypertrophied health sector budget or about specific interventions.

The second goal was to extract from the available reports of health promotion writ large (i.e., mostly including integrated prevention projects), those activities, programs and interventions that seem to be effective in order to group them in user-friendly retrieval systems. It is this kind of goal that is actively pursued both in Cochrane collaborations and in the CDC Guide to preventive services. The intention is to provide authoritative arguments in favor of interventions in order to improve specific health promotion practices by providing data on the outcomes empirically associated with a variety of practices. "The Community Guide summarizes what is known about the effectiveness, economic efficiency, and feasibility of interventions to promote community health and prevent disease. The Task Force on Community Preventive Services makes recommendations for the use of various interventions based on the evidence gathered in the rigorous and systematic scientific reviews of published studies conducted by the review teams of the Community Guide. The findings from the reviews are published in peer-reviewed journals and also made available on this Internet website" (Guide to Community Preventive Services, 2008). In order to contribute to this goal, evaluation is implicitly defined as a tool to improve health promotion through coding, standardization and dissemination of its best practices.

In most of these endeavors the role of health promotion evaluation has always been implicitly or explicitly situated as being "external" to health promotion itself. In most instances, because the role of evaluation is often conceived as instrumental for decisions made outside of health promotion practice, the latter is also objectified. The relationship between evaluation activities and health promotion practice is one in which the former objectively studied the latter. It is generally understood that, in most instances, evaluation does not have a significant role in the implementation and effectiveness of the programs being evaluated. While in some instances, mainly associated with process evaluation, it is acknowledged that local health promotion practice can be transformed by specific evaluation, the reverse is never considered, mainly because when conceived primarily as a tool kit of scientific methods and techniques, evaluation cannot be influenced by its object of investigation.

Purpose of This Book

In response to the limited capacity demonstrated to date by evaluation endeavors to contribute solid evidence to both the overall value of health promotion and to some of its specific interventions, the purpose of this book is to explore the specificity of health promotion evaluation, developing the argument that, over and above a methodological kit, evaluation is a practice that seeks to transform the social reality of interventions (Schwandt, 2005). This book answers the question whether health promotion evaluation should be approached differently from other evaluation endeavors, with a clear *yes*. Contributors, who are either evaluators or health promotion practitioners from the three Americas, were asked to reflect on how it can be done and the challenges associated with such an enterprise and to report on the practical solutions they implemented in real health promotion evaluation projects.

All contributors to the book are associated with health promotion evaluation in North, Central or South America. Narrowing down our discussion of health promotion evaluation to experiences from the New World was a deliberate choice. We think that it gives us the opportunity to present a diverse yet still very coherent perspective on health promotion evaluation. Diverse because it encompasses realities of countries that represent all stages of economic development and a variety of public health issues. Diverse also because contributors are from various cultural backgrounds, bringing together the richness of the Latin and Anglo-Saxon understanding of the world.

Taking up the task where the WHO-EURO book of 2001 has left it, this book aims to explore how health promotion's unique characteristics influence the conduct of evaluation research. In line with the most recent development in the field of evaluation our definition of evaluation encompasses much more than research design and methods to collect and analyze scientific data. We conceive evaluation as a social and research practice, which, like all professional practices, represents rational attempts to transform or reproduce the world. Having programs and interventions as objects of inquiry, evaluators' practices shape the way decision makers and public policy advisors conceive programs. This is one of the great lessons of the decisive work of Carol Weiss and later Michael Patton on the utilization of evaluation results.

We think that health promotion evaluation in the Americas is unique and challenging enough so as to require a book in which evaluators would describe, and reflect on, their way of doing evaluation: their evaluation practice (Schwandt, 2005). The main challenge of health promotion evaluation rests chiefly with the openly value-oriented nature of health promotion. In our discussion of the Ottawa Charter, the founding document of health promotion, we have a tendency to retain only that it proposes five strategies of action for health promotion: creating supportive environments; building public health policy; strengthening community actions; developing personal skills; and reorienting health systems. We rarely mention that it also proposes a set of values and principles that would characterize the way these strategies should be implemented. Indeed, health promotion has spelled out a set of humanistic values and principles to guide public health intervention.

In our reading of the WHO-EURO Working Group on Health Promotion Evaluation (1999) report on health promotion evaluation, we identify seven values and principles that seem to form the core of health promotion. Two of these values, participation and empowerment, are more largely associated with health promotion than the others. A closer examination of the Ottawa Charter would show that values of equity and sustainability are also very much present as well as principles of intersectoral action, multi-strategy and contextualism, understood as embedding interventions into local circumstances. For some people, values and principles are incompatible with the notion of scientific rigor and health promotion should therefore be evaluated with the sole preoccupation of implementing rigorous methods.

Like many evaluators preoccupied with the use of their evaluation results, the editors and contributors of this book do not believe that scientific rigor in evaluation is incompatible with humanitarian values and principles. After all, what is evaluation about if it is not about value? And the past three decades of work in the domains of sociology and anthropology of sciences (Campbell, 1984; Latour, 2001 Toulmin, 2001) have shown that any scientific project is crowded with arbitrary decisions that more or less impact on the methodological rigor and on the validity of the results. In our conception, those decisions are characteristic of the scientific practice associated with certain fields and disciplines. We further argue that the practice of health promotion evaluators should be informed by the same values as that of health promotion practitioners, and this is exactly what this book is about. We first want to demonstrate that despite, and probably in part because of, its rigor, evaluation is a practice that can be informed and shaped by the same values and principles that underlie health promotion.

This project was conceived by a group of practitioners and evaluators from South and North America who believe that there is something distinctive to be described about the region of the Americas. The manner in which health promotion is practiced, and the challenges encountered in evaluating health promotion in the context of the Americas deserves a unique space for reflection, and the editors aim to provide structure for this examination through this book. The six editors, who hail from Brazil, Colombia, the United States and Canada, began meeting in 2003 to engage in a dialogue about whether there are differences in this region compared to the rest of the world, and what these differences might imply for the practice of health promotion, the practice of evaluation, and what might be learned from this reflection. Certainly the various professional histories and practical experiences of the editors have shaped their beliefs about the uniqueness of the region, as well as the forces shaping the fields of health promotion and evaluation. Yet, all agreed that the values and principles examined are essential elements for the practice of evaluation as it relates to health promotion in the Americas. Once these values were chosen, the editorial group searched the region for practitioners in the field whose work reflects these values in practice and selected those few who appear in this book.

Contributions to the book were written in the author's native language and were translated for the book. In some cases native Portuguese speakers paired with native French speakers, and the translation process has an inevitable impact on the process and the product. Translators and editors made monumental efforts to maintain as much of the text as close to literal translation as possible. However, some meaning has inevitably changed from the original due to the necessity to present the book in a single language. Through the process of editing, the editors have discovered that the cultural mindset going with the language is of ultimate importance, and every attempt was made to maintain this mindset.

The Book

The book is constructed in three parts. In the first part, as editors, we present and defend our conception of health promotion as a value- and knowledge-driven enterprise and of health promotion evaluation as a practice whose underlying values could be aligned with those of its object. In the second part we discuss four nexus of an evaluation practice where this alignment of values and principles with health promotion seems to be more crucial. Finally for the third part, we asked contributors who have developed a practice of evaluators or health promotion evaluators to analyze and reflect on their practice and to draw the lessons on what they do and implement to realize this alignment between their evaluation practice and the values and principles of health promotion.

The third section of the book, which provides a series of chapters that reflect on the practice of evaluation, is meant to illustrate the challenges to, and lessons learned from, evaluating according to certain health promotion values. For example, the chapter by Strickland et al. demonstrates the challenges posed by participation, as well as the necessity to acknowledge cultural values in the evaluation process in order to increase empowerment. For some of the values, namely context and equity, only a single chapter is presented exploring these values through the process of evaluation. This may perhaps reflect the difficulty that exploring these values presents in true health promotion practice. Authors in this section were given the charge of describing their evaluations in a manner not often seen, which calls for a reflection on the practice, rather than a presentation of the results. Authors were asked to reflect upon the process of evaluation as a social practice, which is value-laden, and that is intended to reinforce the values of health promotion. We believe that the collection of analyses presented here currently cannot be found elsewhere.

We think that a wide variety of audiences will be attracted by this book. First of all, graduate students will be able to develop their own thinking and critical appraisal of health promotion evaluation practices. Health promotion practitioners will find inspiration and arguments in their dealing with evaluators. Public health decision makers and policy people will be interested in examining how this alignment of scientific rigor with practical values and principles is possible and can be operated. Finally, we think that evaluators in all fields of evaluation will be interested in our work, perhaps particularly those interested in the Americas. In the late 1990s, the New York-based Aspen Institute published two books that dealt with the practical challenges of conducting community-based project evaluations. These books were the product of the reflection conducted by the Roundtable on Comprehensive Community Initiative for Children and Families appointed by the Institute "with the goal of helping resolve the lack of fit that exists between current evaluation methods and the need to learn from and judge the effectiveness of comprehensive community initiatives" (Connell, Kubisch, Schorr, & Weiss, 1995, p. viii). The outcome of the work of this roundtable had a significant impact in the field of evaluation in that it explicitly positioned evaluation as a practice that affects the way social betterment interventions are planned and implemented. The two books from the Aspen Institute (Connell et al., 1995; Fulbright-Anderson, Kubisch, & Connell, 1998) are already more than ten years old. In the continuity of this work, the present book is an excellent example of the enormous potential for health promotion evaluation to lead the way to important innovations in the general field of evaluation.

References

Breslow, L. (1999). From disease prevention to health promotion. *JAMA, 281*, 1030–1033.

Campbell, D. T. (1984). Can we be scientific in applied social sciences? In R. F. Connor, D. G. Altman, & C. Jackson (Eds.), *Evaluation studies review annual, Vol 9* (pp. 26–48). Beverly Hills, CA: Sage.

Campbell, D. T. (1986). Relabeling internal and external validity for applied social scientists. *New Directions for Program Evaluation, 31*, 67–77.

Connell, J. P., Kubisch, A. C., Schorr, L. B., & Weiss, C. H. (Eds.) (1995). *New approaches to evaluating community initiatives. Concepts, methods, and context.* New York: Aspen Institute.

Cook, T. D., & Campbell, D. T. (1979). *Quasi experimentation: Design and analysis issues for field settings.* Boston: Houghton Mifflin.

Fulbright-Anderson, K., Kubisch, A. C., & Connell, J. P. (Eds.) (1998). *New approaches to evaluating community initiatives. Volume 2: Theory, measurement, and analysis.* New York: Aspen Institute.

Green, L. W., & Lewis, F. M. (1986). *Measurement and evaluation in health education and health promotion.* Palo Alto CA: Mayfield.

Guide to Community Preventive Services. (2008). *The community guide.* Retrieved in January 2008 from: www.thecommunityguide.org/about/

International Union for Health Promotion and Education. (1999). *The evidence in health promotion effectiveness. Shaping public health in a new Europe.* Part two. Evidence book. Paris: Jouve Composition & Impression.

Kickbusch, I. (2003). The contribution of the World Health Organization to a new public health and health promotion. *American Journal of Public Health, 93*, 383–388.

Kickbusch, I. (2007). Health promotion: Not a tree but a rhizome. In M. O'Neill, A. Pederson, S. Dupéré, & I. Rootman (Eds.), *Health promotion in Canada. Critical perspective* (pp. 363–366). Toronto: Canadian Scholar's Press.

Latour, B. (2001). *L'espoir de Pandore. Pour une version réaliste d el'activité scientifique.* Paris: La découverte.

McQueen, D.V. (2001). Strengthening the evidence base for health promotion. *Health Promotion International, 11*, 261–268.

McQueen, D. V. & Jones, C (Eds.) (2007a) *Global perspectives on health promotion effectiveness.* New York: Springer.

McQueen, D. V., & Jones, C. (2007b). Global perspective on health promotion effectiveness. An introduction. In D. V. McQueen, & C. Jones (Eds.), *Global perspectives on health promotion effectiveness* (pp. 3–11). New York: Springer.

National Public Health Partnership. (2000). *Public health practice in Australia today: A statement of core functions.* Downloaded in January 2008 from: http://www.nphp.gov.au/publications/phpractice/phprac.pdf

Neiman, A., & Hall, M. (2007). Urbanization and health promotion: Challenges and opportunities. In D. V. McQueen & C. Jones (Eds.), *Global perspectives on health promotion effectiveness* (pp. 201–224). New York: Springer.

Potvin, L., Gendron, S., Bilodeau, A., & Chabot, P. (2005). Integrating social theory into public health practice. *American Journal of Public Health, 95*, 591–595.

Reddy, S. (2002). Cardiovascular diseases in the developing countries: Dimension, determinants, dynamics and directions for public health action. *Public Health Nutrition, 5*, 231–237.

Rootman, I., Goodstadt, M., Hyndman, B., McQueen, D. V., Potvin, L., Springett, J., & Ziglio, E. (Eds.) (2001). *Evaluation in health promotion. Principles and perspectives.* Copenhagen: WHO Regional Publications, European Series, No. 92.

Rychetnik, L., Frommer, M., Hawe, P., & Shiell, A. (2002). Criteria for evaluating evidence on public health interventions. *Journal of Epidemiology and Community Health, 56*, 119–127.

Schwandt, T. A. (2005). The centrality of practice to evaluation. *American Journal of Evaluation, 26*, 95–105.

Shadish, W. R., Jr., Cook, T. D., & Leviton, L. C. L. (1991). *Foundations of program evaluation.* Thousand Oaks CA: Sage.

Springett, J. (1998). *Practical guidance on evaluating health promotion.* Copenhagen, WHO Regional Office for Europe, 1998 (unit document, Integrated Health Development).

Susser, M. (1995). The tribulation of trials – intervention in community. *American Journal of Public Health, 85,* 156–158.

Swedish National Committee for Public Health. (2000). *Health on equal terms. National goals for public health.* Stockholm: Fritzes Offentliga Publikationer.

Toulmin, S. (2001). *Return to reason.* Cambridge Mass: Harvard University Press.

Waters, E., Doyle, J., Jackson, N., Howes, F., Brunton, G., & Oakley, A. (2006) Evaluating the effectiveness of public health interventions: the role and activities of the Cochrane Collaboration. *Journal of Epidemiology and Community Health, 60,* 285–289.

Windsor, R. Baranowski, T., Clark, N., & Cutter, G. (1984). *Evaluation of health promotion, health education programs.* Mountain View: Mayfield.

Winkleby, M. (1994). The future of community-based cardiovascular disease intervention studies. *American Journal of Public Health, 84,* 1369–1372.

WHO European Working Group on Health Promotion Evaluation. (1998). *Health promotion evaluation: Recommendations to policy-makers.* Retrieved in January 2008 from: http://www.euro.who.int/document/e60706.pdf

World Health Organization. (1986). *The Ottawa Charter for health promotion.* Downloaded in January 2008 from: http://www.who.int/healthpromotion/conferences/previous/ottawa/en/

World Health Organization. (2005). *The Bangkok Charter for health promotion in a globalized world.* Retrieved in January 2008 from: http://www.who.int/healthpromotion/conferences/6gchp/bangkok_charter/en/

Zaza, S., Briss, P. A., Harris, K. W. (Eds.) (2005). *The guide to community preventive services. What works to promote health?* New York: Oxford University Press.

Ziglio, E. (1997). How to move towards evidence-based health promotion interventions. *Promotion & Education, IV,* 29–33.

Part I
Health Promotion Evaluation
in the Americas

Chapter 2
Health Promotion in the Americas: Divergent and Common Ground

Ligia de Salazar and Laurie M. Anderson

Practitioners and theorists in health promotion have tried to identify the conceptual basis and principles of practice that distinguish the health promotion field (McQueen, 2007a). Interchangeable use of the terms health promotion, social medicine, public health, collective health, disease prevention, and health protection suggests little distinction. Yet health promotion has distinct historical roots. Across the Americas, diverse political forces have shaped health promotion practice from North to South. Attempts to identify a universal set of principles of health promotion practice are confounded by the divergent sociocultural contexts in which health promotion occurs. In this chapter we explore some of these historical developments in health promotion across the Americas to see where shared ground exists and where differences emerge.

North American Development in Health Promotion

Most would agree that an international understanding of health promotion was solidified under the 1986 Ottawa Charter (WHO, 1986). Earlier work contributed to this culmination of convictions in the field of health promotion. The 1974 Lalonde Report, "A New Perspective on the Health of Canadians", set the stage by raising questions about the likelihood of achieving major gains in the health of Canadians by focusing solely on the biomedical sphere: e.g., physician services, hospital care, pharmaceuticals, medical technologies (Lalonde, 1974). A few years later the World Health Organization's International Conference on Primary Care again focused on the failure of medicine to address underlying determinants of health and health inequalities (WHO, 1978). The Declaration of Alma-Ata in 1978 affirmed that individuals and communities had the right to fully participate in their health care; that health is essential to sustained economic and social development; and that primary care should be universally available to reduce inequalities in health among developing and developed countries to achieve "health for all by 2000."

L. de Salazar
Universidad del Valle, Cali, Colombia

L. Potvin, D. McQueen (eds.), *Health Promotion Evaluation Practices in the Americas*,
DOI: 10.1007/978-0-387-79733-5_2, © Springer Science+Business Media, LLC 2008

U.S. Healthy People Objectives for the Nation

In the late 1970s, the release of a national agenda for disease prevention in "Promoting Health/Preventing Disease Objectives for a Nation" influenced health promotion in the United States (U.S. Department of Health and Human Services, 1980). This national agenda explicitly recognized the importance of lifestyle in promoting health. It was based on the recognition that the greatest potential for improving the health of the population lay in health promotion and disease prevention, rather than medical care, and it became the framework for public health practice in the United States. Two hundred and twenty-six specific, measurable health objectives were identified as targets for improvement in health status, risk reduction, public and professional awareness, health services and protective measures, and surveillance and evaluation. As a consequence of this new national focus, the field of health education gained prominence and provided impetus to the health promotion movement in the United States (Cottrell, 1999).

WHO-Europe Healthy Cities Movement

In the mid-1980s the WHO-Europe Healthy Cities movement gained momentum and helped shape health promotion practice in Canada and the United States (Duhl, 1996). Based on the premise that people are healthy when they live in nurturing environments and are involved in the life of their community. Participatory strategies were fundamental (Hancock, 1993). Local community action was seen as the means to tackle sociocultural determinants of health by alleviating poverty and social exclusion, improving living conditions and opportunities for care and social support, and by improving community environments through sustainable urban planning. Intersectoral approaches were necessary to change unhealthy environments. If communities were to gain control over the institutional and socioeconomic factors that affect their lives and subsequent health, multiple strategies were needed: policy development, organizational change, community development, legislation, advocacy, education and communication.

Ottawa Charter for Health Promotion

The Ottawa Charter for Health Promotion was issued at the first WHO International Conference on Health Promotion in Ottawa, Canada in 1986 (WHO, 1986). It defined health promotion practice as "the process of enabling people to increase control over, and to improve, their health." The Ottawa Charter's broad mandate moved health promotion practice beyond the health sector and beyond a sole focus on healthy life styles. It insisted that social and personal resources were necessary for health and well-being. Prerequisites for health were: peace, shelter, education, food, income, a stable eco-system, sustainable resources, social justice, and equity.

Strategies for health promotion included: (1) advocacy for political, economic, social, cultural, environmental, behavioral and biological conditions favorable to health; (2) enabling control over resources – supportive environments, access to information, opportunity for healthy choices – that promote health; and (3) mediation between different interests in society – governmental, social and economic institutions, non-governmental and voluntary organizations, industry and the media – in the pursuit of health (WHO, 1986). The Ottawa Charter became the cornerstone for health promotion practice in North America and Europe.

After the 1986 conference in Ottawa, a series of WHO international health promotion conferences were held (Adelaide (1988), Sundsvall (1991), Jakarta (1997) Mexico (2000), and Bangkok (2005)) each focusing on issues fundamental to health promotion practice: healthy public policy, supportive environments, investment for healthy development, building healthy alliances, and closing the equity gap. Increasingly health promotion advocates recognized that many determinants of health lie beyond the control of individuals, communities, or even nations. They recognized that the population demand for finite natural resources was degrading environments globally. Excessive consumption by wealthy countries was imposing disproportionate harm on poorer countries. These problems spanned national borders and required international solutions. Also, global cooperation was needed to quell emerging communicable, non-communicable, and man-made threats to human health.

Bangkok Charter for Health Promotion

In 2005, the 6th Global Conference on Health Promotion was held in Bangkok, Thailand. At the conference, the Bangkok Charter for Health Promotion was released to respond to the determinants of health in a globalized world (WHO, 2005). Its stated aim is to close the health gap between rich and poor by making the promotion of health "central to the global development agenda; a core responsibility for all of government; a key focus of communities and civil society; and a requirement for good corporate practice" (WHO, 2005). Since the Bangkok conference there has been some debate that the legal and economic discourse of the Bangkok Charter departs from the social justice discourse in the Ottawa Charter (Porter, 2006a; Mittlemark, 2008). It is probably fair to say that the Ottawa Charter remains the cornerstone for health promotion around the world (Mittlemark, 2008).

Latin American Developments in Health Promotion

Social Medicine

While the principles of health promotion set forth in the Ottawa Charter resonate in Latin America, the historical foundations of health promotion differ. A long tradition of social medicine provides philosophical and theoretical underpinning to Latin American health promotion practice, which is absent, to a large degree, in the

North. Latin American intellectual traditions recognized the contribution of political and economic conditions to social inequalities in health (Tajer, 2003). In the late 1930s, Salvadore Allende, Chilean Minister of Health, advanced the idea that poor health resulted from deprived social conditions (Allende, 1939). In Europe during the second half of the 19th century, similar ideas were voiced by Rudolf Virchow in Germany, and Edwin Chadwick in Britain, among others (Brown, 2006; Jones, 1931). In the United States, too, were those who argued that economic conditions had a manifest relation to health (Warren, 1918; Winslow, 1948). But the political milieu in the United States was generally unsupportive of social medicine, instead favoring free markets and a peripheral role for national government (Birn, 2003).

In the Latin American context, ideas about social conditions and health took root and developed in ways not seen to the North. For example, Allende proposed state measures to redistribute income and insure adequate housing, food and clothing to address root determinants of poor health resulting from underdevelopment (Waitzkin, 2001). In the 1950s, as a senator, Allende spearheaded legislation that created the Chilean nation health service to provide universal access to healthcare. At the same time, in the United States, the American Medical Association was strongly opposed to popular efforts to achieve a national system of health care (Birn, 2003). Later movements in the Latin American region, such as the Cuban revolution, the Nicaraguan revolution, Frei Betto's liberation theology in Brazil, and Paulo Freire's empowerment strategies in education in Brazil, reinforced the principles of equity and social justice (Waitzkin, 2001). Addressing socially determined health inequalities has been at the core of Latin American public debate for decades (Laurell, 2003).

Health Reforms in Latin America

In the early 1970s proponents of social medicine recognized the failure of regional economic growth strategies that promised, but did not produce, improvements in health for the entire population (PAHO, 1998). The external debt crisis faced by Latin American countries in the 1980s, followed by fiscal adjustment policies, changed the scope of health promotion initiatives and operational strategies. The countermeasure to long term social debt from the health and welfare sectors was structural adjustments to increase productivity and competitiveness (OIT, 2006). Health reforms in several Latin American countries, intended to increase economic efficiency, led to less emphasis on population-wide health promotion goals (Stein, 2006).

As Latin American countries moved towards decentralized and privatized health services, financing and policy authority for these services was shifted from the national to regional levels of accountability. Local governments, ultimately responsible for the people's health, faced major challenges assuming responsibility for health services, and, at the same time, demonstrating high productivity and efficiency in healthcare system (PAHO, 2000). In Colombia, health reforms resulted in fragmentation of health system structures: debilitation of health information systems; deterioration of the quality of health services; and emphasis on efficiency instead of equity (Gomez, 2005). In Nicaragua, a decentralization policy resulted in dismantling of a system of universal primary care (Birn, 2000). During this time, health spending cuts favored curative over preventive services, privatization and the promotion of user fees, and confusion over lines of accountability.

Downsizing and decentralizing the health sector in Latin America resulted in several different systems of care across the region and, in many places, lack of trained personnel to provide the minimum infrastructure needed, particularly in rural areas (PAHO & WHO, 2006). The shortage of trained health professionals was exacerbated by proximity to the United States where professionals were drawn away from their countries of origin. This left regional governments without mechanisms to support professional education and to sustain a well-organized use of human resources for an adequate health system (Arroyo, 2005).

Increasing Health Inequalities

Latin American inequities in health status grew in the 1980s and 1990s. A gap in life expectancy between the richest and the poorest countries approached 30 years (PAHO, 2002). Neoliberal health reforms, endorsed by the World Bank and the International Monetary Fund during times of economic crisis, accentuated problems in health systems by calling for privatization without sufficient attention to the infrastructure needed to regulate a complex health sector (Homedes, 2005). The consequences of these reforms are still being debated (Laurell, 2003). At odds in the debate are those who envision a universal, public healthcare system and those who favor commodified health care.

Proponents of social medicine gained momentum in response to growing inequalities in health. Incorporating Marxist intellectual traditions, social medicine focused on the role of social, political, economic and ideological processes as determinants of health and disease. Situated in the social sciences, more than biomedicine, the use of theory to guide practice and the production of knowledge was considered key for the field (Laurell, 1989). Compared to Latin America, North America and Europe had focused more on the biological and behavioral rather than the social components of health. Little attention was given to the social aspects of conditions like cancer or occupational illness because of the absence of explicit theories of the production of health in North American medicine (Laurell, 1989). While in Latin America, a combination of theory and political action – praxis – was seen as a practical way to deal with the sociopolitical and structural changes needed to improve health (Waitzkin, 2001). The Latin American Association of Social Medicine, established in 1984, endorsed a political vision for equity in all aspects of life which recognizes health as an essential human right that the State is obligated to protect and support (Tajer, 2003).

The late Juan Cesar Garcia is considered as an influential force in Latin American social medicine (Waitzkin, 2001). Trained in medicine in Argentina and sociology in

Chile, Garcia worked for the Pan American Health Organization from the mid-1960s to the mid-1980s overseeing grants and fellowships for public health programs and training in Latin America. Theory and research in social science and health were advanced in these programs and the scientific foundation for social medicine was considerably strengthened.

Women's Movement and Gender Equality

The women's movement in Latin America drew attention to social and health inequalities. The United Nation's Decade for Women, 1976–1985, was an outgrowth of the International Women's Year conference in Mexico City in 1975. The women's movement focused on the conditions and position of women in sociocultural, political, and economic spheres. It elucidated the profound inequities that existed in women's relationships as a consequence of powerlessness and subordination, and as products of a military, patriarchal culture (Diniz, 2003). Examining the health of women using a gender focus brought attention to the relationship between biology and the social environment. The women's health movement reframed female gender to include more than a reproductive focus. Human sexuality and conditions like cancer, depression, and violence were examined from a feminist perspective. The United Nations Decade for Women served as a platform for political action to promote social justice and equity through improvements in education, employment opportunities, equality in political and social participation, and increased access to health and welfare services.

Pratice in a Sociopolitical Context

From the landmark Ottawa Charter to the recent Bangkok Charter, the ramifications of global markets, rapid information and communication technologies, commodification of health services, and emphasis on evidence-based approaches and cost-effectiveness has prompted a reflection on health promotion theory, core principles and strategies.

Collective Health

The Latin American notion of the collective health, seen as historical interactions between the social and biological spheres, is a useful analytical approach for investigating the social production of human health (Laurell, 2007). As a theoretical construct, collective health provides a framework to test hypotheses concerning social processes that transform biological processes. As a scientific inquiry, the social and historical nature of human biological processes can be observed empirically in different patterns of morbidity and mortality in societies and in social classes. In North America, the construct of embodiment in epidemiology considers historically contingent social and biological processes that generate population health patterns, and resembles Latin American theories of collective health (Krieger, 2004). However, this construct is less well-developed and less influential than the construct of collective health in Latin America. Risk factor epidemiology continues to be the dominant paradigm in North America, with a focus on changing individual behaviors rather than addressing the social and structural determinants of health (Porter, 2006b).

Social Conditions and Social Solutions

National and regional boundaries that existed between sociocultural, political and economic systems have increasingly diminished in the Americas, as well as the rest of the world (Labonte, 2003). It is argued that forces of globalization are dominated by affluent countries; governments and citizens of poorer countries have less control over the conditions shaping their opportunities for health and well-being.(Mehta, 2005). A holistic perspective on determinants of health is thwarted by fragmentation of health and social services into increasingly competitive enterprises. While an expansive North American literature examines the social conditions that contribute to poor health outcomes, there is a paucity of literature on upstream social solutions (Raphael, 2006). The national health objectives for the United States, Healthy People 2010, identify two overarching goals: increasing the span of healthy life and reducing health disparities (US Department of Health and Human Services, 2000). Although the importance of underlying social determinants of health is explicitly recognized in the document, little emphasis is given to systematically addressing social determinants of health within a public health intervention framework.

In 2006 the International Society for Equity in Health, Chapter of the Americas, issued a report on the consequences of health reforms in the region. The report describes policy reform as focusing primarily on efficiency criteria and less on comprehensive approaches to organize the healthcare system towards a pro-equity model (Flores, 2006). As a result, health reforms in the region have contributed to inequity in health. In spite of the historical focus on social determinants of health in Latin America, there still exists a contradiction between recognizing social causality of disease and healthy public policy actions (Pellegrini, 2000).

Principles of Practice and Politics

Political, economic and social conditions have changed since the Ottawa Charter was issued. Across the Americas, level of national debt, economic growth trajectories, levels of employment, distributional and social welfare policies, administrative and financial decentralization, and economic liberalization policies have influenced social determinants of health over time. These factors, in turn, have shaped trade agreements, social and health policies, and the degree of citizen participation in decision-making processes. Each country in the Americas presents a different context for health promotion practice. Few countries, North or South, have been able to realize the fundamental principles and values of health promotion outlined in the Ottawa Charter. Health promotion interventions continue to deal mostly with activities to control and prevent proximal causes of morbidity and mortality. Citizens and communities are not fully participating in the decisions that affect their lives (Abma, 2005)

Migration of populations to urban areas is changing the landscape of health promotion (De Mattos, 2000; Cariola, 2003). Almost 76% of the population of Latin America lives in urban settings and, by 2020, that number is predicted to be 81% (Mehta, 2005). Similarly, in the United States 80% percent of the population lives in metropolitan areas (Auch, Taylor, & Acevedo, 2004). But benefits from an urbanized and globalized economy have had differential impacts across countries, and among social groups within countries (Navarro, 2003). Urban slums and growing inequality in income and wealth have marginalized the most vulnerable people (Sclar, 2005). In much of Latin America, attracting foreign investment for economic development has required trade liberalization in agriculture and industrial products. Government-directed economic approaches have given way to privatizing state-owned industries and utilities; removing trade restrictions and deregulating domestic markets; and downsizing government bureaucracy. The result has been a shift in emphasis from social and environmental protection systems to competition and private ownership (Sainz, 2006).

There is no single solution to improving people's health, yet the guiding principles in health promotion – empowerment, participatory, holistic, intersectoral, equitable, sustainable, and multi-strategy – suggest strategies for incremental and long-term change (Rootman, 2001). How health promotion practice is informed by these principles may differ, not only in Latin America and North America, but across all regions of the world. Gauging progress in health promotion is not a simple task (McQueen, 2007b). Changing social conditions may require a shift in thinking from technical solutions to ones that employ political action for social change (Milio, 2005). Fair trade agreements, worker protection rules, environmental and cultural preservation policies, and health and social welfare policies are potential legal tools. Communication technologies and mass media systems can be conduits for an engaged society to draw attention to existing inequalities and locally relevant solutions. Economic markets can be subject to safety net regulations and human rights records can serve as criteria for investment. Whether macro-level or community-based actions or whether philosophical traditions of Latin America, North America, or elsewhere, the ideal of social justice provides a common ground for health promotion practice.

Conclusion

Is a Pan-American approach to health promotion possible or even desirable in a hemisphere characterized by diversity? We have pointed out divergent views on the role of the individual versus the collective or social determinants of health; and there are historical differences in public versus private provision of health care and other basic resources. Economic conditions differ; Latin American countries have had more difficulties maximizing their economic resources than the United States or Canada, contributing to greater poverty, instability and foreign hegemony. There are also converging trends in the North and South: widening health inequalities within and across countries; a growing gap in income between the most wealthy and the poor; the movement of people into impoverished conditions in urban centers; degradation of the environment as a consequence of unsustainable consumption; and vulnerability to global economic forces that shape people's opportunities for health and well-being, yet are governed by no single country or region.

Progress in promoting people's health will benefit from knowledge gained from diverse perspectives on what it means to practice health promotion. Thinking of the Americas as a whole, and recognizing that health across and within countries is the consequence of a larger common experience over time, may move us towards collectively generating new knowledge to improve the conditions that enable people to increase control over, and to improve, their health.

References

Abma, A. (2005). Tineke. Responsive evaluation: its meaning and special contribution to health promotion. *Evaluation and Program Planning, 28*, 279–289.

Allende, S. G. (1939). La Realidad Medico-Social Chilena, Ministerio de Salubridad. *American Journal of Public Health, 2003*, 93.

Arroyo, H. (2005). Health promotion in latin america. In A. Scriven, & S. Garman (Eds.), *Promoting health global perspectives*. New York: Palgrave Macmillan.

Auch, R., Taylor, J., & Acevedo, W. (2004). Urban growth in american cities: Glimpses of U.S. urbanization. U.S. Department of the Interior, U.S. Geological Survey.

Birn, A., Zimmerman, S., & Garfield, R. (2000). To decentralize or not to decentralize, is that the question? Nicaraguan health policy under structural adjustment in the 1990s. *International Journal of Health Services, 30*, 111–128.

Birn, A., Brown, T. M., Fee, E., & Lear, W.J. (2003). Struggles for nation health reform in the United States. *American Journal of Public Health, 93*, 86–91.

Brown, T.M., & Fee, E. (2006). Rudolf carl virchow: Medical scientist, social reformer, role model. *American Journal of Public Health, 96*, 2104–2105.

Cariola, C., & Lacabana, M. (2003). Globalizacion y desigualdades socioterritoriales: la expansion de la periferia metropolitana de Caracas. *Revista eure, 29*, 5–21.

Cottrell, R. R., Girvan, J. T., & McKenzie, J. F. (1999). The history of health and health education. *Health Promotion and Education* (pp. 32–67). Needham Heights, MA: Allyn & Bacon.

De Mattos, C. (200) Santiago De Chile, globalizacion y expansion metropolitana. Lo que existia sigue existiendo. Sao Paulo Em Perspectiva. 14.

Diniz, N. M. F., Lopes, R. L. M., Couto, T. M., Gomes, N. P., Alves, S. L. B., & de Oliveira, J. F. (2003). Conjugal violence and its implication in STD/HIV prevention (Portuguese). *Revista Enfermagem UERJ, 11*, 80–84.

Duhl, L. (1996). An ecohistory of health: the role of 'Healthy Cities'. *American Journal of Health Promotion, 10*, 258–261.

Flores, W. (2006). *Equity and health sector reform in Latin America and the Caribbean from 1995 to 2005: Approaches and limitations*. Report Commissioned by the International Society for Equity in Health, Chapter of the Americas.

Gomez, R. D. (2005). Efectos de la Ley 100 sobre la institucionalidad de la salud en Columbia. Universidad de Antioquia.

Hancock, T. (1993). The evolution, impact and significance of the healthy cities/healthy communities movement. *Journal of Public Health Policy, 14*, 5–18.

Homedes, N., & Ugalde, A. (2005). Why neoliberal health reforms have failed in Latin America. *Health Policy, 71*, 83–96.

Jones, D. (1931). *Edwin Chadwick and the early public health movement in england, Vol. 9: University of Iowa studies in the social sciences.* Iowa City, University of Iowa

Krieger, N. (2004). Embodiment: a conceptual glossary for epidemiology. *Journal of Epidemiology and Community Health*, 59, 350–355.

Labonte, R. (2003). From the global market to the global village: "free" trade, health and the World Trade Organization. *Promotion and Education*, 10, 23–27.

Lalonde, M. (1974). *A new perspective on the health of canadians.* Ottawa, Canada.

Laurell, A. C., (1989). Social analysis of collective health in Latin America. *Social Science and Medicine*, 28, 1183–1191.

Laurell, A. C. (2003). What does Latin American social medicine do when it governs? the case of the Mexico City government. *American Journal of Public Health, 93*, 2028–2031.

Laurell, A, C. (2007). Social analysis of collective health in Latin America. *Social Science and Medicine*, 28, 1183–1191.

McQueen, D. V., Kickbusch, I., Potvin, L., Pelikan, J. M., Balbo, L., & Abel, T. (2007a). *Health and modernity: The role of theory in health promotion.* New York: Springer.

McQueen, D. V., & Jones, C. M. (Eds.) (2007b). *Global perspectives on health promotion effectiveness.* New York: Springer.

Mehta, D. (2005). Health promotion in an urbanizing world. Presentation at the 6th Global Conference on Health Promotion. Bangkok.

Mittlemark M. (2008). Setting an ethical agenda for health promotion. *Health Promotion International 23*, 78–85.

Milio, N. (2005). Ideology, science, and public policy. *Journal of Epidemiology and Community Health, 59*, 814–815.

Navarro, V. (2003). Equity: a challenge for the future in a multi-cultural world. *Promotion and Education, 10*, 114–117.

OIT. (2006). Programa Regional de Empleo para America Latina y el Caribe. de lat Organizacion Internacional del Trabajo.

PAHO. (1998). La Salud en las Americas, Volumen 1. 569. 1998. Organizacion Panamericana de la Salud.

PAHO. (2000). *Multicenter study – Inequities in health status, Access and expenditure: using secondary data to inform policy making.* Washington DC, Pan American Health Organization.

PAHO, & WHO. (2006). Human resources for health – critical challenges for the regions of the Americas – roundtables. CD47/19. 2006. Washington, DC.

Pan American Health Organization. (2002). *Health in the Americas: Volumes 1 and 2.* Washington D.C.: PAHO.

Pellegrini F. A. (2000). Ciencia en Pro de la Salud: Notas sobre la Organizacion de al Actividad Cientifica Para el Desarrollo de la Salud en America Latina y el Caribe. Washington DC, Pan American Health Organization. Science for Health. Notes on the Organization of Scientific Activities for Health Development in Latin America.

Porter, C. (2006a). Ottawa to Bangkok: changing health promotion discourse. *Health Promotion International, 22*, 72–79.

Porter, D. (2006b). How did social medicine evolve, and where is it heading. *PLoS Medicine, 3*, 1667–1672.

Raphael, D. (2006). Social determinants of health: present status, unanswered questions, and future directions. *International Journal of Health Services, 36*, 651–677.

Rootman. I., Goodstad, M., Hyndman, B., McQueen, D. V., Potvin, L., Springett, J., et al. (2001). Evaluation in Health Promotion: Principles and Perspectives. WHO Regional Publication, European Series, No.92.

Sainz, P. (2006). Equity in Latin America since the 1990s. ST/ESA/2006/DWP/22. New York, United Nations Department of Economic and Social Affairs. 10-27-0006.

Sclar, E. D., Garau, P., & Carolini, G. (2005). The 21st century health challenge of slums and cities. *Lancet, 365*, 901–903.

Stein, E. M., Tommasi, K. E., Lora, E., & Payne, M. (2006). *The politics of policies: economic and social progress report 2006.* Cambridge: International Development Bank and Harvard University Press.

Tajer, D. (2003). Latin American social medicine: roots, development during the 1990s, and current challenges. *American Journal of Public Health, 93*, 2023–2027.

US Department of Health and Human Services. (1980). Promoting health/preventing disease: objectives for the nation. Washington, DC

US Department of Health and Human Services. (2000). Healthy People 2010, 2nd ed. Washington, DC: US Government Printing Office.

Waitzkin, H., Iriart, C., Estrada, A., Lamadrid, S. (2001). Social medicine then and now: lessons from Latin America. *American Journal of Public Health*, 91, 1592–1601.

Warren, B. S., Sydenstriker, E. (1918). The relation of wages to public health. *American Journal of Public Health, 8*, 883–887. Reprinted in (1999). *American Journal of Public Health, 89*, 1641–1643.

WHO. (1986, November 21). Ottawa charter for health promotion. *First International Conference on Health Promotion*, Ottawa.

WHO. (1978, September 6–12). *Primary Health Care: Report on the International Conference on Primary Health Care, Alma-Ata, USSR*, Geneva.

WHO, (2005, August). Bangkok charter for health promotion in a globalized world, Bangkok, Thailand.

Winslow, C. E. A. (1948). Poverty and health. *American Journal of Public Health Nations Health, 38*, 173–184.

Chapter 3
Practical Dilemmas for Health Promotion Evaluation

Louise Potvin and David V. McQueen

There are many interesting parallels to make between the field of evaluation and that of health promotion. Both are relatively new areas of activity in the broadly defined domain of empirical applied research. Both emerged within the last quarter of the twentieth century mostly related to government administrations. Finally both appear as applied fields in search of theories (see McQueen (1996) and McQueen, Kickbusch, Potvin, Pelikan, Balbo and Abel (2007) with regard to health promotion and Christie (2003), King (2003) and Shadish, Cook, and Leviton (1991) for evaluation).

For many authors (O'Connor, 1995; Rossi & Freeman, 1993; Shadish et al., 1991) evaluation started to become a distinct and institutionalised field of empirical research in the late 1960s. This process was fuelled in part by the explosion of the U.S. Government demand for evaluation following the Johnson Administration adoption of the "Planning-Programming-Budgeting System" in all executive branch agencies (O'Connor, 1995) as a rational budgeting approach to his War on poverty. This system calls for each agency to establish a process for "setting goals, defining objectives, and developing planned programs for achieving those objectives as integral parts of preparing and justifying budget submission" (Bureau of the Budget, 1965, p. 1, cited in O'Connor, 1995, p. 30). According to O'Connor (1995) the process of assessing how those programs were meeting their objectives became increasingly handled by a separate division permanently staffed by specialized social scientists. This was paralleled by the publication of the first evaluation textbook by Suchman (1967). Interestingly, Suchman was a sociologist working in the field of public health, known for his efforts to adapt "the standard epidemiological model (of host, agent and environment) to research on action programs in the field of health" (Suchman, 1967, p. 199). As for health promotion, the Ottawa Charter (WHO, 1986) published in 1986 was the result of 10 years of work and international discussions in which the European office of WHO played a major leading role (Kickbusch, 2003).

L. Potvin
Department of Social and Preventive Medicine, Université de Montreal, Québec Canada

L. Potvin, D. McQueen (eds.), *Health Promotion Evaluation Practices in the Americas*,
DOI: 10.1007/978-0-387-79733-5_3, © Springer Science+Business Media, LLC 2008   25

Despite the existence of apparent numerous similarities, these two fields have not met very often. Each has developed its own stream of journals and professional associations, with few overlaps. In essence, only five textbooks (Green & Lewis, 1986; Hawe, Degeling, & Hall, 1990; Nutbeam & Bauman, 2006; Valente, 2002; Windsor, Baranowski, Clark, & Cutter, 1984), one of which is now in its third edition (Windsor et al., 1984; Windsor, 1994; Windsor, Clark, Boyd, & Goodman, 2003), have been published during the past twenty years in attempts to import into health promotion methods, debates, and theoretical issues that make the fabric of evaluation as a field of inquiry. These books largely center their discussion of evaluation on methodological issues mainly promoting approaches based on the experimental and quasi-experimental tradition of evaluation with an integration, however, of the field's preoccupation with implementation issues. There is, however, much more to be learned from the burgeoning debates in the evaluation literature about practical and theoretical issues (Hawe & Potvin, forthcoming). Many of the thorny questions health promotion evaluators are struggling with such as the integration of qualitative and quantitative data, the nature of evidence, the limits of a strictly experimentalist approach in evaluation, the pros and cons of participatory approaches to evaluation, and many others have been regularly discussed in the evaluation literature in the past 25 years.

To account in detail for the lack of focus on evaluation in health promotion requires a historical examination beyond the scope of this chapter. However discussions and debates arising earlier from the publication of *Evaluation in Health Promotion* (Rootman, Goodstadt, Hyndman, McQueen, Potvin, Springett, & Ziglio, 2001), which argued for all health promotion interventions and programs to set aside

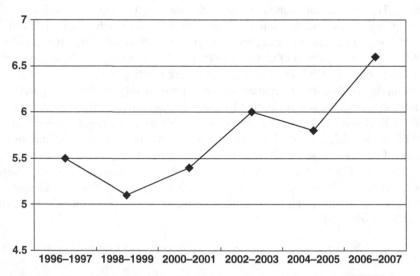

Fig. 3.1 Proportion of articles reporting on evaluation research projects in health promotion specialised journals

financial resources for evaluation, coupled with more recent debates centered on the reconsideration of the Ottawa Charter in conferences, classrooms and papers (Hills & McQueen, 2007), have identified the seeming lack of concern for evaluation in the Charter itself. Perhaps, as a founding document for the field, it was necessarily focused on the concepts and principles of health promotion, largely ignoring issues of underlying theory and the evaluation of practice. But as a seminal document it did not urge the field to be critical of its practice.

It is difficult to judge how the field of health promotion has reacted to the various urges for conducting evaluation projects. Figure 3.1 presents the results of a Medline search conducted on articles published between January 1996 and July 2007 in eight leading health promotion specialised journals. The list of journals surveyed includes: American Journal of Health Promotion, Health Promotion International, Health Promotion Journal of Australia, Health Promotion Practice, Health Education and Behavior, Health Education Quarterly, Health Education Research, and Promotion & Education. Although other public health general venues regularly publish the results of prevention and health promotion interventions this inquiry was restricted to health promotion specialised journals in order to get a more precise assessment of the importance of evaluation research within the more institutionalised health promotion discourse. Although the proportion of articles reporting on the evaluation of a health promotion intervention[1] has grown steadily during this period, it remains very small varying from 5.1% to 6.8%. So, despite various urgent calls for health promotion to develop a strong evaluation agenda (Rootman et al., 2001; Nutbeam, 2004) and various projects aiming at synthesizing the results of prevention and health promotion interventions, it seems that authors who lament the paucity of health promotion evaluation studies are right (Potvin, 2006).

The field badly lacks the empirical basis on which pleading for effectiveness or even for successful implementation. The recognition of this was one of the chief reasons the International Union for Health Promotion and Education (IUHPE) set out at the close of the twentieth century to take on evaluation of effectiveness as a major scientific endeavour of the organization. The history of this effort is described in detail in the monograph edited by McQueen & Jones (2007). There are two chief characteristics of this endeavour that are pertinent here: (1) at its best the Global Programme on health Promotion Effectiveness of IUHPE has been plagued by lack of adequate funding and (2) it has clearly revealed at a global level that evaluation of practice is equally, if not less so, not on the agenda of most health promotion practices.

In the many discussions taking place about evaluation, one rarely finds critical examination of the role evaluation could or should play in advancing the field of health promotion. It is generally taken for granted that evaluation is vitally important

---

[1] We kept articles in the title and abstract of which appears the word evaluation in its various forms. We deleted from this pool all articles presenting psychometric evaluation of measurement instruments, articles presenting and discussing evaluation designs, frameworks or methods without reporting of empirical study results, and editorials and general advocacy papers.

and is the means by which health promotion can prove itself worthy of the use of scarce public health resources. Also linked to that kind of contribution is the coding and standardisation of health promotion through the constitution of inventories and catalogues of practices and programmes (best practices) from which health promotion practitioners could or should borrow to intervene on local problems. In both cases what is at issue is the ruling of local health promotion practice from an objective, centralised and institutionally controlled set of criteria, in a typically "top down" institutional approach to intervention and problem solving.

The intention of many is to base health promotion practice and decision making about program and policy on evidence derived from a scientific model of research. Because health promotion borrows knowledge and theory from such diverse sources as biomedical and social sciences, much of the debate surrounding health promotion evaluation has been centred on two questions that ultimately explore how to retrofit so called soft research into the objectivistic agenda of classical hard research. This is largely based on the belief of many that hard research, that is research springing from the natural sciences, particularly physics, is chiefly concerned with reliability, generalizability, and universality of knowledge, that is the physics that works in the Western world is the same physics for the whole world. This more traditional view argues for as little room as possible for subjective and interpretative, local knowledge. Of course this translates into a methodological question and pertains to the nature of evidence that should be searched for, collected and synthesised for health promotion evaluation. This debate includes discussions regarding the relative value of several types of inquiry as well as the integration of qualitative and quantitative data. The second question is more procedural and concerns the rules and techniques to be applied in order to draw evidence-based conclusions out of the synthesised data.

In this book in general and in this chapter in particular, we argue that there is another very important role for evaluation research to play in health promotion. Indeed, to the extent that health promotion is also based on a set of values and principles in addition to scientific knowledge about the production of health, it should be expected that any activity linked to health promotion, such as health promotion evaluation, should also relate to its general goals, or at least not interfere with their pursuit. In order to play such a role, evaluation, as a scientific activity, needs to be defined much more broadly; it cannot only be in reference to a set of methods and procedures. We argue that defining health promotion evaluation as social practice expands on the meaning and range of activities that could legitimately be developed and implemented in health promotion evaluation. We will also propose that it is only through that kind of expansion that health promotion evaluation can fulfil its role of fully participating in the very broad health promotion agenda, primarily in two ways: first by promoting the values and principles of health promotion and second by providing tools to reflect on, value, and reproduce health promotion practices that are developed and experimented locally in response to local needs and circumstances. In short, we argue for a concept of health promotion evaluation that is in itself health promoting.

The Practice of Evaluation

The main thesis underlying this chapter is that evaluation is a social practice and as such not only does it have an impact on the object of evaluation, but it is also transformed through its interaction with the interventions that are evaluated. So, because of its coupling with specific interventions and in order to maintain its significance as a general type of inquiry and the relevance of its conclusions for those directly involved in health promotion, health promotion evaluation also has to be responsive to the specific features of health promotion while maintaining its general characteristics that will still make it evaluation. In our definition evaluation is the assessment of the transformative action of social actors upon social structure that constrains their practice. Sharing with all evaluation practices, health promotion evaluation is characterised by a high scientific content and by the fact that its object is another form of practice, intervention, program or policy that aim at social betterment (Mark, Henry, & Julnes 2000). Specific to health promotion evaluation, is the fact that its object, health promotion practice, is deeply rooted in values and principles as well as in scientific knowledge (McQueen & Anderson, 2001). Contrary to most techno scientific innovations, health promotion makes remarkable efforts not only to acknowledge the important role of values underlying its practice but also to render those values increasingly transparent through public debate. Thus, values are intrinsic to evaluation; there is no independent, value-free evaluation in health promotion.

What is a practice? Most contemporary sociologists define practice as the transformative work of a social actor upon his or her environment. It involves the deployment of causal powers in order to produce an outcome (Giddens, 1984), with the intention of either making a difference or reproducing a given situation. A practice is always situated, meaning that the identity of the actor as well as specific structural opportunities and constrains influence the practice. The process however is recursive. Through their mutual interactions actors and social structures acquire and maintain their identity for the former and get transformed for the latter. Importantly this transformation may be seen as continuous. That is transformation doesn't necessarily have an end product. The interaction is, in effect, always transforming as the practice continues.

Putting this notion of practice at the core of evaluation has implications for knowledge production. "Regarding practice primarily as a matter of the local and situational goes hand in hand with the view that the kinds of scientific knowledge that are provided to practice must somehow be adjusted or adapted to fit circumstances" (Schwandt, 2005, p. 98). Developments in the field of sociology throughout the twentieth century have highlighted the social nature of knowledge.

The influential albeit controversial work of the anthropologist of science Bruno Latour, has shown that scientific activity is much more than the application of a scientific method, it corresponds to the characteristics of a social practice as defined above. His anthropological work in science laboratories has unveiled the social processes that lead from empirical observations and measurements to the construction of scientific facts (Latour, 1987). Knowledge does not lie within objects of nature. It is the result of deliberate actions that involve the interaction between previous knowledge and theory, measurement or inscription devices that cumulate the scientific knowledge at specific points in time, an active knowledge seeker who uses this previous knowledge and inscription devices to create situations that can render visible some features of the mechanism and of course the mechanism itself that can only be known through those mediated interactions. Scientific activity is not simply a reflection upon the world or observations made by neutral observers. It is the systematic, deliberate and informed transformations of elements of the world in order to render evident other features of the world (Latour, 1993). It is the result of the scientist work upon the world.

Well before Bruno Latour's publications and in a book that had been long forgotten before being rediscovered by Kuhn (1962), the physician, Ludwick Fleck has highlighted the social nature of scientific activity. Using the complex case of the history of syphilis, Fleck demonstrates that scientific facts are elaborated within communities of scientists whose work and methodology define and form collective ways of thinking. Within each of these communities, sets of norms as well as specific bodies of knowledge and instrumentations not only determine scientific practice but also the content of the scientific production (Fleck, 1935, 1979 for the English translation). Nearly 50 years later, a pioneer in the field of evaluation and the inventor of the quasi-experimental design , Donald T. Campbell described how science validity systems are not methodological in nature but rest essentially on social mechanisms of verification and mutual criticism operated by scientists themselves within such communities (Campbell, 1984).

Thus we would argue that the search for evidence and the conduct of evaluation is a social practice. Therefore knowledge produced by evaluation depends upon the evaluator's: (1) point of view; (2) training; (3) view of science; and (4) context. Point of view relates to the whole conceptual basis on which one frames one's ideas, concepts, values and self-meaning. It is essentially abstract and not easily translated to others. In essence it is similar to the Meridian idea that meaning is buried within the individual and is not really transferable out of the individual. From a practical evaluation standpoint it implies that these deeper meanings are not readily or even possibly transparent to other participants and stakeholders in the evaluation. Yet a field such as health promotion is highly promulgated on values that are deeply held. For example, if one deeply values respect for the values of others, this deeply held value cannot help but have impact on the meaning of the evaluation practice.

With regard to training, we often tend to disregard one's training in the academic world. Nevertheless many in public health are quick to refer to the clinical mentality or the social science perspective. These mentality metaphors are indeed direct products of years of academic training that shape our perspective. It is obvious that when a person trained for years in biochemistry and medicine thinks of body chemistry that a whole cascade of years of learning formulae and obsequious learning of body parts and interactions is forthcoming. Similarly, when a sociologist hears a term used like social class, it evokes years of reading from Hegel to Marx to Weber to Veblen, etc. Social class is not just a variable; it is a torrent of reflection on years of academic scholarship. Science can loosely be described as the best understanding of phenomena at any given point in time. Aristotle was a great scientist, but he was not Einstein. However, their view of physics at the time was state of the art. Now both are ancient scientists. The point is that science as a pursuit, like evaluation, is transformational. Despite the evaluator's point of view, training, or view of science, the context of the person's work cannot be dismissed in the evaluative process. We have noted the role of government in the search for evaluation of health promotion. Those who sit in governmental agencies have a dual responsibility, one to demand the best evaluation and one to protect the public's purse. Those who sit in academe feel other pressures, publication, and academic recognition. Still those in practice want things that work, projects that transform, and they are dependent for support from academe and governments. In short, evidence does not exist independent of the observer; it is not a thing in itself. Therefore evaluation is a very social discovery process.

To reiterate, in applied sciences the objects of knowledge and scientific inquiries are not objects or mechanism of nature but products of human activity. There is a further distinction to be made between social sciences and applied sciences. In social sciences the object of inquiry is the social and society also resulting from human activity. We will make the case that in social science the object of inquiry is not necessarily a deliberate construction of human beings, that many of its features are unperceived by human beings. The general concept of social structure concerns such objects. In applied science the objects of inquiry are deliberate and wilful artefacts of human action. They can be generally labelled as technical objects the features of which are deliberately designed to perform specific functions. So health promotion evaluation is an applied scientific activity since its objects are interventions designed and put together by social actors. It is not a social science, it is not about theorising social structures, it is about creating knowledge and meaning about deliberate human actions seeking transformation of population health and its determinants.

Health promotion evaluation can thus be conceived as a set of actions carried out to render evident features of another set of human actions, an intervention. So in order to produce knowledge about the latter, the former has to get into some kind of interaction with the intervention and this interaction implies social actors who carry their own problematization of the overall situation, their own power differentials and their own interests over the situation. So the evaluation situation is not only scientific in that it implies science-related activity, it is also social in that it involves interactions between social actors who assign different meanings to the situation, and it is also political in that social actors involved do not necessarily pursue the same interests in the situation and some of those interests can be imposed upon other actors. Evaluation thus becomes a practice through which, actors involved work upon their environment to create meaning out of it, and to reproduce and transform it. So the practice of health promotion evaluation is one that implies: (1) the manipulation of instruments for scientific inquiries with regard to sets of actions, interventions, (2) the creation of meaning about the interactions that take place between all actors involved in the intervention, including intervention staff, funders and beneficiaries and (3) the mediation of potentially conflicting interests.

Any discussion of evaluation that focuses only on one of those features would be incomplete and potentially misleading.

Building on Anselm Strauss' distinction between sociology of health and sociology in health, we will also discuss the distinction to be made between evaluation of health promotion and evaluation in health promotion. The former refers to an evaluation perspective situated outside the field of health promotion. A perspective that takes as its object the whole activity of health promotion using methods and paradigms that belong to the outside perspective from which the field is being evaluated. The various current exercises aiming at providing evidence for health promotion effectiveness are to be included in evaluations of health promotion. In that sense, it is paradoxical that so many people from inside the field of health promotion are advocating for, and contributing to, the evaluation of health promotion. Evaluation in health promotion is the borrowing and adaptation by health promotion of conceptual and methodological tools developed in other scientific domains to enhance its own capacity to better understand its own object. The adaptation process usually aligns the new concepts and methods to the existing science base. Evaluation in health promotion is the use of evaluation methods to improve health promotion. This position is the one defended by those who argue that because health promotion is a social practice, evaluation is among basic scientific activities through which knowledge about health promotion is produced (Potvin & Goldberg, 2007).

Four Challenges for the Practice of Health Promotion Evaluation

There exist many definitions of evaluation. Some are focusing on the managerial and instrumental aspects of evaluation whereas others insist on methodological features. For this book we think it is important to align our definition with one that is of current use in the general evaluation literature. This will facilitate the elaboration of a shared language and perspective between health promotion evaluators and evaluators in general. For Mark et al. (2000, p. 3) "evaluation assists sense making about policies and programs through the conduct of systematic inquiry that describes and explains the policies' and programs' operations, effects, justifications, and social implications."

According to this definition, three characteristics distinguish evaluation research from other activities. (1) The object of evaluation is one of several features of an intervention, program or policy that includes a diversity of practice and activities. (2) Evaluation methodology is systematic and scientific. (3) The aim of evaluation is to produce knowledge to support action from a variety of social actors bearing a diversity of interests in the evaluated intervention. When a systems of action is situated as an object of inquiry as it is the case in program evaluation (Potvin, Gendron, & Bilodeau, 2006) there are necessarily interactions taking place between the intervention and the evaluation systems and these interactions affect both systems. In the particular case of health promotion interventions based on empowerment and participation and that essentially aim at transforming local and general conditions relevant to health, the obligation to develop evaluation discourse and practice that encompasses more than data collection and analysis methods is even more critical. Because they are explicitly founded on a value system, we believe that health promotion interventions represent particular challenges for evaluation. These challenges pertain to (1) defining the object to evaluate, (2) using methods that are both appropriate to the object and rigorous, (3) producing results that can be synthesized and (4) producing relevant knowledge for action.

Challenge 1: Defining the Object to Evaluate

There is confusion in terms when one tries to label systems of action that are operated in health promotion. Indeed, notions such as program, intervention, project, initiative are often used interchangeably. Despite some serious efforts (Levesque et al., 2000), nobody has ever been able to propose a taxonomy founded on generally agreed upon ontological distinctions. For reasons of simplicity, in this book we prefer the term "program". Taking from Dab (2005), we define a program as a mode of planning and organisation for collective action that aims at producing a desirable transformation.

When so defined, programs constitute a complex social reality (Potvin, Haddad, & Frohlich, 2001) that operate as systems. Programs are systems of actions in which actors mobilise knowledge, activities, networks and resources in order to produce some change. Programs do not change conditions in and of themselves. It is the people operating within the parameters defined by the program and using resources made available through it who create the events that are thought to activate the desired changes. Like all other complex systems a program becomes intelligible only through a representation or a model of its formal aspects situated in time and context (LeMoigne, 1977). Indeed, like all complex objects a program intelligence cannot be captured by a series of instructions or by a work plan. Any program representation or model is necessarily partial and biased in order to highlight specific features to support specific interests.

In evaluation in general and in health promotion evaluation in particular there is a strong emphasis on the importance of logic models in the conduct of evaluation (McLaughlin & Jordan, 1999). There are mainly two criticisms to be made related to this. First, what is often described in logic models is a linear set of relationships that obliterates a fair number of features of the open system reality in which programs are implemented. In open systems, found in the real world, relationships are recursive that is there is not a single direction of causality. In open systems, the borders between the inside and the outside are blurred and can only be defined arbitrarily in reference to a set of external criteria. Open systems create and are created through their interactions with their environment. This criticism addresses the narrow nature of the conception of knowledge that is often found in health promotion evaluation. The other criticism is more fundamental and concerns the fact that in addition to modeling the chain of events that are involved in an intervention, evaluation should also be concerned with modeling the symbolic relations in which actors are engaged through the interventions through a social model but also with modeling the power relationships involved through a political model. We could also think of an economical model that would be concerned with the exchange relationships between the actors. The point here is to note that logic models concentrate on events that are stripped of their social significance because actors, their interest and the symbolic significance they bring to the intervention is rarely taken into account in such models. This is precisely where evaluators' viewpoint, training, view of science, and context become relevant.

In addition, representations such as logic models emphasise a perspective in which programs are created outside of their implementation context and are then grafted to the life of local actors without the latter being actively involved as if programs were totally new entities inside a given context. Logic models are blind to social actors who carry action and operate programs. Such an objectification of social actors is at odds with fundamental values and principles in health promotion (Potvin, Gendron, Bilodeau, & Chabot, 2005). Indeed in addition to strategies that imply a strong contextualisation of programs such as strengthening community actions, and creating supportive environment, the Ottawa Charter for Health Promotion (WHO, 1986) identifies values and principles in support of creating processes such as participation and empowerment that are framed as being as important as the expected health results. We concur with others that the values and principles identified in the Ottawa Charter are parameters of efficacy for health promotion evaluation (Rootman, Goodstadt, Potvin, & Springett, 2001).

Program is a mode of collective action and as such does not have a pre-defined and objective reality. It is not a thing in itself. It is not the program that makes things change, it is the people within the program who make things happen. Health promotion rhetoric suggests that loaded with value and meaning, program operations aim at creating strong and meaningful linkages between programs' ends, apparatus and actors on the one hand and the context in which it is implemented on the other hand (Dooris et al., 2007). Establishing, maintaining and reinforcing such linkages is only possible through a strong embeddedness of the program within implementation context and a conceptualisation of the co-evaluation of the program within its context. This leads to defining health promotion program as a dynamic social system in which a diversity of actors' interests meet and confront. The more programs resemble the ideal of the Ottawa Charter the less they maintain characteristics that would make them distinct objects objectively defined from their context. Changing social systems rather than lifeless apparatus programs with their changing contours sensitive to situated actors, pose highly critical definitional problems to evaluators.

With contingent contours and definitions of what is in and what is out (Potvin, 2007), programs as evaluation objects are not totally objective facts. One important early task for health promotion evaluators is to propose a program definition or representation that is acceptable and judged adequate by social actors involved in the evaluation project (see Chap. 8 for a complete discussion of the role of models in participatory evaluation). Without such a shared representation, which like all complex system models aim at increasing the system's intelligence while occulting some features to highlight others, it is impossible to agree on which relevant question the evaluation should provide answers. Even more, such a representation is necessary to identify all relevant constituents that should take part in defining the evaluation questions. This process of program modeling that can be done through methods of systematization (see Chap. 14 for an illustration of method of systematization and its role in health promotion evaluation) is an essential component of evaluability assessment (Thurston & Potvin, 2003).

As dynamic systems that evolve through time, programs pose additional definitional problems to evaluators. Indeed program adaptation to local conditions and context is necessarily associated with program changes as discussed in Chap. 17. Those changes can be relatively trivial but as partners turn over with new alliances being negotiated, new interests become at play in a program's social space and can radically alter its orientation and direction. Bisset and Potvin (2007), showed how successive alignments of program objectives and resources that accompany the development of new partnerships elaborated in response to environmental constraints and opportunities, slowly but inexorably transform the orientation of collective action. It is thus crucial to factor in time and evolution in the definition of the program to evaluate in order to alleviate the risk to attribute observed results to an idealised program that is different than the one that has been effectively implemented.

Finally, defining a program as a social system in which interests are at play makes a program a political entity. It is because they see a program as an opportunity to pursue their interests that social actors will become involved in the program space (this is true for all actors, from funders, staff, and volunteers to beneficiaries) making them strategic actors (Crozier & Friedberg, 1977), and this includes the evaluator. We believe that the stakes represented by the evaluation and for which the evaluator is spokesperson influence and shape the evaluation project (Brown, 1995). In a potentially controversial space in which legitimacy might be questioned it will be extremely difficult for the evaluator to deploy rigorous methods to control for confounding variables that at the same time constrain practices of other actors. Thus, health promotion evaluators have to create a space for dialog with local actors in order to develop an evaluation project that takes into account often diverging projects from a diversity of actors (Schwandt, 2005).

Challenge 2: Balancing Relevance and Rigour in the Choice of Methods

In this particular context of dynamic and changing environments crowded with potentially conflicting interests, the challenge that consists in designing and implementing rigorous research methods is key. Indeed research rigour is always contingent to a disciplinary perspective (McQueen & Anderson, 2001). Each discipline that composes the field of human scientific knowledge has developed its own corpus of procedures and techniques. These are essential to assist in the reciprocal critique that founds most apparatus that ensure scientific rigour (Campbell, 1984). In addition to insuring rigour, this strong association between disciplines and methods facilitates the development of a coherent body of observations to support theoretical knowledge development.

Having its origins mainly in the efforts of the WHO EURO to develop a strategy in the pursuit of the objectives of "Health for All by the Year 2000" (Kickbusch, 2003), health promotion is an integral part of the more general field of public health (Potvin & McQueen, 2007). The methodological discourse in public health is largely dominated by epidemiology (Mcqueen, 1988; Potvin & Chabot, 2002). Positioned in the conceptual and discursive universe of public health, health promotion is doomed to justify its research procedures relatively to epidemiological criteria, itself founded on positivist and classical empiricist paradigm (Rothman, 1986). This paradigm suggests that experimentation in a controlled situation that allows one to isolate the relationship between a putative cause and an expected effect independently of all other confounding factors is the gold standard to establish causality (Baskhar, 1978). The nine criteria for causality identified by Hill (1953) are indeed ways of mimicking experimental conditions in situations where they cannot be implemented. In the field of public health, laboratory studies which are very useful to establish causality are of limited value to study many of the phenomena that shape population health, and the interventions implemented to address them. In this case and following the tradition long established by Claude Bernard in experimental medicine, epidemiology proposes that treatment manipulation "in vivo", while controlling as much as possible for contextual elements constitutes the golden route to demonstrating causality between an intervention and its hypothetical effects. But, random assignment of study subjects to the various treatments to be compared in a study is the only way to insure the necessary statistical equivalence between the study groups in order to establish causality (Rubin, 1974). This methodological paradigm that requires, at least in principle, a strong control over the experimental situation and the objectification of study subjects is, a priori, not compatible with the values of participation and empowerment that underlie the Ottawa Charter. Consequently there are essentially two options to ensure rigour in health promotion evaluation studies whether the objective is to establish a causal relation between an intervention and hypothetical effects or to understand the transformation dynamic between a program and its context. The first option consists, within the epidemiological paradigm, in identifying and defining program elements that are under the evaluator's control and to conduct the analysis accordingly. The second option is to get out entirely of the epidemiological paradigm and implement research methods that satisfy rigorous criteria elaborated in disciplines that have taken social transformation processes as their research object.

Hawe, Shiell and Riley (2004) developed the argument that experimentation in health promotion should not be conceptualised as the prescription of specific activities and operations. For them the essence of health promotion intervention does not lie in any specific kit of activities but in functions that practitioners implement and operate through activities that are adapted to local conditions. For example, in a community development program a function to implement could be a mechanism that facilitates dialog and exchanges between various key actors. The exact form such mechanism takes as well as the specific identity of the local actors are to be adapted to local conditions. According to Hawe et al. (2004), causal relations can then be established between such health promotion functions and observed results when resources to develop such functions are randomly assigned to organisational (cluster) units such as schools, burrows, enterprises, even if there is no control over the local dynamics interplay in the shaping of the local activities and operations.

Whereas this proposition of randomised cluster design allows dealing with causality, it nonetheless puts on the evaluator the onus of closely monitoring experimental units, first to ensure the implementation of the assigned functions and second to understand the processes that lead to specific results. There are two serious flaws with this design. The first is the presence of higher order interactions that experimental designs are ill equipped to deal with unless the number of experimental units, in this case clusters, is very large. Indeed the causal pathways between functions, activities and results will be shaped by the interactions with local conditions. To the extent that these will be higher order interactions and that local conditions will vary to such an extent that the number of units per cell is going to be too small to test these interactions, causality will be difficult to establish. The second is the definition of specific outcomes of interest. Indeed, because activities are free to vary across experimental units, it is unlikely that pre-defined specific health outcomes will be achieved throughout a large spectrum of units. It is well known that general health indicators such as all cause mortality or overall perceived health are more stable and less likely to be affected by specific interventions than more specific indicators. The question of how to balance the need to predefined specific health outcomes of interest and the necessary local freedom in implementing health promotion function remains unanswered. The essential problem is that the complexity in health promotion programs is essentially ignored.

From this empiricist paradigm we should retain that causality is a narrow concept the establishment of which requires very rigid conditions that are costly to establish, both in terms of resources and in loss of adaptability to local conditions. In epidemiology those rigid conditions are known as Hill causality criteria (Hill, 1953). To the extent that health promotion evaluation criteria are formulated in terms of causality it is very difficult to move away from epidemiological criteria for scientific rigour. One can always innovate in the application of those criteria in health promotion evaluation, keeping in mind however that those adaptations add up another layer of limitations to a program's internal validity.

The second option available to health promotion evaluators is to move away from classical empiricist paradigm and epidemiology and to mobilise conceptual and methodological instruments that are more adequate for the study of complex social systems like health promotion interventions. Social sciences have developed a whole range of methodologies that have been successfully implemented to study social change processes and to evaluate programs. For a long time evaluators were caught in a dilemma of choosing to work in a structuralist/positivist perspective of causality and a phenomenologist/relativist horizon of representations and intentions, both equally unsatisfactory but to different audiences. Wherein a paradigm of causality satisfies, in principle decisions need to be made based on generalizable evidence to solve objectively defined problems, whereas practitioners have more appetite for contextualised interpretations of the live experience of program actors in order to develop more relevant practice. We believe that simply juxtaposing those two perspectives into a single study does not constitute a satisfying solution. "Consensus is not possible or desirable, because it masks power struggles and it restricts development of innovative solutions through informed dialogue and compromise. Moreover, professionals and practitioners who try to implement social-change programs rarely find conceptual tools pertinent to their practice in the evidence-based discourse. They rightly argue that generalizable estimates constitute only one of many indicators that reflect on their practice." (Potvin et al., 2005, p. 593).

Social transformation processes are to be conceptualised within the structure-agency debate that has characterised theoretical progress in the disciplines of the social sciences throughout the twentieth century. In a nutshell, this debate opposes those who believe that humans are free subjects who construct their life based on their preferences and whose decisions and actions are unconstrained expressions of those preferences and those who believe that human agency or capacity for single individuals to exercise causal power upon their environment is almost entirely determined by structural forces that are objectively situated outside of the reach of any single individual (Williams, 2003). A lot of recent theoretical work in sociology has been dealing with this debate trying to find a way out of this impossible dilemma, whose extreme positions are not tenable anyway. The notion of practice has been elaborated by post-structuralist sociologists such as Giddens (1984) and Bourdieu (1972) as an interface of the duality between structure and agency. Although these authors differ in their specific conceptualisation of how this interface comes about and operates, both suggest that practice is the structurally constrained expression of human agency through which social structures are constantly reproduced and transformed.

We believe that this debate is of utmost importance for public health in general and health promotion programs in particular because what is essentially at stake in health promotion is individual and collective health related practices and the conditions that constrain and enable them. Very often, the task of health promotion evaluators is to make sense of how actions aimed at deliberately modifying structural conditions are associated with practice changes. Fundamentally one can conceive of health promotion as being situated outside or inside the local context, as a force that operates independently of, or in close conjunction with, local instances. A dualist conception of the structure/agency dilemma leads to locating health promotion inside of a local context as being one of many other agents that exercise transformative power in a situation (Potvin, 2007). This bears enormous epistemological implications. Indeed, situated inside the intervention context, health promotion is necessarily affected itself by its transformative intentions regarding structural conditions. As proposed by McQueen (2007a), reflexivity and contextualism are thus intrinsic features of health promotion that affect research theoretical and methodological options. From the point of view of health promotion evaluation practice the key question then becomes whether evaluation can itself be conceptualised as being located outside of the intervention context posing upfront the epistemological question of the reflexivity of health promotion evaluation.

Resolving this question requires that evaluation closely follows the actions that objectively characterise program implementation (Potvin et al., 2006). However, following action where it takes place requires that hypotheses and observations be anchored in strong theoretical propositions (Barnes, Matka, & Sullivan, 2003). This is where social sciences methodology takes its strength but also its weaknesses for an applied field such as public health, in which the tendency is to consider that data bear intrinsic objective meaning and consequences (McQueen & Anderson, 2001).

Challenge 3: Synthesising Evaluation Results into Meaningful Indices

Synthesising knowledge has become an essential research function in an era where research is increasingly valued by its capacity to be useful for decision makers and practitioners. Being able to summarise in synthetic indices whole bodies of research conducted on related subjects using comparable methods appears as a powerful instrument to promote rationality in practice and evidence-based decision making. As a heuristic device to facilitate directions of action synthetic indices are in increasing demand. The range of interventions for which evaluations are being reviewed and synthesised is widening to include now health promotion interventions.

Documenting program efficacy also poses the question of the normalisation and standardisation of professional practices or the prerequisites to reproduce relevant practices. To the extent that effective practices are to be reproduced or disseminated there is a need to characterise more precisely what constitute the essence of those practices to facilitate transferability or translation in other contexts. Interestingly recent attempts to codify and standardise reporting of evaluation and applied research such as CONSORT (Moher, Schulz, & Altman, 2001) and more recently STROBE (Elm et al., 2007) are driven in most parts by knowledge synthesis enterprises that can better and easily apply their report analysis grid when the evaluation studies are reported in a standardised manner. In general interventions are subjected to synthesising processes in order to identify principles of action that could be transferred to address similar situations as part of a collection of best practices. The aim is to derive synthetic effectiveness indices. Those indices are meaningful only to the extent that implementation variations are smoothened or judged as irrelevant.

In the case of health promotion evaluation the difficulty of synthesising evaluations that take a large account of local adaptations, context and variations has been noticed in each of the projects that were developed to synthesise health promotion evaluation research results. Empirical evidence cannot be easily summed up when there is enormous uncontrolled implementation variation among programs for which evaluations are being synthesised. One solution indeed is to attempt to classify interventions according to the mechanisms that are thought to be triggered and operated through the interventions. Critical realist syntheses are being developed to

achieve such an objective (Pawson, 2000). Trying however to empirically and inductively identify such mechanisms through synthesis projects is highly exploratory
and the probability that the ex post models derived from those enterprises bear any
potential of transferability or generalizability remains tenuous.

We believe that theory has been underused as a heuristic device for synthesising
evaluation results (Green, 2000; Potvin, 2006). Indeed, a chronic lack of theory
in our field has been lamented by numerous commentators on health promotion
(McQueen et al., 2007). This inevitably leads to the question of which theories are
appropriate in health promotion. For McQueen et al. (2007) the potential contribution of social sciences to frame theories of and theories in health promotion is
yet to be realised. A good theory of health promotion would allow practitioners to
better define the objects of their interventions and not only the strategy, values and
principles by which such objects should be addressed. In counterparts, good social
theories in health promotion would highlight how health promotion interventions
as social systems interact in any given social context to produce whatever health
promotion is geared to produce.

Challenge 4: Producing Relevant Knowledge

Given the difficulty to delineate the reality of programs to evaluate and considering
the dilemmas associated with the selection of appropriate methods, the fourth challenge for evaluation consists in producing results and knowledge that is relevant and
contributing to health promotion objectives. In this perspective, evaluation fulfils
two functions. One is to document program efficacy to produce a desired outcome
and the other is to assist in the development of innovative health promotion practice
(Potvin & Goldberg, 2007; Schwandt, 2005).

Evaluation is often associated with the former perspective of documenting program efficacy. Recent knowledge synthesis projects led by the International IUHPE
(McQueen & Jones, 2007) and by the US Centers for Disease Control (Zaza,
Briss, & Harris, 2005) in order to justify health promotion interventions for health
sector decision makers are examples of enterprises in line with such objectives.
Indeed, in their attempts to locate evaluation studies of interventions designed and
implemented in response to specific problems, to isolate and identify the effective
components of these interventions and to combine observed results into synthetic
indices, the aim of these projects is clearly to assemble empirical arguments composed of scientific evidence in order to consolidate public investments in health
promotion. Another consequence of those projects is to propose collections of best
practices that not only guide but also standardise accepted and acceptable practice
in health promotion.

In addition to the problem of defining what constitutes evidence in a field
that is largely developed outside of explicit and precise theoretical propositions
(McQueen, 2007b), there is a paradox in the creation of such collections. Indeed,
notions such as efficacy and effectiveness are empty shells that are useful only to the

extent that a higher end is explicitly defined. Efficacy for what? This is certainly the next logical question but unfortunately it has rarely been given adequate attention in health promotion (see Chap. 15). In the field of public health pursuing objectives of increasing DALY or QALY independently of their distribution, or of improving conditions that shape population health, or increasing equity in the distribution of health outcomes, or strengthening community action independently of their ends are all legitimate objectives of action. Although these outcomes are not necessarily incompatible, their respective pursuits may require actions that are conflicting with one another (Potvin, Mantoura, & Ridde, 2007). Fundamental texts such as the Ottawa Charter do not give definitive answers to such questions. To be really relevant, efforts to document health promotion efficacy should be coupled with an in-depth reflection to clarify and prioritise objectives to which it contributes.

Another use of evaluation results is to support innovation in practice rather than their reproducibility and transferability. When conceived as a reflexive apparatus for a system of collective action, evaluation produces information that allows the system a better positioning of its interactions with its environment and eventually to better understand its co-evolution with its context (Potvin & Goldberg, 2007; Schwandt, 2005). This refined understanding of lived experience allows program stakeholders to continuously create the necessary micro adjustment in order to address controversies that arise from action (Potvin, 2007). Evaluation provides the objective empirical basis that makes reflexivity possible. Because health promotion is founded and moved by normative system composed of values and principles that are often better defined than its objectives, this function of reflexivity fuelled by evaluation is crucial in order to avoid ideological confusions (McQueen, 2007a). This reflexivity that characterises reasoned and reasonable professional practice is essential to avoid dogmatic pitfalls of a practice founded on the narrow ideology of its reproduction at all cost. A mirror for health promotion action, evaluation thus becomes not only a key component to support innovation but also a safeguard to maintain a rational direction for action.

Conclusion

Health promotion evaluation faces challenges that extend well beyond technical and methodological difficulties associated with the scientific nature of evaluation projects. Health promotion evaluators should expect to enter a dynamic and political arena the contours of which are continuously changing. In addition to scientific expertise health promotion evaluators need to think of their trade as a social practice the aim of which is to contribute to the betterment of our collective capacity to intervene on the determinants of population health. As the main operators of a scientific device functioning in a politicised space, health promotion evaluators face dilemmas and challenges the solution of which bears potentially enormous consequences for the field of health promotion. In this book we defend the thesis that as a practice, health promotion evaluation cannot implement activities that have the potential to undermine the pursuit of health promotion objectives whatever these are. More explicitly, since health promotion is generally defined by a core set of values and principles, health promotion evaluation has to account for those values and eventually even participate to their implementation. Like any scientific endeavour, evaluation is not a value neutral enterprise (Latour, 2004). In most cases, evaluation activities can be conceptualised as activities in the intervention space. If one undermines the potential effect of programs by conducting evaluation, then health promotion will never be able to be assessed fairly. Because the field of health promotion is openly and deliberately oriented by specific values, we believe that adequate and relevant practice in health promotion evaluation should attempt to align criteria of research rigour with those values and principles underlying health promotion.

The next section of this book is composed of four chapters, each one elaborating on the four dilemmas that were just outlined above. Written mostly by this book's editors, these chapters explore the content of what constitutes the practice of health promotion evaluators. That we have more questions than answers should not be of any surprise. Indeed health promotion is still struggling in attempts to define its proper theoretical foundations. Taken together however, these four chapters indicate possible directions for development and practical reflection in health promotion evaluation.

References

Barnes, M., Matka, E., & Sullivan, H. (2003). Evidence, understanding and complexity. Evaluation in non-linear systems. *Evaluation, 9*, 265–284.
Baskhar, R. (1978). A realist theory of science. Londres: Haverster Wheatsheaf.
Bisset, S. L., & Potvin, L. (2007) Expanding our conceptualization of program implementation: Lessons from the genealogy of a school-based nutrition program. *Health Education Research, 22*, 737–746.
Bourdieu, P. (1972). *Esquisse d'une théorie de la pratique*. Genève: Librairie Dorz.
Brown, P. (1995). The role of the evaluator in comprehensive community initiatives. In J. P. Connell, A. C. Kubisch, L. B. Schorr, & C. H. Weiss (Eds.), *New approaches to evaluating community initiatives. Concepts, methods and contexts* (pp. 201–225). New York: Aspen Institute.
Campbell, D. T. (1984). Can we be scientific in applied social science? In: R. F. Connor, D. G. Altman, & C. Jackson (Eds.), *Evaluation studies review annual, Vol 9* (pp. 26–48). Beverly Hills CA: Sage.
Christie, C. A. (2003). What guides evaluation? A study of how evaluation practice maps onto evaluation theory. New *Directions for Evaluation, 97*, 7–35.
Crozier, M., & Friedberg, E. (1977). *L'Acteur et le système*. Paris: Seuil.
Dab, W. (2005). Reflections on the challenges of health programs. *Promotion & Education, Suppl. No 3*, 74–77.
Dooris, M., Poland, B., Kolbe, L., De Leuuw, E., McCall, D., & Wharf-Higgins, J. (2007). Healthy settings. Building evidence for the effectiveness of whole system health promotion – Challenges and future directions. In D. V. McQueen & C. M. Jones (Eds.), *Global perspectives on health promotion effectiveness* (pp. 327–352). New York: Springer.
Elm, E. von Altman, D. G., Egger, M., Pocock, S. J., Gotzsche, P. C., Vandenbroucke, J. P. for the Strobe initiative (2007). Strengthening the reporting of observational studies in epidemiology (STROBE) statement: Guidelines for reporting observational studies. *British Medical Journal, 335*, 806–808.

Fleck, L. (1979). *Genesis and development of a scientific fact. (originally published in German in 1935)*. Chicago: University of Chicago Press.

Giddens, A. (1984). *The constitution of society: Introduction to the theory of structuration*. Berkeley CA: University of California Press.

Green, J. (2000). The role of theory in evidence-based health promotion practice. *Health Education Research, 15*, 125–129.

Green, L. W., & Lewis, F. M. (1986). *Measurement and evaluation in health education and health promotion*. Palo Alto CA: Mayfield.

Hawe, P., Degeling, D. & Hall, J. (1990). *Evaluating health promotion: A health worker's guide*. Sydney Australia: MacLennan.

Hawe, P., & Potvin, L. (Forthcoming). What is population health intervention research? *Canadian Journal of Public Health*.

Hawe, P., Shiell, A., & Riley, T. (2004). Complex interventions: How "out of control" can a randomized control trial be? *British Medical Journal, 328*, 1561–1563.

Hill, A. B. (1953). Observation and experiment. *The New England Journal of Medicine, 248*, 995–1001.

Hills, M., & McQueen, D. V. (Eds.) (2007). The Ottawa Charter for health promotion – A critical reflection. *Promotion & Education, Suppl. 2*.

Kickbusch, I. (2003). The contribution of the World Health Organization to a new public health and health promotion. *American Journal of Public Health, 93*, 383–388.

King, J. A. (2003). The challenge of studying evaluation theory. *New Directions for Evaluation, 97*, 57–80.

Kuhn, T. (1962). *The structure of scientific revolutions*. Chicago: University of Chicago Press.

Latour, B. (1987). *Science in action: How to follow scientists and engineers through society*. Cambridge MA: Harvard University Press.

Latour, B. (1993). *We have never been modern*. Cambridge MA: Harvard University Press.

Latour, B. (2004). *Politics of nature. How to bring science into democracy*. Cambridge MA: Harvard University Press.

LeMoigne, J-M. (1977). *La théorie du système général. Théorie de la modélisation*. Paris: Presses universitaires de France.

Levesque, L., Richard, L., Duplantie, J., Gauvin, L., Cargo, M., Renaud, L., et al. (2000). Vers une description et une évaluation du caractère écologique des interventions en promotion de la santé: le cas du Programme de la Carélie du nord. *Rupture, revue transdisciplinaire en santé, 7*, 114–129.

McLaughlin, J. A., & Jordan, G. B. (1999). Logic models: A tool for telling your programs performance story. *Program Planning and Evaluation, 22*, 65–72.

McQueen, D. V. (1996). The search for theory in health behaviour and health promotion. *Health Promotion International, 11*, 27–32.

McQueen, D. V. (1988). Directions for research in health behaviors related to health promotion: an overview. In R. Anderson, J. K. Davies, I. Kickbusch, D. V. McQueen & J. Turner (Eds.), *Health behaviour research and health promotion* (pp. 251–265). Oxford: Oxford University Press.

McQueen, D. V. (2007a). Critical issues in theory for health promotion. In D. V. McQueen, I. Kickbusch, L. Potvin, J. M. Pelikan, L. Balbo, & T. Abel (Eds.), *Health & modernity. The role of theory in health promotion* (pp. 21–42). New York: Springer.

McQueen, D. V. (2007b). Evidence and theory. Continuing debates on evidence and effectiveness. In D. V. McQueen & C. M. Jones (Eds.), *Global perspectives on health promotion effectiveness* (pp. 281–303). New York: Springer.

McQueen, D. V., & Anderson, L. M. (2001). What counts as evidence: Issues and debates. In I. Rootman, M. Goodstadt, B. Hyndman, D. V. McQueen, L. Potvin, J. Springett, & E. Ziglio (Eds.), *Evaluation in health promotion. Principles and perspectives* (pp. 63–81). Copenhague: WHO regional publications. European series; No 92.

McQueen, D. V., & Jones, C. M. (Eds.) (2007). *Global perspectives on health promotion effectiveness*. New York: Springer.

McQueen, D. V., Kickbusch, I., Potvin, L., Pelikan, J. M., Balbo, L., & Abel, T. (2007). *Health & modernity. The role of theory in health promotion.* New York: Springer.

Mark, M. M., Henry, G. T., & Julnes, G. (2000). Evaluation: An integrated framework for understanding, guiding, and improving policies and programs. San Francisco: Jossey Bass.

Moher, D., Schulz, K. F., & Altman, D. G. (2001). The CONSORT statement: Revised recommendations for improving the quality of parallel-group randomised trials. *Lancet, 285,* 1191–1194.

Nutbeam, D. (2004). Getting evidence into policy and practice to address health inequalities. *Health Promotion International, 19,* 137–140.

Nutbeam, D., & Bauman, A. E. (2006). Evaluation in a nutshell: A practical guide to the evaluation of health promotion programs. New York: McGraw Hill.

O'Connor, A. (1995). Evaluating comprehensive community initiatives: A view from history. In J. P. Connell, A. C. Kubisch, L. B. Schorr, & C. H. Weiss (Eds.), *New approaches to evaluating community initiatives: Concepts, methods, and context.* (pp. 23–63). Washington D.C.: Aspen Institute.

Pawson R. (2000). Evidence-based policy: The promise of Realist Synthesis. *Evaluation, 8,* 340–358.

Potvin, L. (2006). Should we worry about the enthusiasm toward evidence-based health promotion practices? *Promotion & Education, 13,* 228–229.

Potvin, L. (2007). Managing uncertainty through participation. In D. V. McQueen, I. Kickbusch, L. Potvin, J. M. Pelikan, L. Balbo, & T. Abel (Eds.), *Health & modernity. The role of theory in health promotion* (pp. 103–128). New York: Springer.

Potvin, L., & Chabot, P. (2002). Splendour and misery of epidemiology for evaluation of health promotion. *Revista Brasileira de Epidemiologia, 5*(Suppl. 1), 91–103.

Potvin, L., Gendron, S., Bilodeau, A. (2006). Três posturas ontológicas concernentes à natureza dos programas de saúde: implicações para a avaliação. In M. L. M. Bosi & F. J. Mercado (Eds.), *Avaloaçao qualitative de programas de saude. Enfoques emergentes* (pp. 65–86). Petropolis, Brazil: Vozes Editorial.

Potvin, L., Gendron, S., Bilodeau, A., & Chabot, P. (2005). Integrating social science theory into public health practice. *American Journal of Public Health, 95,* 591–595.

Potvin, L., & Goldberg, C. (2007). Two roles of evaluation in transforming health promotion practice. In M. O'Neill, A, Pederson., S. Dupéré & I. Rootman (Eds.), *Health promotion in Canada. Critical perspective,* Second edition (pp. 347–360). Toronto: Canadian Scholar's Press.

Potvin, L., Haddad, S., & Frohlich, K. L. (2001). Beyond process and outcome evaluation: A comprehensive approach for evaluating health promotion programmes. In I. Rootman, M. Goodstadt, B. Hyndman, D.V. McQueen, L. Potvin, J. Springett, & E. Ziglio (Eds.), *Evaluation in health promotion. Principles and perspectives* (pp. 45–62). Copenhague: WHO regional publications. European series; No 92.

Potvin, L., & McQueen, D. V. (2007). Modernity, public health and health promotion. A reflexive discourse. In D. V. McQueen, I. Kickbusch, L. Potvin, J. M. Pelikan, L. Balbo, & T. Abel (Eds.), *Health & modernity. The role of theory in health promotion* (pp. 12–20). New York: Springer.

Potvin, L., Mantoura, P., & Ridde, V. (2007). Evaluating equity in health promotion. In D. V. McQueen & C. M. Jones (Eds.), *Global perspectives on health promotion effectiveness* (pp. 367–383). New York: Springer.

Rothman, K. L. (1986). *Modern epidemiology.* Boston: Little, Brown and Company.

Rootman, I., Goodstadt, M., Hyndman, B., McQueen, D. V., Potvin, L., Springett, J., et al. (Eds.) (2001). *Evaluation in health promotion. Principles and perspectives.* Copenhague: WHO regional publications. European series; No 92.

Rootman, I., Goodstadt, M., Potvin, L., & Springett, J. (2001). A framework for health promotion evaluation. In I. Rootman, M. Goodstadt, B. Hyndman, D.V. McQueen, L. Potvin, J. Springett, & E. Ziglio (Eds.), *Evaluation in health promotion. Principles and perspectives* (pp. 7–38). Copenhague: WHO regional publications. European series; No 92.

Rossi. P. H., & Freeman, H. E. (1993). *Evaluation. A systematic approach.* Newbury Park CA: Sage.

Rubin, D. B. (1974). Estimating causal effects of treatments in randomized and non randomized studies. *Journal of Education Psychology, 66,* 688–701.

Schwandt, T. A. (2005). The centrality of practice to evaluation. *American Journal of Evaluation, 26,* 95–105.

Shadish, W. R., Jr., Cook, T. D., & Leviton, L. C, L. (1991). *Foundations of program evaluation.* Thousand Oaks CA: Sage.

Suchman, E. A. (1967). *Evaluation research.* New York: Russel Sage Foundation.

Thurston, W. E., & Potvin, L. (2003). Evaluability assessment: A tool for incorporating evaluation in social change programs. *Evaluation, 9,* 453–469.

Valente, T. W. (2002). *Evaluating health promotion programs.* New York: Oxford University Press.

WHO. (1986). *The Ottawa Charter for heath promotion.* Downloaded in November 2007 from: www.phac-aspc.gc.ca/ph-sp/phdd/pdf/charter.pdf

Williams, G. H. (2003). The determinants of health: structure, context and agency. *Sociology of Health & Ilness, 25,* 131–154.

Windsor, R. A. (1994). Evaluation of health promotion, health education and disease prevention programs. Mountain View CA: Mayfield.

Windsor, R. Baranowski, T., Clark, N., & Cutter, G. (1984). *Evaluation of health promotion, health education programs.* Mountain View: Mayfield.

Windsor, R. A., Clark, N. M., Boyd, N. R., & Goodman, R. M. (2003). *Evaluation of health promotion, health education and disease prevention programs* (3rd edition). New York: McGraw Hill.

Zaza, S., Briss, P. A., & Harris, K. W. (2005). *The guide to community preventive services. What works to promote health.* New York: Oxford University Press.

Part II
Issues in Health Promotion Evaluation: Fitting Evaluation Practice to Health Promotion

Chapter 4
Developing Evaluation Questions: Beyond the Technical Issues

Ligia de Salazar and Mary Hall

This chapter is a contribution to the evaluation debate in health promotion. It explores the strategies for, and main concerns in, identifying and formulating relevant and answerable evaluation questions. Unlike many previous texts discussing what is involved in developing evaluation questions, in this chapter we argue that a wide range of contextual and highly political factors contribute to the framing of evaluation questions. Furthermore, we strongly believe that the same intervention can lend itself to a variety of different evaluation questions depending upon the stage of intervention development at which the evaluation is conducted. Finally, we contend that the evaluation question or set of questions should reflect the ever-changing context of the intervention, as well as the stage if the intervention, if evaluation is to be truly useful for health promotion.

The Cochrane Collaboration defined the relationship of health promotion and public health in this way: "health promotion and public health encompasses the assessment of the health of populations formulating policies to prevent or respond to health problems promoting healthy environments and generally promoting health through the organized effort of society. Public health promotes societal action to invest in living conditions that create, maintain and protect health. This covers an extremely wide range of interventions aimed at improving health, with various levels and types of interventions included" (EPPI – Centre, 2006). Health Promotion expands upon the definition of health by addressing the complexity of social changes, reiterating the importance of acting not only on the issue of demedicalization and reorientation of health services and practices, but especially in the sphere of local development and empowerment. Carvalho, Bodstein, Hartz, and Matida (2004) discussed political and economic determinants of the health-disease process, reaffirming health as an ethical imperative and a citizen's right.

There are many elements common to the numerous different definitions of evaluation available in the literature. These include describing, comparing and assessing the value of programs and interventions in the pursuit of specific aims and, increasingly, incorporating lessons learned into the decision-making process (OECD, 1998). Other authors conceive of evaluation as a process of systematic and

L. de Salazar
Universidad del Valle, Cali, Colombia

L. Potvin, D. McQueen (eds.), *Health Promotion Evaluation Practices in the Americas*,
DOI: 10.1007/978-0-387-79733-5_4, © Springer Science+Business Media, LLC 2008

objective appraisal of a project, program or policy (Shadish, Cook, & Leviton, 1995). According to Hawe, Degeling, Hall, and Brierley (2003) evaluation is a judgement about something. These authors assert that the way in which these judgments are made depends upon expectations, past experiences, and what relevant actors believe to be important. For (Battista et al., 1999), evaluation reinforces the critical link between science and policy, and attempts to reconcile those two worlds, which operate within different paradigms. While Western science often adopts a positivist paradigm that assumes the existence of truth, policy-making is an interpretive process oriented toward the integration of various factors into operating decisions.

In addition to assessing interventions' success, evaluations are also oriented toward obtaining information in order to interpret what has happened in interventions, particularly through participatory processes and techniques. They take various forms, including process evaluation, participatory evaluation, formative evaluation, empowerment evaluation, and illuminating evaluation (MacDonald, Veen, & Tones, 1996).

Effectiveness evaluation has been highly debated in recent years, and the term is loaded with many connotations. As a particular type of outcome evaluation (Weiss, 1998) effectiveness evaluation is increasingly considered to be an accepted standard for health promotion evaluation (McQueen & Jones, 2007). Issues and criticism regarding effectiveness evaluation are often related to the question: *Do we need evidence of effectiveness to make decisions in order to accomplish health-promotion objectives?*

Potvin, Haddad, and Frohlich (2001) have discussed the fact that evaluation questions need to reflect a comprehensive understanding of health promotion programs they are intended to address. This paper takes this argument a step further and discusses the wide range of other factors that influence and shape the process by which evaluation questions are identified and formulated.

Many issues related to evaluation in health promotion have been raised over the years. Discussions pertaining to the definition of the subjects and objects of the evaluation, the criteria for selecting and developing appropriate evaluation questions; the variables and indicators for measuring and rating success; the various methodological approaches to data collection; and the relationship between evaluators and decision-makers or between policy and research, can all be found in the health promotion literature. In this chapter our aim is to bring together new and old arguments in favor of focusing health promotion evaluation on a variety of relevant aspects of health promotion interventions in order to strengthen health promotion theory and practice.

The issue of where to focus the evaluation is often perceived as simply a matter of the stage of the intervention, or decision-makers' needs for information. Developing and formulating an evaluation question goes far beyond the technical aspects of formulating an answerable question. We argue that it is essentially a practical issue; it is a complex process, iterative in nature, which involves negotiation among the various stakeholders. This negotiation is most often political in nature, and requires trade-offs and compromises on the scope of the evaluation, the methodological approaches required and the political relevance of the information produced by the evaluation.

The iterative aspect of identifying and formulating an evaluation question reflects the constantly changing context of the intervention, and consequently, the evaluation. Different questions can be formulated during the life cycle of the healthpromotion intervention, which are influenced by the context, the evolution and the changing nature of the intervention, as well as by the demands of decision-makers or other stakeholders. This point is illustrated in Chapter 12 of this book in the discussion of the challenges of evaluating intersectoral initiatives.

Practical Isssues in Formulating an Evaluation Question

Fomulating an evaluation question is a practical, rather than a technical issue. Developing the evaluation question or questions is not solely a matter of fitting a research question with available data collection methods. It is rather an inherently political matter affected by, and impacting numerous factors. Those factors that shape the process of developing the evaluation question include: the purpose of the evaluation, the interests of the various stakeholders, their beliefs and representations about the intervention, and the criteria for success or failure. Furthermore, developing evaluation questions has to do with the improvement of health promotion interventions as well as the use of results to improve health conditions and promote population health. A poorly formulated question could have negative impact on present and future health; therefore this activity bears political, ethical and economic consequences.

The evaluation of health promotion interventions has traditionally been driven by academic interest rather than by the information needs of those responsible for managing and allocating resources or by community people who benefit from those decisions. Whose point of view should be considered when defining evaluation questions? Is it feasible to reach an agreement, and if so, how?

Several factors drive the process of identifying relevant evaluation questions. These are: (1) the theoretical and operational definition of the intervention being evaluated, (2) the meaning and scope of evaluation for the health promotion practitioners involved, (3) the purpose of the evaluation, (4) the criteria by which stakeholders will judge intervention effectiveness, (5) the decision-making context and (6) the feasibility of producing the expected results within a reasonable timeframe. Each of these factors presents different challenges to the evaluation of health promotion, and may carry different weight depending on the intervention and the persons involved. A discussion of the impact each has on selecting the evaluation question follows.

Theoretical and Operational Definition of the Intervention Being Evaluated

One of the key aspects to keep in mind when evaluating health promotion interventions is the changing nature of the context in which they are implemented and the effects these transformations have on interventions and their potential outcomes. Interventions can, and must, be adjusted to real situations according to demands and needs, even those that were not foreseen when planning the intervention. Therefore, it is of utmost importance to define, in practical terms, what is the intervention that is going to be evaluated, and to achieve agreement on this matter among the various stakeholders, including those who are responsible for the evaluation. Context, defined as the characteristics of the setting into which the health promotion intervention is implemented, can act both as a factor influencing the implementation of the intervention and as an effect modifier of the intervention.

The elements and parameters that constitute the operational definition of the intervention (the way it is implemented) vary according to the sociopolitical context in which the intervention is implemented, the availability of certain conditions to make implementation feasible, and the beliefs and values of practitioners involved. Conducting evaluation of those projects is also dependent on these factors. The principles and values that support health promotion action are not always in agreement with the political system in which they operate, making it difficult to find appropriate implementation strategies.

An example of how the definition of the intervention can impact the evaluation is provided by the issue of equity, a key principle of health promotion. Unequitable distribution of resources in a community, and the way it affects both risks and outcomes, are important issues to be considered in the evaluation. It has been recognized (Waters, Doyle, & Jackson, 2006) that inequities are related not only to the risk of developing an adverse condition but also with the effectiveness of the intervention. Therefore, if socioeconomic status is associated with the implementation of the intervention, and if socioeconomic status is unevenly distributed among the population targeted by the intervention, these probabilities affect the effectiveness of the intervention.

We recognize that the task of characterizing and simplifying what are actually complex multi-component interventions is often very difficult and challenging. This is made even more difficult by the need to think of causes not as properties of agents, but as results of systems in which the population phenomena of health and disease occur, and to conceive of populations as organized groups with relational properties rather than mere aggregates of individuals (Loomis & Wing, 1990). However challenging the task, a clear description of the intervention must be achieved before formulating evaluation questions in order to draw any meaningful conclusions from the evaluation.

Meaning and Scope of Evaluation in Health Promotion Interventions

Evaluation in health promotion should consider, among other things, the fact that health promotion initiatives respond to dynamic processes that are participatory, multifactorial, political and multidimensional. Health promotion involves concomitant and diverse interventions oriented to reach specific but complementary objectives. It focuses on groups and communities rather than individuals. It has short and long-term effects, as well as intangible benefits. It is articulated toward development and intersectoral planning more than the health sector alone. These distinctive characteristics of health promotion are important, as they influence the conduct of evaluation. Because of these characteristics there is a need to articulate knowledge stemming from political, social and biologic sciences in the analysis and interpretation of evaluation results. Also related is the challenge of defining in measurable terms the health promotion principles and values that are effective in an intervention. Finally, the potential need for, and difficulty in, generalizing evaluation results can also be linked to these unique characteristics.

Evaluation in health promotion also involves a trade off between credibility, opportunity, relevance, replicability of evaluation results, as well as diverse, and at times, conflicting interests of stakeholders. It is important to keep in mind that, as health promotion interventions are inherently dynamic and are the product of a permanent reflection-action process, the risk of evaluating something other than what was supposed to be evaluated, remains significant.

Evaluation Purpose

In addition to defining the intervention to be evaluated, those conducting the evaluation must reach agreement concerning the purpose for the evaluation. The reasons for engaging in health promotion are highly varied, and depend to a great degree on the interest of the stakeholders. Questions about the intervention and goals for the evaluation must therefore be explicitly addressed.

What exactly should be evaluated? Should the focus be on the design, process (implementation), impact or results of intervention? What are the variables and indicators of success for each of these components? Answers to these questions drive the types of evaluation questions to be asked, and have significant impact on the success of health promotion evaluation projects.

Evaluators often face conflicting situations when they have to decide on the type of evaluation, bearing in mind the need to produce timely, accessible and relevant information according to technical, managerial, and political considerations. Defining the right question, at the right time, within a particular context, depends on several factors, some of which have already been mentioned. It is important to include also: the availability of technical and financial resources, access to reliable sources of information, the requirements of the funding agencies and planners, and the decisions that will be made using the evaluation results.

There exist a variety of reasons for which we conduct evaluation, including scientific interest, and the need for information to decide how or whether to improve, expand, extend or replace a determined intervention. Evaluation questions orient the selection of the appropriate evaluation study design. Two categories of questions will be considered in the following discussion. The first one pertains to the process and intermediate results of the implementation of the intervention. The purpose in this type of inquiry is to identify the characteristics of the intervention life cycle, the interrelations among actors, the strengths and limitations, the changes or intermediate results, and their contributing factors. It responds to questions as to what and how social changes occur within the intervention. The second category addresses the need for decision-makers to determine whether the intervention should be extended expanded or replaced, and answers the question whether the intervention produced the desired outcomes.

Process evaluation is a means to strengthen health promotion practice, and to improve intervention planning and execution. When integrated within intervention planning, implementation and follow up, process evaluations significantly improve interventions. In this cycle, planning, implementation, follow-up and evaluation are not independent events but are designed to continually feed back and provide new information inputs in the process. As stated earlier, the dynamic nature of health promotion intervention requires that questions and evaluation designs take this dynamic process into account, and more importantly, make explicit the mechanisms that produce those transformations. This is achieved through a monitoring system that constantly documents and analyzes the intervention as implemented. Such a system can be achieved by conducting a systematization analysis (de Salazar, 2002), using qualitative research methods appropriate to understand complex phenomena.

Systematization requires that process oriented questions are asked, so that the intervention can be continually improved. Did public opinion change over time? Did changes in opinion, if any, have an impact on policymaking? What was the media opinion as reflected in news coverage? How feasible is it to measure values? (Diez-Roux, 1998) These are the kind of questions addressed in this type of evaluation.

Another type of evaluation, in which the purpose is to make sound recommendations for decision-making, requires that we ask the question: how much do we know about the intervention we are evaluating? And if the intervention is not well defined, then what are we going to recommend? These types of evaluation questions are also useful to identify the necessary conditions for the intervention to produce the desired effect and that constitute requirements for future intervention deployment.

What is at stake in this type of evaluation is whether the intervention produces the desired effects. The emphasis is on identifying what changed as a result of the intervention and how much. Although these two types of evaluation – process and effectiveness – respond to different interests and purposes, they are complementary.

Criteria to Judge Effectiveness

Effectiveness evaluation has been conceived in this chapter as the description and measurement of intervention indicators of success or failure and the establishment of empirical associations between their variations and the intervention. In effectiveness evaluation there is interest in establishing whether the intervention worked and if it achieved the outcomes for which it was designed. It responds to what, how much, and how questions regarding changes produced by the intervention.

The political and ethical issues raised by effectiveness evaluation have been discussed by Ray and Mayan (2001). They raise questions such as who determines what counts as evidence, and what are the right indicators and appropriate standards in effectiveness evaluation research? Another concern is how different stakeholders, with vastly different expectations, can reach an agreement about criteria to establish effectiveness of an intervention that benefits them in different ways and to varying degrees.

For health promotion interventions, it is essential not only to inquire about the effectiveness of a given intervention, but about the process through which the intervention achieved the desired outcomes in the short, medium, and long term. This is paramount in order to understand how interventions work, and to increase their relevance and responsiveness to local conditions and contexts (WHO, 2001).

One important aspect in judging intervention effectiveness is the integration of the evidence yielded by evaluation into health promotion theory and practice. The evaluation purpose must be made clear at the outset, in order to determine how it can contribute to health promotion theory and practice. Being aware of whether the evaluation is seen as a contributor to strengthen health promotion theory or practice, or as a research tool to support decisions, or as merely a means to justify decisions already made will help put the evaluation results into a proper perspective.

Another important issue in judging an intervention's effectiveness is related to the type of information valued by the relevant stakeholders. Depending on the rationale supporting the decision-making process and the definition of evidence held by stakeholders what is judged as relevant knowledge varies. According to Lomas (WHO, 2005) scientific evidence can be categorized into context free (absolute truth), and context sensitive but conversely, Oxman (WHO, 2005) argues that all evidence is context sensitive since all observations are made in a specific context. Both science-based and non-scientific information, when properly translated, have potential strategic value. Interventions in which the change process has been documented and a permanent reflexive process has been implemented in order to understand the nature of the changes occurring and the factors that facilitate those changes as well as the influence of various actors on those processes, provide examples of the usefulness of various types of evidence.

The above implies that "evidence is plural and that the implementability of good global evidence must be triangulated with local knowledge" (WHO, 2005). This raises other issues, such as how useful, generalizable and amenable to standardization should health promotion evidence be? Should the criteria for judging effectiveness be adjusted according to the type of inquiry, to the context where decisions will be made? Or is evidence, by definition, not suited to the judgement of effectiveness of complex social interventions and to the information needs of decision-makers?

The critical issue raised by such questions pertains to the contextual factors that influence evidence of effectiveness. Are they the same in health promotion as in other types of public health interventions? It is expected that context-sensitive evidence is influenced by political and social factors, whereas personal and institutional factors are more associated with scientific evidence. Although most definitions of evidence cover qualitative and quantitative indicators, the term evidence is often restricted to quantitative facts derived from large-sample, randomized experimental studies that are ill-equiped to capture the inherent complexity of health promotion (McQueen & Anderson, 2000). Madjar and Walton (2001) argue that a broad notion of evidence also includes qualitative evidence in the form of lived experiences, case histories and stories. This kind of evidence is important because it enhances the understanding of human behaviour; it promotes holistic thinking, offers contextual qualitative data, and is more than just mere opinion because it is generated in a systematic way.

Our purpose here is not to debate about the meaning of evidence in health promotion, as many authors have discussed this issue elsewhere (Kemm, 2006; Madjar & Walton, 2001; Marmot, 2004), but rather to mention the theoretical and practical underpinnings of the term evidence as linked to effectiveness in the context of decision- making.

If evaluation is considered a means to strengthen health promotion practice, it should be accepted that the evaluation studies should not only document intervention effects but they should also contribute to a better understanding of, and make explicit, the mechanisms that produce them (de Salazar, 2002). These two goals require that different types of questions are formulated, and it is important to make these explicit at the outset of the evaluation.

Health promotion interventions are supposed to be adapted according to stakeholders' needs and expectations and to the context in which they are developed. Thus, beyond etiological explanations obtained in controlled situations, evaluation in health promotion must account for changes occuring in real situations. Evaluation questions should therefore be oriented toward identifying, quantifying and explaining these changes, and also understanding the processes that produce them, giving meaning to the associations between intervention and changes.

Decision-Making Context

A precise and profound knowledge about the context in which interventions are being implemented and evaluated is necessary to define appropriate and relevant evaluation questions as well as the manner in which those questions should be answered. Information about context includes: information related to the life cycle of the intervention; degree of intervention acceptance among stakeholders, decision-makers, and beneficiaries; the current policies and programs influencing the intervention; and the interests of decision-makers and practitioners regarding terminating or extending the intervention.

The health promotion literature reflects a growing interest in linking knowledge, policy and action. There is, however, little discussion on how such linkage can be accomplished (Stivers, 1991). It is only recently that public health researchers in developing countries have become aware of the importance of working more closely with policy-makers and the public to implement their findings into policy arenas. Brint (1990) illustrates how scientifc studies may stimulate new ways to conceive policy problems and solutions. A number of ancillary questions can guide the exploration of the decision-making context.

Who Are the Decision-Makers?

The interests of the main users of evaluation help define the scope of the evaluation, so their identification is important, as well as the identification of their interests, needs and perceptions with regard to the intervention. There are different users of evaluation results. Stakeholder is the label for those groups whose interests are, or are perceived to be affected by a change in interventions and policy. Stakeholders include elected or bureaucratic officials as heads of committees, parties, and bureaus as well as commercial, scientific, medical and voluntary nonprofit entities, including public interest groups (Feldstein, 1996; Jasanoff, 1993).

Evaluation results have the potential to influence the agenda of policy makers when they respond to their needs and interests in a timely manner. Should health promotion evaluation therefore be driven by policy-makers' needs, given the political nature of health promotion endeavors? What is at issue here is how to combine the interests of different parties, given that most of the time interventions involve a variety of people at different levels and from various sectors.

What Are the Needs and Interests of Decision-Makers and Other Stakeholders?

It is important to inquire about what results are needed and by when, and to determine how to formulate evaluation questions that correspond to users interests without losing relevance and accuracy. The rationale and perspectives with which evaluators appraise interventions do not necessarily correspond to those of decision-makers, so evaluators are well advised to ask themselves whether the information required by decision-makers to take action can be translated into a researchable question. Evaluators must also ask if, in fact, scientific research is the most appropriate manner to obtain evidence, or if evidence is needed at all for policy-makers to take action.

It is important to ask and find answers to questions such as: What do we want to know? Which information do we hope to obtain with the evaluation? For what purposes are we evaluating this intervention? What will we do with the information? Who requires the evaluation? This information is of great utility in defining the scope of the evaluation, the degree of precision needed, and the most appropriate evaluation study design.

There are significant differences in the type of questions deemed relevant by those implementing the intervention, the sponsors, the public and the intervention staff. Implementers may be more interested in the performance of the intervention and in understanding the implementation process in order to make adjustments.

Sponsors funding agencies and staff may have greater interest in knowing the outputs and the benefits to special groups. Funders' evaluation questions tend to pertain to the worth of society to allocate financial, human or other resources to particular interventions (PAHO, 2007).

How Is the Evaluation Perceived?

According to CIID (2001), evaluation is an integral part of program and project management. It is an organizational learning tool oriented toward strengthening institutional responsibility. Milio (1990), on the other hand, argues that policy evaluation studies seek to assess the gaps between what is, and what ought to be, in terms of policy objectives and results, between means and ends (Brewer & de Leon, 1983).

Evaluation is considered a multidisciplinary and applied field intended to address real-world issues in a timely fashion. Its audiences include a wide range of non-scientific groups, such as policy-makers in legislatures and administrative bodies, advocacy groups, and organizations' governing bodies (Benjamin, Perfetto, & Greene, 1995).

How to Adapt Evaluation Questions to the Interests of Users Without Losing Relevance and Accuracy?

The answer to this question is: through negotiation. But to do this, good information must be available. Evaluation is conducted in a political environment, a fact that is sometimes not fully recognized by evaluators. In some instances, insufficient, untimely, and irrelevant information is provided to decision-makers and the public. Such unfortunate evaluation outcomes can be attributable to various causes such as: the way evaluation studies are designed, the type of questions formulated, the manner in which evaluation results are presented, insufficient knowledge about the context, deficiencies in evaluator's abilities to deal with decision-makers and insufficient management and negotiation skills from the evaluator.

It is well known that decisions are supported not only by information about effectiveness, but also by information about when and how the intervention works, and the conditions that influence the intervention effects. Additional information required for decision-making includes the characteristics of the life cycle of the intervention, the interrelations among actors, the strengths and limitations of the evaluation study design, and factors that are responsible for outcomes. In addition to those evaluation related factors, evaluators should be cognizant of what is at stake for the various stakeholders affected by the decision. In other words, context-bounded knowledge is necessary to judge the replicability or extension of an intervention (Milio, 1990). Even when policy analyses show health benefits, the decision to support an intervention may be negatively influenced by factors related to the environment in which the evaluation and negotiations were conducted.

Evaluators must be aware of the conditions and context in which evaluation is required and conducted. Evaluators often face conflicting situations when they must decide on the type of evaluation question to be pursued, considering the need to produce timely, accessible and relevant information according to technical, managerial, and political conditions. They should consider the trade-offs between the validity and utility of evaluation results and between evidence of effectiveness versus evidence of social profitability. To respond to information needs in an opportune and accurate manner, the process of developing and formulating an evaluation question and deciding on the scope of the evaluation has to be conducted with the decision-making context in mind.

The Feasibility of Producing the Expected Evaluation Results Within a Reasonable Timeframe

Evidence of effectiveness is also bound by time considerations. For those implementing an intervention, it is rather counterproductive to wait until the end of the intervention before obtaining evaluation results. So, questions related to intermediary results are often appropriate and constitute important input for making decisions regarding intervention implementation.

Type of Questions and Methodological Issues Practical Issues in Defining Evaluation Questions

In social and complex phenomena, like in most health promotion interventions where adaptations to specific conditions could mean significant changes in the conceptual framework, implementation and scope of the intervention, there is a big risk in attempting to evaluate plans that have not in fact been implemented. On the other hand, if the evaluation is conceived of as contributing to intervention improvement and a political tool to induce intervention changes through negotiation, this should be taken into account in the formulation of the evaluation questions.

Different methodological approaches support the definition of appropriate and sound evaluation questions. In general there are two interrelated categories of questions: those related to understanding social changes, or changes in social practices of social agents, including the relationships among actors within the intervention; and those that account for the results and effects of interventions.

There is a wide range of foci and methodologies to assist or orient the identification and definition of evaluation questions, and therefore also a range of study designs that can be implemented. The first category of questions is supported by the practice of documentation and systematization of interventions, and by practices such as responsive and participatory evaluation and outcome mapping (Jara, 2000; Francke & Morgan, 1995; Chilean Government, 2004, de Salazar, 2004; de Salazar, Diaz, & Magaña, 2002).

Undertaking the development of evaluation questions with the following principles in mind may facilitate the evaluator's task.

• Recognize the complexity of developing a theoretically sound series of questions that relate the multiple levels of action in health promotion interventions.
  This complexity is likely to be a better reflection of reality than the simpler
  multicausal models prevalent today (Loomis & Wing, 1990). Evaluations that
  are guided by complex sets of questions provide information to understand the
  process, enhance the understanding of human behaviours, promote holistic thinking, offer contextual information and bring to the forefront the perspectives and
  preoccupations of the community or target groups;
• Develop questions that are oriented to identifying and understanding the
  processes of change, and the intermediary results of those changes. Even when
  questions are derived from the goals and intentions of policy-makers, they
  should pertain to issues relevant to as many stakeholders as possible, including
  policymakers, managers, practitioners, community and target groups (Guba &
  Lincoln, 1981, 1989; Lincoln & Guba, 1985; Stake, 1975; Stake & Abma,
  2005).
• Develop permanent procedures that facilitate communication among the various interventions' stakeholders. The interface between knowledge and practice
  should be facilitated as well as with the context, that is the social, organizational,
  and political settings in which the intervention is implemented. Such a procedure
  is vital to identify the meaning and scope of the intervention in the real world;
  the needed changes in protocol design, and their justifications.
• The evaluation questions should address the preoccupations and interests of
  the people that are close to the intervention (Chilean Government, 2004; Earl,
  Carden, & Smutylo, 2001; Jara, 2000, de Salazar, 2004; de Salazar et al., 2002).
  Evaluation questions are ideally derived through a process of documentation-
  reflection that involves intervention stakeholders. It is a product of the dynamics
  and interests present within the intervention.
• Interest and evaluation questions are associated with intervention's success. They
  increase the probability of learning about how to improve the effectiveness of
  an intervention. In this case the danger of not discovering the hidden contribution is eliminated, when feedback is focused on improving rather than proving,
  understanding instead of making responsible, and creating knowledge instead of
  contributing merits for itself (Smutylo, 2001).
• Ideally, evaluation criteria used to asses interventions' effectiveness are not only
  derived from the goals and intentions of policy-makers, but include a wide range
  of issues from as many stakeholders as possible, including policy-makers, managers, practitioners, community and target groups. Evaluation questions are formulated through partnerships among the sectors and actors committed to the
  intervention, contributing to an active and permanent participation into the evaluation, picking up perceptions, interests, contributions and points of agreement.
• Negotiation of the evaluation questions and study design has to be undertaken
  considering the overall intervention complexity. Ideally, the evaluator takes on

the role of facilitator, interpreter and creator of conditions for the interaction and negotiation between participants in a sharing and learning environment.

References

Abma, T. A. (2005). Responsive evaluation: Its meaning and special contribution to health promotion. *Evaluation and Program Planning, 28*, 279–289.

Battista, R. N., Lance, J. M., Lehoux, P., Régnier, G. (1999), "Health Technology Assessment and the Regulation of Medical Devices and Procedures in Quebec", in International Journal of Technology Assessment in Health Care, vol. 15, pp: 593–601.

Benjamin, K., Perfetto, E., & Greene, R. (1995). Public policy and the application of outcomes assessments: Paradigms vs politics [Suppl.]. *Medical Care, 33*(4), AS299–AS306.

Brewer, G., & de Leon, P. (1983). *Foundations of policy analysis.* Homewood, IL: Dorsey.

Brint, S. (1990). Rethinking the policy influence of experts: From general characterizations to analysis of variation. *Sociological Forum, 5*(3), 361–385.

Carvalho, A., Bodstein, R. C., Hartz, Z. & Matida, A. (2004). Concepts and approaches in the evaluation of health promotion. *en Ciência e Saúde Coletiva, 9*(3), 521–529.

de Salazar, L. (2002). *Municipios y Comunidades Saludables. El reto de la Evaluación. Centro para el Desarrollo y Evaluación de Políticas y Tecnología en Salud Pública*, Colombia. Cedetes. Universidad del Valle.

de Salazar, L. (2004). Efectividad en Promoción de la Salud. Guía de Evaluación Rápida. Capítulo 8: La Sistematización de Experiencias en Promoción de la Salud. CEDETES – Universidad del Valle. Cali, Colombia.

de Salazar, L., Díaz, C., & Magaña, A. (2002). Municipios y Comunidades Saludables. El reto de la Evaluación. Cali, colombia, Cedetes, Universidad del Valle.

Diez-Roux, A. V. (1998). Bringing context back into epidemiology: variables and fallacies in multilevel analysis. *American Journal of Public Health, 88*(2), 216–222.

Earl, S., Carden, F., & Smutylo, T. (2001). Outcome mapping: building learning and reflection into development programs, International Development Research Centre.

EPPI – Centre (2006). "Cochrane Health Promotion & Public Health Field" [en línea], disponible en: http://eppi.ioe.ac.uk/cms/Default.aspx?tabid=269, recuperado: 4 de febrero de 2008.

Feldstein, P. (1996). The Politics of Health Legislation. An Economic Perspective. Chic: Health Administration Press.

Francke, M., & Morgan, M. (1995). La sistematización: Apuesta por la generación de conocimientos a partir de las experiencias de promoción. Lima, Materiales Didácticos No 1. Escuela para el desarrollo.

Chilean Government, Programa Orígenes (2004). Estudio sistematización participativa de experiencias de salud intercultural en las comunidades Mapuche y establecimientos de salud existentes en las comunas focalizadas por el programa desarrollo integral de comunidades indígenas.

Guba, E. G., & Lincoln, Y. S. (1981). *Effective evaluation.* Beverly Hills:Sage.

Guba, E. G., & Lincoln, Y. S. (1989). *Fourth generation evaluation.* Beverly Hills: Sage.

Hawe, P. Degeling, D., Hall, J. & Brierley, A. (2003). *Evaluating health promotion: A health worker's guide.* Sydney, Australia: Maclennan and Petty Ltd.

Jara, O. (2000). Tres posibilidades de sistematización: comprensión, aprendizaje y teorización, Sistematización de experiencias, Aportes. Bogotá, Colombia Dimensión Educativa.

Jasanoff, S. (1993). *The fifth branch: Science advisors as policymakers.* Cambridge: Harvard University Press.

Kemm, J. (2006, June). The limitations of 'evidence-based' public health. *Journal of Evaluation in Clinical Practice, 12*, 319.

Lincoln, Y. S., & Guba, E. G. (1985). *Naturalistic inquiry.* Beverly Hills: Sage.

Loomis, D., & Wing S. (1990). Is molecular epidemiology a germ theory for the end of the twentieth century? *International Journal of Epidemiology, 19*, 1–3.

MacDonald, G., Veen, C., & Tones, K. (1996). Evidence for success in health Promotion: Suggestions for improvements. *Health Education Research. Theory and Practice, 11*(3), 367–376.

McQueen, D. V. & Anderson, L. (2000). What counts as evidence? Issues and debates on evidence, relevance to the evaluation of community health promotion programs.

McQueen, D. V. & Jones, C. (2007). Global Perspective on Health Promotion Effectiveness. An introduction. In D. V. McQueen & C. Jones (Eds.), *Global Perspective on Health Promotion Effectiveness* (pp. 201–224). New York: Springer.

Madjar, I. & Walton, J. A. (2001), What is problematic about evidence? In J. M. Morse, J. M. Swanson, and A. J. Kuzel (Eds.), *The nature of evidence in qualitative research*. Thousand Oaks, CA: Sage.

Marmot, M. (2004). Evidence-based policy or policy-based evidence? *British Medical Journal, 328*,906–907

Milio, N. (1990), Nutrition policy for food-rich countries: A strategic analysis. Baltimore: Johns Hopkins University Press.

Organisation for Economic Co-operation and Development (OECD) (1998). Review of the DAC Principles for Evaluation Development Assistance, [en línea], disponible en: http://www.oecd.org/dac/evaluation, recuperado: 5 de enero de 2004.

Pan American Health Organization (PAHO). (2007). *Guide to Economic Evaluation in Health Promotion*, Washington, PAHO.

Potvin, L., Haddad, S., & Frohlich, K. L. (2001). Beyond process and outcome evaluation: A comprehensive approach for evaluating health promotion programmes, in I. Rootman, et al. (Eds.), *Evaluation in health promotion. Principles and perspectives* (pp. 45–62). Copenhague: WHO regional publications. European series; No 92.

Ray, L. D. & Mayan, M. (2001). Who decides what counts as evidence? In J. M. Morse, J. M. Swanson, & A. J. Kuzel (Eds.), *The nature of evidence in qualitative research* (pp. 50–73). Thousand Oaks: Sage.

Shadish, W. R., Cook, T. D. & Leviton, L. C. (1995). *Foundations of Program Evaluation. Theories of Practice, newbury Park*. London & New Delhi: Sage.

Smutylo, T. (2001). Impacto latente, atribución oculta: Cómo superar las amenazas al aprendizaje en los programas de desarrollo, Unidad de Evaluación, Centro Internacional de Investigaciones para el Desarrollo, IDRC, Ottawa, Canadá.

Stake, R. E. (1975). To evaluate an arts program. In R. E. Stake (Ed.), Evaluating the arts in education: A responsive approach, Colombus Ohio, Merrill, 13–31.

Stake, R. E., & Abma, T. A. (2005). Responsive evaluation. In S. Mathison (Ed.), *Encyclopaedia of evaluation* (pp. 376–379). Thousand Oaks: Sage.

Stivers, C. (1991) The politics of public health: The dilemma of a public profession. In T. Litman & S Robins, (Eds.), *Health politics and policy* (pp. 356–369). Albany, NY: Delmar Pub.

Waters, W., Doyle, J., Jackson, N., Howes, F., Brunton, G. & Oakle, A. (2006, April). Evaluating the effectiveness of public health interventions: the role and activities of the Cochrane collaboration. *Journal of Epidemiology and Community Health, 60*, 285–289.

Weiss, C. H. (1998). Have we learned anything new about the use of evaluation? *American Journal of Evaluation, 19*(1), 21–33.

World Health Organization (WHO). (2005, October 10–12). *Bridging the "Know–Do" Gap Meeting on Knowledge Translation in Global Health*. Geneva, Switzerland: WHO.

World Health Organization (WHO). (2001). *Evaluation in health promotion. Principles and perspectives*. I. Rootman et al. (Ed.), WHO Regional Publications, European Series, No 92.

Chapter 5
There Is More to Methodology than Method

Louise Potvin and Sherri Bisset

There is much more to evaluation than collecting, analyzing, and interpreting scientific data in order to compare the outcomes of vious treatments. For the past 40 years, method-related discussions in the field of program evaluation have evolved to include models and reflections on the complex and multiple roles associated with the practice of evaluation. In fact, for Shadish, Cook, & Leviton, (1991), the knowledge basis which pertains to the practice of evaluation must consider issues related to the evaluator's roles as well as to the design of evaluation. Thus, evaluation practice requires both the methodological and technical competencies for systematic inquiry, in addition to a whole set of interpersonal and negotiation skills, identified by Brown (1995) as ranging from pedagogical to political. Conceiving evaluation as a practice, as we do in this collection of essays, is based upon the premise that evaluators are more than good and rigorous scientists, implementing empirical inquiry devices to study programs and interventions. While there is clearly more to the evaluator's role than data-related activities, how do these two aspects of practice which are inherently part of program evaluation, come together and build knowledge of evaluation practice? To address this question, we propose revisiting the teleological, epistemological and ontological foundations upon which evaluation roles are defined.

Consistent with the orientation of this book, we define evaluators' roles vis-à-vis a program as framed by one's evaluation practice. We suggest that evaluation practice does not however simply represent a repertoire of roles from which the evaluator may (more or less) arbitrarily choose from in order to define themselves and their evaluation activities (i.e. their methodological tool kit). In this chapter we argue that the evaluator's role vis-à-vis programs stakeholders and the approach taken to identify, describe, and measure a program and its effects, form an evaluator's practice, which is consistent and coherent across the contexts of their work. We will also argue that a practice, like a paradigm, constitutes an organized rationality (Crozier & Friedberg, 1977) common to groups of individuals that allow

L. Potvin
Department of Social and Preventive Medicine, Université de Montreal, Montreal, QC, Canada

L. Potvin, D. McQueen (eds.), *Health Promotion Evaluation Practices in the Americas*,
DOI: 10.1007/978-0-387-79733-5_5, © Springer Science+Business Media, LLC 2008

those groups to identify, structure, interpret and solve practical problems identifiable through the lens of a practice or paradigm (Kuhn, 1962).

Four Dimensions of Practice

Methodology is one of four dimensions that characterize a practice (Levy, 1994). Practices like paradigms have a coherent organization such that, as taken together these four dimensions are highly related to each other and constitute a rational and coherent set of propositions that connect a practitioner to the world through her practice. Those four dimensions are labeled: teleological, ontological, epistemological, and methodological.

The teleological dimension relates to the ultimate goal of the practice: what the practitioner is setting herself to achieve through her work and activities. It is this dimension that defines intentionality and relates to the overarching project and vision underlying the practice. It provides meaning to action by identifying the possible worlds the practice is contributing to. This dimension is often taken for granted and rarely openly discussed and critically reviewed in the field of evaluation. Typical of a practical field, however, evaluation results are often described as having to be usable and contributing to some transformation project (Mark & Henry, 2004). Evaluation is often defined as providing scientific data in support of decision-making. Such an instrumental use of evaluation results in program-related decisions constitutes the ultimate criteria by which a great majority of evaluators describe the raison d'être of their field (Preskill & Caracelli, 1997). Such an instrumental use however is rarely attained (Patton, 1997) and many theorists of evaluation have proposed other types of uses for evaluation results (see Hartz, Denis, Moreira, & Matida, 2008; Chapter in this book for a more complete discussion of evaluation use) such as enlightenment, that is the contribution of evaluation results to theoretical explanations about the functioning of the world (Weiss, 1998). For Mark, Henry and Julnes (2000) all those specific uses of evaluation results can be subsumed to contribute to social betterment in light that "even in the absence of direct use, evaluation results often appeared to help shape people's assumptions, beliefs and expectations, and in turn they appear to influence subsequent decisions about programs and policies, sometimes distant in time and place from the original evaluation" (Mark et al., 2000, p. 22). For these authors in order to contribute to social betterment, evaluators take the following responsibilities with regard to their study results. First, evaluators determine which results can best contribute to support the deliberations, decisions and actions carried out by institutions, since institutions represent the legitimate agents of societal regulation and transformation in democratic societies. Second, they take responsibility for the quality of information derived from the actual evaluation studies. Third, they ensure that results are disseminated in the relevant practitioner and decision-maker networks.

The second dimension of practice is related to its object. Considering that a practice is the transformative work of a practitioner upon her world, this work focuses on a specific class of objects. There is no practice without the objects which a practice seeks to regulate, reproduce or transform. This is the ontological dimension of practice. With the exception of Weiss (1998) there is very little discussion about the ontological reality of the programs and policies that are usually presented as objects of evaluation (Potvin, Gendron, & Bilodeau, 2006). Almost nobody ever asks questions about what programs are made of. As discussed in Chapter 3 of this book (Potvin & McQueen, 2008), most discussions and representations of programs are devoid of actors, taken in the sense of agents who exercise causal power in a situation; actors whose actions induce a reaction in other actors. In the rare occasions where actors are discussed together with material objects, such as in Weiss (1998), the articulation and connections between human and nonhuman program elements are not well developed. Representing programs as series of actions or events in the absence of actors who operate those actions puts the onus of the action in the technical and material dimensions of programs. In this chapter we argue that evaluators' conceptions about the nature of programs and what constitutes their reality bear fundamental influence on evaluation practice, and ultimately define the other dimensions of practice.

Defining practice as the work of a practitioner on an object implies the presence of a rapport between the practitioner and the class of objects that characterizes the practice. The epistemological dimension of practice is about this relationship between practitioners and the object of her practice. It asks the question of the kind of rapport that should exist between a practitioner and the world in order for the former to influence transformations or regulation on the latter. For an evaluator this dimension is about the relationship between herself and programs or policies to evaluate. Often simplified as an opposition between outside or inside evaluation (e.g. participatory versus non-participatory research, participant versus non-participant observation), a proper answer to this question requires the evaluator as a subject to position herself with regard to the program. Evaluation practice can range from a simple subject-object rapport in which the evaluator as a subject controls the circumstances of the program ideally conceived as devoid of power in the relationship (evaluator's decisions are not influenced by the program), to a much more complex subject-subject-project rapport in which both the evaluator and the program are active agents in the evaluation, and in which, this rapport is also conceived as being an active ingredient in the evaluator's practice. We have shown that when evaluation is designed to be responsive to the various phases through which a program evolves, both the program and the evaluation influence each other and become increasingly ingrained in the context in which the program was initially developed (Potvin, Cargo, McComber, Delormier, & Macaulay, 2003). For the research base practice of evaluation, this epistemological dimension which ultimately poses the question of the status of the evaluator with regard to the program, is concerned with how knowledge about programs is possible given their nature.

Finally the methodological dimension of a practice refers directly to the type of actions practitioners undertake to achieve their goal. For an evaluator, the methodological dimension of practice is primarily, but not exclusively, related to how knowledge about programs is produced but it cannot be reduced to this sole aspect. Indeed, to the extent that the finality pursued by an evaluation expands beyond the mere production of scientific knowledge, the methodological dimension of evaluation practice may include a wide range of actions that pertain principally to evaluability assessment which defines the evaluation question and project (Thurston, Graham, & Hatfield, 2003; Thurston & Potvin, 2003) and to knowledge use (Mark & Henry, 2004; Patton, 1997).

Three Ideal-Types of Evaluation Practice

A practice is the operationalization of a coherent set of positions regarding the four dimensions described above. This coherence is the foundation of practice, and is observed as a consistency and continuity of practice across time and space. Although it is conceivable that the various combinations of answers practitioners provide to those four questions could produce an infinite variety of practices, we believe that there exist inherent correlations between these dimensions, thus limiting variations in the types of evaluation practice. In this respect, Weber's notion of ideal-type is useful (Weber, 1952). An ideal-type is a mental construction of a social phenomenon that combines and simplifies characteristics usually not to be found in any single instantiation, but which provides an exemplary case representative of a whole category of social phenomena. There exist, many taxonomies of evaluation ideal-types, depending on the features one wants to highlight. In this section we present three ideal-types of evaluation practices that emphasize the methodological consequences of three coherent evaluation paradigms as presented in Table 5.1.

Note that some well-known evaluation ideal-types practices such as utilization-focused evaluation (Patton, 1997), or participatory evaluation (Springett, 2001) are

Table 5.1 Three ideal-types of evaluation practice

	Teleological	Ontological	Epistemological	Methodological
Evaluation as Experimentation	Testing causal hypotheses about programs' effects on context	Programs as technical entities with an objective reality	Objective distance between evaluator and programs	Experimentation; ruling out plausible rival hypotheses
Evaluation as Negotiation	Improve program by increasing programs actors awareness about their actions	Programs as representations that describe and/or guide actors' actions	constructivist subject–subject co-construction of program representation	Constructing program's theory through actors' representations and hermeneutic circles
Evaluation as Organized Reflexivity	Understanding the mediating role of programs in social transformations	Programs as systems of actions that connects entities	Reflexive transformation of subject-object-project	Following programs actions and the connections they operate

not directly circumscribed within our typology, mainly because such practices are not primarily discussed in terms of their methodological implications. The former is generally presented with regard to the teleological dimension of evaluation, i.e., its use by decision-makers, whereas the latter is mostly presented in relation to the epistemological question of the relative value of various forms of knowledge. In this light however, participatory evaluation can also be understood as a form of negotiation.

The main caveat about the use of ideal-types to characterize health promotion evaluation practice is that because they do not necessarily exist in reality, ideal-types are simplistic representations. As a heuristic device, an ideal-type cannot render all the subtleties and nuances of the social reality it represents. It is called upon mainly to contrast social phenomena by exacerbating their differences on a limited number of dimensions. A practice is much richer than any ideal-type that can be constructed to represent it. This is why this chapter has to be complemented by the chapters composing the fourth section of this book, in which colleagues from the Americas, North and South report and discuss practical issues of conducting health promotion evaluations that also contribute to the health promotion agenda.

Evaluation as Experimentation

According to Pawson and Tilley (1997) this ideal-type of evaluation practice has been the hallmark of evaluation since the early time of this field. "Underlying everything in the early days was the logic of experimentation (. . .) The practitioner, policy adviser, and social scientist are at one in appreciating the beauty of the design. At one level it has deepest roots in philosophical discourse on the nature of explanation as in John Stuart Mill's *A system of Logic*; at another it is the hallmark of common sense, ingrained into advertising campaigns telling Washo is superior to Sud" (Pawson & Tilley, 1997, p. 4).

Evaluation as experimentation practice is characterized by the finality of testing causal hypotheses about program's effects in the environment into which they are implemented. This finality is deeply rooted in the field of evaluation. As early as 1967, in one of the first books published with the word evaluation in the title, Suchman (1967) explained that evaluation is ultimately a hypothesis testing mechanism whereby demonstrating a positive effect of a program designed to solve a problem is providing evidence of the validity of the theory underlying the program. In practice, as hypothesis testers, evaluators are also often academic researchers, deeply involved in program design and planning. Programs as treatments are seen as devices to test theoretical propositions about disease etiology. This was the case with the first cardiovascular disease community intervention trials such as the Stanford Five City Project (Farquhar et al., 1985), the Pawtucket Heart Health Program (Carleton, Lasater, Assaf, Lefebvre, & McKinlay, 1987), and the Minnesota Heart Health Program (Blackburn et al., 1984). In these programs, as in those that were designed and evaluated in their aftermath according to the same evaluation paradigm, there is a strong involvement of researchers/evaluators in the definition and design of the program that usually stops just short of implementation, keeping evaluation at arms length from implementation issues, but not from the stakes of demonstrating a program effect.

As exemplified by those programs designed by academic researchers and which encompass the most update scientific knowledge about disease etiology and prevention, in evaluation as experimentation, programs are conceived of as generalizable solutions to objectively defined problems. The origin of the program lies outside the problematic situation, that is, the program is assumed to come after the problem and after potential solutions have been named. It is this externality that bears generalizability. Programs are thus essentially conceived of as technical solutions that incorporate scientific knowledge in response to a problematic situation, without reference to the social actors involved with the problem, its definition, or its solution. The paradigm of reference is that of drug development (Flay, 1986). In this paradigm programs are made of material objects arranged according to a stable and predictable set of procedures. Contextual and implementation variations are noise to be eliminated or controlled for as much as possible (see Chapter 17 of this book, Poland, Frohlich, & Cargo, 2008) for an in-depth refutation of this proposition). Here, the causal mechanisms that produce changes are not understood as being between the actors who operate the program, or in the relationships that they develop with other actors and non-human components of the implementation context. Instead, actors are instruments whose role is defined in the program's description and logic model.

When programs are primarily conceived as technical arrangements, usually, the agency of the concerned actors is likewise regarded as being quite limited as their interactions with the technical program entities are generally pre-defined by a set of rigid program instructions and rules. This is to ensure maximum fidelity in program implementation and theoretically maximum program effects. Indeed, in the experimentalist language, people who are to benefit from programs effects are often described as program targets. This ballistic metaphor is not benign and this on two counts. First targets are situated exclusively at the receiving end of a transaction. They are meant to be hit by something (i.e., the magic bullet). Second, and most importantly, although targets may be moving, it is not what makes them move that constitutes relevant information. The only important fact about a target's movements is its relative position (distance and direction) in relation to that of the person aiming at that target.

In evaluation as experimentation, relationships between the evaluator and programs, including staff and targets, are usually conceived as being one way. The more specific the hypothesis to be tested by the program and its evaluation, the less flexibility there is in the expression of agency by actors involved. This objectification of programs and their components ideally maximizes control over the treatment and potential confounders. As knowing subject, the evaluator's actions are minimally influenced by the object (program) under study. Conversely, one key hypothesis for external validity – the capacity to generalize the results to other settings and targets –

is that the program is not responsive to evaluator's actions. In other words an evaluated program is not different from a non-evaluated program. The epistemological dimension is thus characterized by maximizing distance and objectivity between the evaluator and the program evaluated.

In this ideal-type practice, methodological choices are fundamentally governed by the experimentalist paradigm. Knowledge is enhanced by one's capacity to manipulate the conditions of production of a phenomenon and reproduce this phenomenon by manipulating the conditions of its emergence, reducing these conditions to the bear essentials. The essence of laboratory science is to isolate, as perfectly as possible, a putative cause and its effect from all other confounding sources. This is done by closing and isolating the experimental situation. Cook & Campbell (1979) have discussed at length the conundrum associated with the emulation of laboratory conditions in research conducted in real life settings where this closure is hardly feasible. In their view, the work of the evaluator in such situations is to try to impose closure to the situation while maintaining the integrity of the experimental treatment. The randomized control trial is one device that allows closure on several but not all aspects of the experimental situation in real-life condition. In fact, according to Campbell (1984), the hard work of an evaluator can be summarized as trying to rule out plausible rival hypotheses in order to remain only with the program under study as an explanation of the observed difference between those who were exposed to it and those who were not. This can be done either by designing studies that automatically rule out some known threats to internal validity (Campbell & Stanley, 1963), like using a control group in order to rule out the possibility that the observed pre-post difference in the exposed group could be due to maturation effect. This can also be done by a post hoc documentation of the low plausibility of such hypothesis, or by statistical control (Cook & Campbell, 1979).

The evaluation as experimentation practice is characterized by a strong concern with the conception and implementation of research devices that ensure optimal internal and external validity of the evaluation results. Ideally, this includes maintaining a proper distance with the program and ensuring that the work and activities serving the evaluation do not interfere with the program's integrity.

Evaluation as Negotiation

Contrary to the previously discussed evaluation as experimentation where emphasis is placed upon the technical identity of the program, the emphasis in evaluation as negotiation is on the social actors who are brought together and form a programmed social space. Recognizing that programs are essentially social systems in which actors' actions and interactions remain the main dimension of interest, evaluators as negotiators focus their practice on the people who are directly concerned by the program. Methodological preoccupations are mainly related to compiling program representations from the perspectives of the various groups of actors. This primacy of social actors and social processes opens up a royal path to social constructivism as a paradigm for program evaluation.

This evaluation ideal-type practice has been mainly, but far from exclusively, advocated by Guba & Lincoln (1989) as the "Fourth Generation Evaluation". Indeed, although the constructivist perspective of Guba and Lincoln is probably the one most acknowledged and cited in the health promotion evaluation literature, some of the well known pioneers in the field of evaluation have also founded their approach on constructivist epistemology. The work of evaluators such as Wholey & Newcomer (1989) or Stake (1975) are well known in the field of evaluation. Both are associated with the fundamental idea that programs as implemented usually differ from the original program planners' intentions; programs are constructed as they go through the various interactions among and between groups of associated actors. One of evaluation's key role is thus to highlight this process by supporting program improvement or simply defining the program on its own terms. By emphasizing the necessity for evaluators to get closer to the action wherever it occurs, both contributed (with others) in the early 1970s to the decline of the quasi-experimental paradigm monopoly over the field of evaluation. Building on the notion that programs are social constructions, their most important contribution was to successfully argue for pluralism of methods and relativism of values when assessing programs.

While there are numerous blends of social constructivism the one that is most often found to underlie constructivist evaluations is rooted in the work, and scholarly tradition of the Chicago School of Sociology, mainly through the work of Anselm Strauss and his methodological propositions, which are embedded within grounded theory type inquiry (Glaser & Strauss, 1967). Although the Chicago School of Sociology is associated with a great number of theoreticians and methodologists in the field of sociology, one of its most critical and relevant innovation for evaluation is the so-called symbolic interactionism. The first and most fundamental proposition of symbolic interactionism is that humans act essentially as a result of their perceptions and interpretations of the meaning they ascribe to others' actions. The second and corollary proposition is that it is through interactions with others that these meanings develop, are transformed, and can be manipulated (Le Breton, 2004). The main driver of action thus is the representation of social situations and those representations are shaped through the social processes of interacting within those situations.

In developing their approach to the "Fourth generation evaluation" Guba & Lincoln (1989) borrowed extensively from symbolic interactionism, from the methodology of the grounded theory, and from the work of Robert Stake (Abma, 2005). They argue that programs can only be understood through the representations that various actors develop and act upon through their social interactions with other program actors.

In both Guba and Lincoln's and in Stake's conception, the evaluators' main task is to support the development of a shared program representation among actors and this is essentially done through negotiation. The teleological dimension in evaluation as negotiation practice is thus to contribute to program improvement as it is being implemented, acknowledging that discrepancies between the program as it is planned, and the program as it is practiced are unavoidable. Here, programs are expected to improve with an elaboration of a common program representation among program's stakeholders, whereby, a common representation is presumed to improve the program through a better coordination and alignment of program's stakeholders' actions. It is the evaluators' main task to develop this shared representation, primarily by feeding back their assessments to program actors thereby permitting the latter to revise their representations in line with those of other program actors.

In line with symbolic interactionism, the ontological dimension of this ideal-type practice lies in actors representations of the program. Thus programs do not have an objective reality in the sense of the primacy of material and technical objects. It is the representations program actors construct of those objects and the symbolic meaning they ascribe to them through their interactions that are orienting individuals' actions in programs' social spaces. So in any program, theoretically, there exist as many representations as there are individuals involved. The evaluator's role is to attempt to reveal those representations and to help achieve consensus among program actors.

This task requires that the evaluator interacts closely with program actors. The epistemology is constructivist, meaning that both the evaluator and program actors are subjects in this construction. There is no prescribed distance between the program and the evaluator. Indeed the program's shared representation resulting from the evaluation can only be collectively constructed and the evaluator's central role is to design and implement the mechanisms through which actors' representations can directly or indirectly confront with one another. For example, mechanisms in the form of feedback derived from discourse, documentation or observational analyses, provide a means for program actors to situate their own interests and interpretations of program events in relation to those of others.

Although there exist variations in the specific technical devices used to collect and analyze data, the methodological dimension in evaluation as negotiation ideal-type practice are essentially concerned with producing the most credible and trustworthy program representation or program theory. In many cases evaluators have referred to the grounded theory methodology as developed by Glaser and Strauss (1967) and later by Strauss and Corbin (1998) in order to inductively create a shared representation from the specific individuals' program representation. Specific data collection and analysis techniques insure a continuous confrontation process between the theory that is emerging from the data and the empirical phenomena which are illuminated by the theory. Guba and Lincoln's (1989), main practical and methodological addition lies in the proposition that Hermeneutic Dialogic Circles should be implemented in order to construct this shared representation. As ultimate negotiators and consensus brokers, evaluators orchestrate dialogs between program actors in order to create a joint construction that comprised as many elements as possible from each individual's program representation.

In health promotion several variations of this ideal-type of evaluation practice have been described as having utmost relevance given the nature of health promotion. Presenting Stake's theory of responsive evaluation, Abma (2005) argues that "Responsive evaluation is not only responsive to the unique feature and emerging ideas in the field of health promotion, it is also synergistic with health promotion" (Abma, 2005, p. 287).

In particular, this approach is touted as having a potential to redress the social processes which maintain health inequalities through the creation of equal partnerships with full participation among health or research experts and community or lay actors. Evaluations then ideally showcase the working relationships or partnerships between various actors as the object of study. Evaluations of community-based programs, for example, describe a set of actors with a range of pre-occupations with community, non-governmental, governmental or research needs as they come together to define a problematic situation and devise corrective strategies. Here, the role of the evaluator is to attempt to trace this process by collecting and interpreting qualitative data in order to capture the perspectives, opinions and lived experiences among the various actors. In the published literature, analytic results from such studies present representations in aggregate where the various actor groups are identified at some level of collective. A collective may be quite general, whereby one overall or encompassing representation is attributed to all the program actors (Lantz, Viruell-Fuentes, Israel, Softley, & Guzman, 2001). Alternatively, representations may be distinct or specific to the various actor groups according to a pre-defined group membership (e.g., community member, health professional) (Schulz et al., 2001). In addition to being organized according to the identity of program actors, data may be interpreted in relation to its correspondence with a stage in the program planning and evaluation (Farquhar, Parker, Schulz, & Israel, 2006) or to a set of concepts which are associated with the guiding principles of the program (e.g., participatory research) (Savage et al., 2006).

More specifically, one initiative, the Detroit Community-Academic Urban Research Center (URC) provides an example where the evaluation plays a role of negotiator by building a collective representations of the partnership building process between a range of actors. Evaluations of this initiative were described at the regional level, where community and academic actors formed a committee (i.e. URC), applied for, and dispersed, funds to local initiatives, and also at the local level where initiatives or projects addressed a particular problem within a particular place. Evaluations at both the regional and the local levels were based upon the representations of the actors with respect to the partnership building process, as well as, the operation of services or acquisition of resources.

The East Side Village Health Worker Partnership (ESVHWP) was one of twelve local projects which was funded through the Detroit Community-Academic URC between 1995 and 1999 (Lantz et al., 2001). Evaluation of this project relied upon the derivation of program representations based upon informant interviews, observations and document review in relation to four stages of program planning process (Farquhar et al., 2006). While data was collected over time, analysis of a given data set within one time period was interpreted according to its reference to four stages of planning (i.e., assessment and problem analysis, goals and objectives, design and implementation, evaluation). The evaluation furthered its role as a negotiation process by feeding back constructed representations to the various program actors, which served both as part of the learning and informed decision-making process and also as a source of legitimization for the lived experiences and representations among the interventionists (i.e., health workers) and steering committee member. For example, by feeding back interpretations of the health worker meetings, the evaluation validated the presence of four distinct problems upon which health workers divided themselves into four subgroups, each with its own focus and set of activities. This approach is somewhat distinct to hermeneutic circle dialogue in that it did not impose a consensual problem statement.

Other evaluations of the Detroit Community-Academic URC (Lantz et al., 2001) and also the ESVHWP (Schulz et al., 2001) identified a diverse range of actors who came together to form a research centre (i.e., URC Board) or a steering committee. Evaluation of the URC Board was based upon a collective representation of the internal and external strength of the partnership, namely how well the partnership was able to move forward as a group toward goals, and how the group encountered conditions which either facilitated or acted as barriers to their public health research goals. Evaluation results were organized into categories which identified the overall satisfaction, perceived benefits, facilitating factors and barriers toward goal attainment. For example, issues which were identified as concerns to the group were time management, resource distribution and balancing community and research needs. Examples of facilitating factors toward goal attainment included community representation on URC Board, trust, relevant knowledge, and organizational support. Alternatively, evaluations derived specifically from the informant interviews provided by the Village Health Workers and the steering committee as part of the ESVHWP, aimed at identifying how the partnership contributed to improving the research, program activities, community relations and participation from community, academic and practice organizations or institutions. Interviews were interpreted according to these over-riding themes and subcategories specific to the themes were induced from the interviews and results were presented as an overall collective representation across both the steering committee and the Village Health Workers. For example, improvements in community relationships were described by stronger social networks among Village Health Workers, stronger relationships between them and steering committee members, and stronger relationships among academic, practice, and community-based organizations. Within these subcategories particular issues, such as trust, power differentials and communication, along with some strategies used to address challenges (e.g., annual picnics, retreats) were presented.

Two criticisms are usually associated with this constructivist paradigm of evaluation. The first is the essentially descriptive nature of the results of such an evaluation practice. That is, while it is possible that consensus can be achieved, as conditions change over time and space, so too may a program's ability to achieve consensus among all program actors. As illustrated above, achieving consensus may not be desirable. This description does not therefore permit knowledge to be garnished from the process by which negotiations or compromises between program actors may have taken place in order to arrive at common or agreed upon goal(s). Indeed, in the renewed version of evaluability assessment, the construction of a shared understanding or representation of the program and its components is only the starting point from which designing the evaluation project begins (Thurston et al., 2003; Thurston & Potvin, 2003). The other criticism relates to the somewhat underestimation of the political influence and power held by evaluators in such processes. As the master negotiator it could be mistakenly understood that the evaluator is neutral in this construction process, which is certainly not the case. The use of formal mechanisms that ensure a fair distribution of roles, resources, and responsibilities in conducting evaluation projects is increasingly seen as a necessary safeguard.

Evaluation as Organized Reflexivity

There is another ideal-type of evaluation practice that is emerging in the evaluation literature and that is slowly making its way into the realm of public health and health promotion program evaluation. Pawson and Tilley (1997) have developed the foundations of a critical realist approach to evaluation (see chapters by Potvin and McQueen (2008); Mercille (2008), and Poland et al. (2008) in this book), based upon the work of the philosopher Roy Bhaskar (1978). "Realist evaluation, as its core, focuses on developing explanations of the consequences of social actions that contribute to a better understanding of why, where, and for whom programs work or fail to work. To this end, realist evaluators place a great deal of emphasis on (a) identifying the mechanisms that produce observable program effects and (b) testing these mechanisms and the other contextual variables . . . that may have impacts on the effects that are observed" (Pawson & Tilley, 2004, p. 359). Working under the realist assumption that programs are but one among many systems of actions that operate simultaneously at any given moment in a context, a realist evaluator's task is ideally to identify the operative program mechanisms and how they interact with contextual conditions (including other programs) to be associated with specific intended and unintended outcome patterns (Pawson & Tilley, 2004). In a complex world of constant interactions, it is through the connections programs are creating and maintaining with contextual conditions that their impacts can be understood and identified. Thus, program evaluators are essentially designers and operators of organized reflexivity devices through which programs' actors can understand how programs contribute to transform peoples' life and conditions.

We propose that the teleological dimension of an evaluation as organized reflexivity practice, is one of understanding the mediations operated by a program in the transformation of the world. The recognition of the inherent complexity of programs and of their operating mechanisms in open systems leads to the critical realist proposition that causality cannot be established solely by the empirical observation of constant conjunctions of events (Bhaskar, 1978). Indeed, in an open system where a multitude of mechanisms are constantly interacting and transforming the system, exact recurring patterns cannot be observed. It is only in controlled conditions where some closure or quasi-closure is exerted on the system that law-like observations can occur. In all other situations, the main role of the scientist is to identify and factor out the effect of irrelevant mechanisms (Cook & Campbell, 1979). In the absence of such closure, empirical observations can only make sense when related to a theory about mechanism-context-outcome pattern configurations that they contribute to strengthen. As operating mechanisms in a context, a program interacting with other existing mechanisms becomes a mediator in the constant transformation of the context. Its presence changes the normal course of events either by reinforcing, or by tempering with, the impact of other operating forces in place.

In this ideal-type practice, programs are conceived of as systems of actions in which human and non-human actors operate the putative program mechanisms through their actions (Potvin, Gendron, & Bilodeau, 2006). Program's ontological reality is thus one of action and interactions. It is what is done by the various program actors, both human and non-human that contribute to transforming the context in the direction expected by program initiators. Thus, the most relevant program reality rests in the actions undertaken in the program space. These, like all actions, involve two types of interacting realities. One type is tangible and objective, and it consists in the peoples, objects, resources, and physical spaces that situate the action and make it possible. It is usually what is subsumed under the work plan and logic models associated with program development. The second type is symbolic and includes the meanings actors assign to actions and the role those actions implicitly and tacitly assign to actors in relation to action. This is what is usually captured by program representations. A realist ontology of program has to encompasses those two types of reality and their interactions.

In order to understand how a program mediates transformations unfolding in a particular space and time, the evaluator has no choice but to follow the actions that are developing and taking place in the name of the program as well as their ramifications and ripples in the program's social context. Following the action is the single most important methodological dimension of a reflexive device. It is through their actions and practice that actors enact their intentions much more than through the discourse they have about their intentions (representations). This is one of the well recognized limits of phenomenology; that one's representation of one's actions is usually blind to the structural conditions that constrain and make this action possible (Bourdieu, 1972). Ideally, it is through description and analysis of the actions that instantiate the program that program actors can critically reflect on the program and rationally make the constant corrections that are necessary to strengthen mechanism-context-outcomes pattern configuration. For example, as practitioners or researchers increase their level of involvement with a group of concerned actors, their representation of what a problem is and how it may be resolved is likely to change. Sometimes, due to the nature of the research, the community or the individuals involved, program plans adapt (Bisset, Cargo, Delormier, Macauley, & Potvin, 2004), other times, however, despite recognizing a need to change or expand upon plans, practitioners latitude is restricted due to an imposed need to stay on course (Hawe & Riley, 2005). Evaluation as organized reflexivity follows why and how transformations of this sort occur, thus providing intelligibility to local adaptations.

The underlying principle upon which a following the action methodology is based, holds that a program is most accurately and comprehensively understood through an in-depth study of the program performers in action. By following the action of program performers, we can obtain a view of the program from its core functioning. This approach contrasts building an understanding of the program based upon accounts of what the program may aim to accomplish and examples of exemplary activities. In the same way that the sociology of association dismisses ostensive definitions of what is social (Latour, 2006), it can similarly be argued that in defining program upon accounts and examples, we side-step the real work of learning about the upkeep of a program, of what brings the program together and makes it operative.

Two distinctive features can be identified with a methodology based upon following the action. First, it does not limit itself to inquiring about actions which are believed to be part of a causal chain of events leading to a pre-defined set of outcomes. While certainly important, these actions, however, capture a limited portion of what practitioners do and assume they share and are driven by a singular model of achievement. Moreover, actions can only be planned to a certain point, after which they become diverted or develop spontaneously given the conditions which arise.

This last point raises a second unique feature of evaluations which follow the action. Following the action requires that the lived experiences occurring inside and outside the typical boundaries of the program be considered. First, actions taking place outside the physical space and time of program delivery form opinions and impressions which impact upon how program participants and practitioners interact with the program. Second, during the given time space of a program, its form is not solely determined by the instructions and materials which are delivered, but rather by the ways in which the various actors that are present, interact with instructions and materials, and with one another.

Finally, the epistemological dimension of this ideal-type practice emphasizes the reflexive position of the actors involved in the program as well as those involved in the evaluation. Indeed, in following the action as it develops and unfolds, the evaluator is necessarily a relevant part of the program's context. As such, one cannot rule out the possibility that the connections between the program and its evaluation that are necessary in order for the latter to follow the actions taking place within the former, are themselves mediating transformations in the program, the context and also in the evaluation. Not only does an evaluated program differ from what it could have been had it not been evaluated, but evaluation projects also differ according to the programs or versions of programs they are coupled with. So an accurate assessment of the mediating role of the program in contextual transformations, takes into account the transformative role of evaluation on the program. Ultimately, evaluation is an intervention on programs (Mark et al., 2000).

Conclusion

In this chapter we have explored three ideal-type practices for evaluation. We based our exploration of those ideal-types on a paradigmatic conception of practice that supposes four underlying coherent dimensions: teleological, ontological, epistemological and methodological, as indicated in Figure 5.1 adapted from Gendron (2001). We deliberately chose the methodological dimension as the main point of entry for our exploration. Certainly, entering this exploration through any other paradigmatic dimension would have led to defining different ideal-types. For example, efforts to highlight the teleological dimension of practices would have led to distinguishing utilization-focused (Patton, 1997) from hypothesis testing/knowledge production practices (Cook & Campbell, 1979), and an emphasize on the epistemological dimension would have contrasted participatory from expert-driven practice. Although there should be some correlations between the outcomes of the various points of entry for exploring evaluation practices (it is more difficult to couple an evaluation as experimentation practice with a participatory practice), we do not think that there is an exact correspondence.

By characterizing evaluation practices through their methodological implications we wanted to emphasize the richness and diversity of the various points of entry that can be used for such an exploration, proposing other dimensions than those usually used from which to define practical issues in evaluation. It is important also to note that we did not discuss the qualitative/quantitative dichotomy. For us, this is not a methodological issue but a technical one that pertains to the nature of the data available rather than to the manner by which a subject can derive knowledge about a given object.

We have shown that all of the three ideal-types described in our paper can be found in the health promotion evaluation literature. All have been used with various frequencies and various levels of success, and we think that there are situations in which health promotion is better served by all three of these ideal-types. We want, however, to point at the interest to consider evaluation as organized reflexivity practice for health promotion evaluation. As a field of practice, health promotion is still very young and cannot rely on an important body of solidly established context-mechanism-outcome pattern configurations. There is therefore a great deal of work to be undertaken in order to create a repertoire of interventions that can be operated efficiently in various contexts. Learning as we go and organizing that knowledge

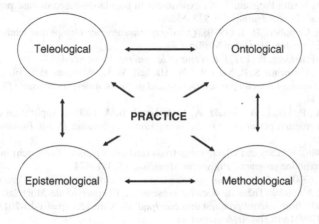

Fig. 5.1 The four inter-related dimensions of practice (Adapted from Gendron, 2001, p. 34)

into coherent intervention theories is certainly a strategy that should be explored and expanded into a proper knowledge base for health promotion. Organized reflexivity as a methodological practice accommodates this strategy of knowledge development. In addition, as shown through several chapters in this book, this ideal-type practice is compatible with many practical and theoretical solutions this book's contributors examined to align the values of health promotion with the scientific rigor of evaluation.

References

Abma, T. A. (2005). Responsive evaluation: Its meaning and special contribution to health promotion. *Evaluation and Program Planning, 28*, 279–289.

Bhaskar, R. (1978). *A realist theory of science*. Hassocks, UK: Harvester Press.

Bisset, S., Cargo, M., Delormier, T., Macauley, A., & Potvin, L. (2004). Legitimizing diabetes as a community health issue: a case analysis of an Aboriginal community in Canada. *Health Promotion International, 19*, 317–326.

Blackburn, H., Luepker, R. V., Kline, F. G., Bracht, N., Carlaw, R., Jacobs, D., et al. (1984). The Minnesota Heart Health Program: A research and demonstration project in cardiovascular disease prevention. In J. D. Matarazzo, N. E. Miller, S. M. Weiss, J. A. Herd & S. M. Weiss (Eds.), *Behavioral health: A handbook of health enhancement and disease prevention* (pp. 1171–1178). Silver Spring, MD: John Wiley & Sons.

Bourdieu, P. (1972). *Esquisse d'une théorie de la pratique*. Genève: Ed. Droz.

Brown, P. (1995). The role of the evaluator in comprehensive community initiatives. In J. P. Connell, A. C. Kubisch, L. B. Schorr, & C. H. Weiss (Eds.), *New approaches to evaluating community initiatives. Concepts, methods and contexts* (pp. 201–225). New York: Aspen Institute.

Campbell, D. T. (1984). Can we be scientific in applied social science? In: R. F. Connor, D. G. Altman, & C. Jackson (Eds.), *Evaluation studies review annual*, Vol 9 (pp. 26–48). Beverly Hills CA: Sage.

Campbell, D. T., & Stanley, J. C. (1963). *Experimental and quasi-experimental designs for research*. Chicago: Rand McNally.

Carleton, R. A., Lasater, T. M., Assaf, A., Lefebvre, R. C., & McKinlay, S. M. (1987). The Pawtucket Heart Health Program: 1. An experiment in population-based disease prevention. *The Rhode Island Medical Journal, 70*, 533–538.

Cook, T. D., & Campbell, D. T. (1979). *Quasi-experimentation; Design and analysis issues for field settings*. Boston: Houghton Mifflin.

Crozier, M., & Friedberg, E. (1977). *L'acteur et le système*. Paris: Seuil.

Farquhar, J. W., Fortmann, S. P., Maccoby, N., Haskell, W. L., Williams, P. T., Flora, J. A., et al. (1985). The stanford five city project: Design and methods. *American Journal of Epidemiology, 122*, 323–334.

Farquhar, S. A., Parker, E. A., Schulz, A. J., & Israel, B. A. (2006). Application of qualitative methods in program planning for health promotion interventions. *Health Promotion Practice, 7*, 234–242.

Flay, B. R. (1986). Efficacy and effectiveness trials (and other phases of research) in the development of -promotion programs. *Preventive Medicine, 15*, 451–474

Gendron, S. (2001). *La pratique participative en santé publique, l'émergence d'un paradigme*. Montréal: Thèse de doctorat présentée à l'Université de Montréal. Retrieved in January 2008 from : http://proquest.umi.com/pqdlink?Ver=1&Exp=01-15-2013&FMT=7&DID=726370931&RQT=309&attempt=1

Glaser, B., & Strauss, A. (1967). *The discoveries of grounded theory: Strategies for qualitative research*. Chicago: Aldine.

Guba, Y., & Lincoln, E. (1989). *Fourth generation evaluation*. Thousand Oaks CA: Sage.

Hartz, Z. A., Denis, J-L., Moreira, E., & Matida, A. (2008). From knowledge to action: challenges and opportunities for increasing the use of evaluation in health promotion policies and practices. In L. Potvin & D. V. McQueen (Eds.), *Health promotion evaluation practices in the Americas: Values and research*. New York: Springer.

Hawe, P., & Riley, T. (2005). Ecological theory in practice: Illustrations from a community-based intervention to promote the health of recent mothers. *Prevention Science, 6*, 227–236.

Kuhn, T. S. (1962). *The structure of scientific revolutions*. Chicago: University of Chicago Press.

Lantz, P. M., Viruell-Fuentes, E., Israel, B. A., Softley, D., Guzman, R. (2001). Can communities and academia work together on public health research? Evaluation results from a community-based participatory research partnership in Detroit. *Journal of Urban Health, 78*, 495–507.

Latour, B. (2006). *Changer de société – Refaire de la sociologie*. Paris: La découverte.

Le Breton, D. (2004). *L'interactionisme symbolique*. Paris : Presses universitaires de France.

Levy, R. (1994). Croyance et doute: une vision paradigmatique des méthodes qualitatives. *Ruptures, revue transdisciplinaire en santé, 1*, 92–100.

Mark, M. M., & Henry, G. T. (2004). The mechanisms and outcomes of evaluation influence. *Evaluation, 10*, 35–57.

Mark, M. M., Henry, G. T., & Julnes, G. (2000). *Evaluation. An integrated framework for understanding, guiding, and improving policies and programs*. San Francisco CA: Jossey-Bass.

Mercille, G. (2008). A realist approach to synthesizing evaluation results. In L. Potvin & D. V. McQueen (eds.), *Health promotion evaluation practices in the Americas: Values and research*. New York: Springer.

Patton, M. Q. (1997). *Utilization-focused evaluation. The new century text*. Thousand Oaks: Sage.

Pawson, R., & Tilley, N. (1997). *Realistic evaluation*. London UK: Sage.

Pawson, R., & Tilley, N. (2004). Realistic evaluation. In S. Mathison (Ed.), *Encyclopedia of evaluation* (pp. 362–367). Newbury Park, CA: Sage.

Poland, B., Frohlich, K. L., & Cargo, M. (2008). Context as a fundamental dimension of health-promotion program evaluation. In L. Potvin & D. V. McQueen (Eds.), *Health promotion evaluation practices in the Americas: Values and research*. New York: Springer.

Potvin, L., Cargo, M., McComber, A., Delormier, T., Macaulay, A. C. (2003) Implementing Participatory Intervention and Research in Communities: Lessons from the Kahnawake Schools Diabetes Prevention Project. *Social Science & Medicine, 56*, 1295–1305.

Potvin, L., Gendron, S., & Bilodeau, A. (2006). Três posturas ontológicas concernentes à natureza dos programas de saúde: implicações para a avaliação. In: M. L. M. Bosi & F. J. Mercado (Eds.), *Avaloaçao qualitative de programas de saude. Enfoques emergentes*. Petropolis, Brazil: Vozes Editorial.

Potvin, L., & McQueen, D. V. (2008). Practical dilemmas for health-promotion evaluation. In L. Potvin & D. V. McQueen (Eds.), *Health promotion evaluation practices in the Americas: Values and research*. New York: Springer.

Preskill, H., & Caracelli, V. J. (1997). Current and developing conceptions of use: Evaluation use topical interest group survey results. *Evaluation Practice, 18*, 209–225.

Savage, C. L., Xu, Y., Lee, R., Rose, B. L., Kappesser, M., Anthony, S. P. (2006). A case study in the use of community-based participatory research in public health nursing. *Public Health Nursing, 23*, 472–487.

Schulz, A. J., Isreal, B. A., Parker, E. A., Lockett, M., Hill, Y., & Wills, R. (2001). The east side village health worker partnership: Integrating research with action to reduce health disparities. *Public Health Reports, 116*, 548–557.

Shadish, W. R., Jr., Cook, T. D., & Leviton, L. C. L. (1991). *Foundations of program evaluation*. Thousand Oaks CA: Sage.

Springett, J. (2001). Participatory approaches to evaluation in health promotion. In I. Rootman, M. Goodstadt, B. Hyndman, D. V. McQueen, L. Potvin, J. Springett, & E. Ziglio (Eds.),

Evaluation in health promotion: Principles and perspectives (pp. 83–105). Copenhagen: WHO Regional Publications, European Series, No 92.

Stake, R. E. (Ed.) (1975). *Evaluating the arts in education: A responsive approach*. Columbus Ohio: Merril.

Strauss, A., & Corbin, J. (1998). *Basics of qualitative research: Techniques and procedures for developing grounded theory*. Thousand Oaks, CA: Sage.

Suchman, E. (1967). *Evaluative research*. New York: Russel Sage Foundation.

Thurston, W. E., Graham, J. & Hatfield, J. (2003). Evaluability assessment a catalyst for program change and improvement. *Evaluation and the Health Profession, 26*, 206–221.

Thurston, W. E., & Potvin, L. (2003). Evaluability assessment: A tool for incorporating evaluation in social change programs. *Evaluation, 9*, 453–469.

Weber, M. (1952). The essentials of bureaucratic organization: An ideal-type construction. In R. K. Merton, A. P. Gray, B. Hockey, & H. Selvin (Eds.), *Reader in bureaucracy* (pp. 18, 21–22). New York: Free Press.

Weiss, C. H. (1998). *Evaluation. Methods for studying programs and policy*, 2nd edition. Upper Saddle River NJ: Prentice Hall.

Wholey, J. S., & Newcomer, K. E. (Eds.) (1989). *Improving government performance : evaluation strategies for strengthening public agencies and programs*. San Francisco: Jossey-Bass.

Chapter 6
A Realist Approach to the Systematic Review

Geneviève Mercille

In clinical medicine, due to the widening gap between the demand and delivery of healthcare services in the 1970s and 1980s, priority-setting in health policies began to focus on efficiency and service costs. This situation, which is frequent in Western societies, led to the emergence of the clinical practice known as evidence-based medicine. This is usually defined as "the conscious, explicit, and judicious use of current best evidence in making decisions about the care of individual patients" (Sackett, Rosenberg, Gray, Haynes, & Richardson, 1996).

Historically, the health promotion field has been slow in embracing the use of evidence, and this hesitation may be connected with the *Ottawa Charter for Health Promotion* (Evans, Hall, Jones, & Neiman, 2007). The Ottawa Charter (World Health Organization, 1986), considered a milestone in the development of health promotion, did not prioritize the use of evidence to measure effectiveness. It was only in 1998 that the World Health Organization launched an appeal to connect health promotion strategies with the production of health promotion evidence (Evans et al., 2007).

In Western societies, where healthcare expenditures account for a large portion of government budgets, there is continuous pressure to demonstrate that health promotion is a good investment (Evans et al., 2007), and this pressure is growing. Evidence is required to lessen the uncertainty of decision-makers and to guide action priorities (Raphael, 2000). In addition, practitioners in the field have a legitimate desire to show that their work brings tangible benefits (McQueen, 2007a). So the health promotion field really has no choice but to continue trying to assess the effectiveness of its interventions.

There is an important gap between interventions that are deemed effective on the basis of evidence and interventions that are actually implemented in practice (Glasgow & Emmons, 2007). For instance, the complexity of health promotion interventions poses significant conceptual and methodological challenges for the assessment and production of results syntheses that would provide a rational basis on which to guide practices. Moreover, users of research results, such as practitioners and decision-makers, raise a broader range of questions than those addressing

G. Mercille
Department of Social and Preventive Medicine, University of Montreal, Canada

L. Potvin, D. McQueen (eds.), *Health Promotion Evaluation Practices in the Americas*,
DOI: 10.1007/978-0-387-79733-5_6, © Springer Science+Business Media, LLC 2008

intervention effectiveness (Glasgow & Emmons, 2007; Petticrew & Roberts, 2003; Rychetnik & Wise, 2004). Among others, they formulate questions concerning the social, political, and economic settings in which the interventions are developed, implemented, and assessed, as well as the development and implementation of the intervention itself, and the conditions required to maintain interventions over time (Armstrong et al., 2008). So how can we respond to the challenge of producing systematic reviews that capture the essence of the practices that are transferable to other contexts (Potvin & McQueen, 2008)? This chapter presents a pragmatic reflection intended for practitioners who must incorporate evidence in their day-to-day decisions. Systematic reviews, which are large-scale projects considered to have high scientific value, also have their limitations. The objective here is to present these limitations and to propose an alternate approach to producing them. The first section describes the paradigm shift in the concept of evidence, which has been under debate for the past fifteen years. Second, an explanation is given for why systematic reviews in this field do not appear to have effectively impacted health promotion practices or policies. Third, we propose four types of criteria to include when assessing systematic reviews in order to encourage transfer of their contents to health promotion practices. In light of these criteria, we suggest a realist approach to the production of systematic reviews. Combining the generation of evidence and social values, it is a promising tool to guide intervention planning and implementation.

The Debate on the Use of Evidence to Assess the Effectiveness of Health Promotion Interventions

The traditional epistemological basis for evidence has been empirical and positivist. Evidence is a final statement formulated after having observed that the variables are causally related to others with a strong probability in a large number of cases (McQueen, 2007b). This positivist tradition is firmly based on the experimental model, which identifies linear cause-and-effect relationships between independent and dependent variables. This type of research prioritizes the analysis of individual factors to the detriment of contextual factors, which are often dismissed as "noise" from which the salient features must be extracted (Raphael, 2000). In clinical medicine, the quality of evidence has largely been determined with hierarchically organized criteria, with study designs ranked according to their strength in terms of internal validity (Petticrew & Roberts, 2003). Internal validity refers to the degree of confidence that the independent variable is the true cause of the change observed in the dependent variable (Fortin, 2006). According to this hierarchy, randomized controlled trials (RCT) and quasi-experimental designs are at the top of the scale (Oxford Centre for Evidence-based Medicine, 2001; Petticrew & Roberts, 2003).

Since the 1980s, the tension between the two poles of the reductionism-complexity continuum has sparked a lively debate on what constitutes effective health promotion (McQueen, 2007a). This debate centers on the dominance of the experimental model in assessing health promotion interventions. Some maintain that the RCT is the best way to assess the effectiveness of such programs (Rosen, Manor, Engelhard, & Zucker, 2006). In opposition, an increasing number of authors are contending that this kind of reductionist approach, which aims to empir- ically demonstrate causal effects by isolating or controlling variables that might interfere with a presumed causal relationship, is inappropriate for the complex and context-sensitive health promotion interventions and programs (McQueen, 2007b; Poland, Frohlich, & Cargo, 2008; Sanson-Fisher, Bonevski, Green, & D'Este, 2007; Victora, Habicht, & Bryce, 2004). Health promotion programs are typically mul- tidimensional, incorporating many simultaneous determinants across integrated, non-medical strategies. They are deployed in an open setting, they are highly integrated with the cultural and social environment, they involve a diversity of actors, and they evolve over time (Raphael, 2000; Potvin & Goldberg, 2007). The emphasis on RCT and quasi-experimental research designs to isolate the effects of specific components ends up placing too much importance on isolated com- ponents, which could yield other types of impacts in the larger, real-life context (McQueen, 2007b; World Cancer Research Fund, & American Institute for Cancer Research, 2007).

A fundamental issue in this debate is the concept of evidence itself. What is evidence, exactly? "At a basic level, the notion of evidence concerns facts (actual or asserted) intended for use in support of a conclusion" (Lomas, Culyer, McCutcheon, McAuley, & Law, 2005, p. 1). For many researchers in public health and health pro- motion, this notion includes, and exceeds, the positivist vision of the experimental model, which considers only observable data (McQueen, 2007b; Raphael, 2000). Conceptually, we can begin by expanding the notion of evidence into a complex mix of observations, experience, and theoretical arguments (McQueen & Ander- son, 2001), including informal knowledge and practical know-how (Mullen & Ramirez, 2006). Evidence basically means the information derived from an evalua- tion study that has assessed the effects and outcomes of interventions and programs (Rychetnik & Wise, 2004). It appears that the ambiguity of the term *evidence* poses another problem.

In the aim of clarifying this concept, the Canadian Health Services Research Foundation conducted a systematic review, the conclusions of which could help elucidate the issue of conclusive evidence and its use (Lomas et al., 2005). This research shed light on two perspectives on evidence: the informal view, prevalent outside the research community, and the scientific view, which is itself divided on the issue. Most decision-makers feel that evidence involves all elements that are used to establish facts or judge something. Thus, informal (also called colloquial) evidence can be provided by multiple sources, including the opinions of experts and practitioners, political values and judgments, and practical and operational interests and considerations (including resources, expertise and experience, habits, and tradi- tions). Informal evidence complements context-sensitive research data and missing data in order to reach conclusions that guide practices and policies.

The scientific view is much more restrictive on the notion of evidence (Lomas et al., 2005). For researchers, evidence is "information generated through a prescribed set of processes and procedures recognized as scientific" (Lomas et al.,

2005, p. 8). This information must be obtained systematically by methods that are transparent and explicitly coded, replicable, observable, plausible, verifiable, and defendable, in short, defined by the methodology.

The divergent opinions on the role of science, which have spurred the above-mentioned epistemological debate, may be summed up in one word: context. Evidence-based medicine emphasizes the seeking of universal truths, which are absolute and context-independent, whereas the applied sciences favor scientific evidence that accounts for the circumstances of its application. An important contribution of this report is the recognition that the methods used to obtain evidence on context factors are equally scientific and rigorous to the methods used to obtain evidence on program effectiveness. Six dimensions of context-related evidence are presented in the literature review published by Lomas et al. (2005): implementation, organizational capacity, ethics, economics/finance, attitudes, and forecasting. The complexity of contextual or setting-based characterization requires a methodological pluralism in order to obtain scientific evidence on each of these six dimensions (Campostrioni, 2007; Lomas et al., 2005; Petticrew & Roberts, 2003). Moreover, empirical research is increasingly adopting more appropriate and varied approaches (Campostrioni, 2007; Hawkins, Sanson-Fisher, Shakeshaft, D'Este, & Green, 2007). Nevertheless, efforts are needed to improve the external validity of contextualized evidence so as to better guide decision-making. We will return to this below with examples of such methods.

In 2004, the World Health Organization released a definition of evidence-based health promotion that expanded on the concept of evidence-based medicine (Smith, Tang, & Nutbeam, 2006; also Rychetnik & Wise, 2004). Thus, evidence-based health promotion consists of "the use of information derived from formal research and systematic investigation to identify causes and contributing factors that contribute to health needs and the most effective health promotion actions to address these in given contexts and populations" (Smith et al., 2006, p. 342).

In sum, the works of Lomas et al. (2005) underscore three sources of evidence: (1) generalizable scientific evidence, emphasizing universal truths through research on effectiveness and inspired by experimental medicine; (2) context-sensitive evidence via research based on the social sciences; and (3) informal evidence via the expertise and viewpoints of a variety of actors. Independently of their sources, what evidence always carries with it some degree of uncertainty, changeability, and complexity, and at the same time it is debatable and rarely complete.

As in clinical medicine, the use of evidence based on research data alone is insufficient for practical effectiveness in health promotion, and it cannot entirely replace the expertise of the practitioners who guide the selection and application of that evidence (Sackett et al., 1996; Smith et al., 2006). Taken together with explanations above, it also appears that scientific methods can generate knowledge that goes beyond program outcomes. Moreover, researchers increasingly prefer the practice/policy-based evidence approach over the evidence-based practice/policy approach, since it is more consistent with the values of participation and health promotion partnerships (Dooris et al., 2007; Glasgow & Emmons, 2007; Green, 2006; Lobstein & Swinburn, 2007). The three essential ingredients of this approach are:

evidence from the scientific literature, informal evidence (via the judgment of various actors), and transparent mechanisms for collaboration (Lobstein & Swinburn, 2007; Lomas et al., 2005). This approach originated with the practitioners/decision-makers, and it considers what could be implemented from the literature, but also what is already being done in the milieu and elsewhere, along with what the decision-makers would like to implement. In research, it translates into study designs that investigate interventions implemented in real-life contexts, thereby generating evidence that better reflects program–context interactions and the circumstances in which the results could be applied (Glasgow & Emmons, 2007). For systematic reviews to properly characterize the essence of practices that could be transferred to other contexts, they must address both potential interventions and context factors.

Producing Systematic Reviews

Because it is difficult to produce valid, context-applicable conclusions based on a complex body of knowledge, a properly conducted systematic review can facilitate understanding of the available evidence (Balk, Lau, & Bonis, 2005). Thus, systematic reviews, i.e., syntheses of research results designed to determine the effectiveness of health promotion interventions, are believed to assist in guiding practices and support the development of public policies (McQueen, 2007b; Potvin, 2006; Waters et al., 2006).

The classic systematic review relies on a rigorous process that systematically identifies studies on a specific issue, assesses them, and presents the main findings and limitations (Balk et al., 2005). The term systematic review is the generic, recognized term to describe this activity. Meta-analysis is a subgroup of the systematic review that uses statistical methods to combine quantitative data into a cumulative index. The main goal is to integrate the empirical research results from a group of studies for generalization to other populations, although all types of literature reviews would benefit from a systematic approach (Mullen & Ramirez, 2006).

The primary requirements of the systematic review are a preliminary specification of the methods by which the reviewed studies are to be identified, selected, and assessed (Rychetnik, Hawe, Waters, Barratt, & Frommer, 2004). It differs from the narrative synthesis and the book chapter in that these are not exhaustive literature reviews, and their selection and interpretation criteria may be biased or lack transparency (Balk et al., 2005; Rychetnik et al., 2004).

A few international initiatives have been organized to conduct evaluative research to produce systematic reviews of health promotion interventions, although such endeavors are much more numerous in the clinical medicine and epidemiology fields. We could even say that the production of systematic reviews has become an enormous scientific business (Mullen & Ramirez, 2006). Among the most well known in the health promotion field are the Cochrane Collaboration (www.cochrane.org), a group specifically dedicated to health promotion and public health (Cochrane

Health Promotion and Public Health Field: www.vichealth.vic.gov.au/cochrane), and the United States CDC Guide to Community Preventive Services (www.thecom munityguide.org). Dating from 1996, these initiatives were among the first and most prolific in the public health and health promotion fields (McQueen, 2007b; Rychetnik & Wise, 2004; Waters et al., 2006).

Albeit different from organizations that produce systematic reviews, we must highlight the efforts of the International Union for Health Promotion and Education (IUHPE) to produce evidence on health promotion effectiveness. Their first review was a report for the European Commission (IUHPE, 1999). This led to the creation of the Global Program on Health Promotion Effectiveness in 2001, a worldwide initiative that resulted in the recent publication of a reference work (McQueen & Jones, 2007).

The task of producing a systematic review is a complex one for researchers, and it requires particular methodological skills. Several organizations such as the Cochrane Collaboration publish guidelines on how to conduct this type of research, and they offer training and support for researchers (Waters et al., 2006). The key steps in the systematic review are similar to those for an original study: develop a protocol, formulate a research question, review the literature, select the studies, combine the results and their interpretations, discuss, and draw conclusions. Developing a protocol minimizes bias and ensures that the synthesis is replicable. The research question must be clearly formulated, and should specify the populations, communities, issues, and interventions. The formation of an advisory committee composed of users who are well versed in the subject is desirable in order to establish the relevance of the research and the extent to which it can identify issues and include different perspectives (Jackson & Waters, 2005). At the literature review stage, the inclusion and exclusion criteria for original studies must be specified in advance to avoid as far as possible arbitrary choices in selecting or rejecting original studies (Lohr, 2004). In clinical medicine, the literature is quite well organized and readily accessible, with enormous bibliographic databases, primarily of scientific journals with peer review committees, and the use of very consistent indexing terms (Waters et al., 2006). The time allotted for this step should be sufficient to allow the most exhaustive possible research. The only drawback is that the number of studies published in English may be insufficient, depending on the topic (Balk et al., 2005; Mullen & Ramirez, 2006). Next, each original study is examined according to the criteria determined for the intervention types, measures, and results (Mullen & Ramirez, 2006). The quality of study design and methodology is assessed for systematic error prevention.

It appears that the publication and diffusion of norms for published articles has helped improve the quality of original studies reported in the literature (Armstrong et al., 2008; Mullen & Ramirez, 2006). For example, for RCT, the adoption of the Consolidated Standards of Reporting Trials – CONSORT (Moher, Schulz, & Altman, 2001) has improved the description of methods and participant flow (Armstrong et al., 2008). Other standards have been developed for other research designs, such as Transparent Reporting of Evaluations with Nonrandomized Designs – TREND, (Des Jarlais, Lyles, Crepaz, & TREND Group,

2004), and more recently, STROBE, for observational epidemiology studies (Elm et al., 2007). There are also guidelines to assist the synthesizing process (Armstrong et al., 2008). Although the usefulness of these standards for RCTs is not at issue, some have blown the whistle about overly strict applications of these standards to exploratory research and the potential danger of limiting future research discoveries (Potvin, 2008).

The methods used to combine results depend on the degree of similarity between studies in terms of population, intervention type, objectives, measures, and results (Balk et al., 2005). For relatively homogeneous quantitative studies, results may be combined and a synthetic index calculated using meta-analysis. Narrative systematic reviews are used to describe the scope of the evidence obtained from heterogeneous studies (Rychetnik et al., 2004).

Other elements come under consideration when qualifying the evidence. The strength and weight of the evidence must be determined as well. The strength of the evidence derives from judgments on the quality of the studies, including the exactitude and reliability of the results, and whether these same results have been found in other studies and in other populations (Lohr, 2004). The weight of the evidence derives from indirect evidence obtained from non-experimental data, practitioner experience, the accumulated wisdom of systematic analyses, and an understanding of the situations and populations to which it may be applied (Green & Glasgow, 2006). According to Green and Glasgow, greater consideration of external validity would add weight to the evidence in the public health field.

The discussion section of published systematic reviews usually explores the heterogeneity of the estimates across studies, but the unexpected and potentially deleterious effects on other population subgroups must be discussed as well, along with alternate interpretations of the study's strengths and limitations. Conclusions must provide an overall assessment of the relevance of the research conducted and the extent to which the results may be transferable to other communities/populations with similar concerns (Balk et al., 2005; Mullen & Ramirez, 2006; Rychetnik et al., 2004).

The Systematic Review in Health Promotion

When producing systematic reviews in the fields of health promotion and public health, we must consider the challenges inherent in characterizing complex, multi-targeted, multi-level interventions, where the emphasis is placed on population levels and not on individual level changes. Among others, a context analysis must consider the involvement of the populations concerned, the intervention implementation process, the resultant local adaptations, and the phasing-in process. Intervention factors can also influence effectiveness: participation, exposure to the intervention, fairness of the intervention for particular populations, allocated resources, delivery skills, and so on (Waters et al., 2006). The variety of assessment methods used, including qualitative and quantitative methods, complicates the selection of studies to include in the production of the systematic review. Moreover, when synthesizing the findings, the data extraction procedure is more complicated due to the diversity of the literature available, the fuzziness of the indexing termi- nology, and the dispersion of public health research, with many relevant studies not published in peer-reviewed journals (Waters et al., 2006). Quantitatively, the pool of evaluative studies in health promotion is still too small to be divided into homoge- neous categories with accurate synthetic indices (Evans et al., 2007; Potvin, 2006).

To illustrate the current limitations of the systematic review in health promo- tion, let us consider an example from an important issue in the field of health pro- motion: interventions liable to reduce health inequalities. While there is general agreement on the priority of working on social determinants to improve equality of opportunities for individuals to achieve their full health potential (Wilkinson & Marmot, 2003), the conclusions of systematic reviews are disappointing. In this respect, Asthana & Halliday (2006) consulted some 125 systematic reviews in order to identify effective interventions addressing processes that engender health inequalities over a lifetime. They found that the best functioning interventions were aimed at adults and targeted individual lifestyle factors (nutrition, physical activ- ity, and tobacco). They concluded that there was little evidence on interventions that affectively addressed these most important determinants. Similar conclusions were reported in the field of obesity prevention in children, where the lack of well designed measures to assess interventions targeting distal factors limits our capacity to consider their contribution as an effective option to complement interventions centered on changing individual behaviors (Summerbell et al., 2005).

An important objective of the systematic review is to inform on the development of practices, policies, and research. However, pitfalls and weaknesses remain. For example, because systematic reviews are based on very strict and restrictive inclu- sion criteria (Glasgow & Emmons, 2007), there is always a very strong possibility that specific evidence-based interventions may have limited applicability, transfer- ability, or generalizability (terms usually considered synonyms of external validity) to other communities (Mullen & Ramirez, 2006; Waters et al., 2006). Another rea- son that the transition from research into practice is slow and incomplete, according to Glasgow, Lichtenstein, and Marcus (2003), is the substantial influence of the methods proposed in the 1980s by Flay (1986), among others, to use the process of drug development and testing to document the effectiveness and population effects of health promotion interventions. Trial efficacy is measured in controlled settings with randomized controlled trials, where program delivery is uniform and the tar- get population is strictly defined. In contrast, population effectiveness involves the overall targeted population and takes into account the accessibility, acceptability, and coverage of the targeted population (Contandriopoulos, Champagne, Denis, & Avargues, 2000). The influence of these methods has led to the publication of a number of trial efficacy studies, but much fewer studies on population effectiveness (Glasgow et al., 2003). Thus, the concept of effectiveness must be qualified in terms of the setting in which the research is carried out (Contandriopoulos et al., 2000). It appears unlikely that interventions that succeed well in a limited, well controlled context can function as well in the real world, where a variety of communities, conditions, and agents come into play. For Potvin (2006), trying to reduce the complexity of the intervention would be tantamount to adulterating the intervention, or widening the gap between its representativeness of the categories of interventions from which it is sampled and the reality of implementation on the ground. There is a need for a science of complex entities to account for the social contexts in which experiments take place.

Although the systematic reviews published in the *Community Guide* have been acknowledged as among the best in the field, it seems that few of their recommendations have been followed (Glasgow & Emmons, 2007; Mullen & Ramirez, 2006). What usually causes inadequate program implementation is a lack of adjustment between a given intervention and the implementation setting, or a discrepancy between the required characteristics and resources and those that are actually available in the community. There may also be a lack of congruence between the information obtained from the research trial and the information sought by the decision-makers (Glasgow & Emmons, 2007; Rychetnik & Wise, 2004). Some systematic reviews may also be criticized for not appreciating the differences between efficacy trials and effectiveness studies, for failing to account for community perspectives in the development of research protocols (Glasgow & Emmons, 2007), or for postulating that pilot projects assessed in certain conditions that facilitate the research process will generate the same benefits in practice (Mullen & Ramirez, 2006).

In conclusion, it appears that systematic reviews produced in health promotion are not exerting any real influence on practices and policies, which are developed in view of a combination of cultural, technical, and political considerations, while evidence concerns technical considerations alone (Mullen & Ramirez, 2006).

Additional Criteria for Assessing Systematic Reviews of Health Promotion Interventions

Systematic reviews should be appraised with the same critical eye as original studies: for their qualities and for the extent to which the results apply to the research question (Balk et al., 2005). Various international groups have produced guidelines for conducting, reporting, and assessing systematic reviews, particularly for RCTs (Lohr, 2004; Mullen & Ramirez, 2006). In general, original studies and data must be reported in sufficient detail for results verification. Four key basic criteria are used to judge the quality of the evidence. These are: the quality of the original studies (traditionally in medicine and epidemiology, depending on internal validity), the number of studies, the coherence of the evidence (do the overall results make sense?), and the consistency of results (similar studies obtained comparable results) (Mullen & Ramirez, 2006; Lohr, 2004). Balk et al. (2005) translated these four criteria into a series of questions for use in interpreting systematic reviews and meta-analyses in clinical medicine. In health promotion syntheses, additional criteria are being formulated. There is strong support for systematic reviews that are more in tune with the needs of users, recognize the importance of context, allow plurality of evidence, and promote greater use of theories (Armstrong et al., 2008; Jackson & Waters, 2005; Summerbell et al., 2005). In this section, we first argue for the use of multiple methods and quality criteria for external validity in empirical research. Next, we take a closer look at theory and shed light on the links between complex interventions and the input of non-researchers in the production of systematic reviews. A better consideration of the criteria presented here could promote the production of systematic reviews that are based more on the quality of the interventions, and not solely on methodological criteria (Asthana & Halliday, 2006).

When synthesizing scientific evidence, the evidence on socioecological interventions is rarely examined for internal validity, since it is unlikely to be gathered using study designs with a strong potential for internal validity, such as randomized controlled trials (RCT). Hence, the portfolio approach, which recognizes the relative strengths and weaknesses of the different study designs, with none in particular predominating, has increasingly been adopted over the hierarchical classification model of research measures (Asthana & Halliday, 2006; Jackson & Waters, 2005; Lobstein & Swinburn, 2007; Petticrew & Roberts, 2003). For instance, this approach was adopted for the recent and prestigious expert report on causes, nutritional risk factors, and physical activity in cancer prevention, and in population approaches to preventing obesity (McNeil & Flynn, 2006; World Cancer Research Fund, & American Institute for Cancer Research, 2007). This approach was also used by the IUHPE in its latest work (McQueen & Jones, 2007). In the words of Lomas et al. (2005), the advantage of methodological pluralism is that it enables the production of absolute scientific evidence for effective research based on medicine and context-sensitive scientific data. Table 6.1 presents examples of some current methods used to gather different types of scientific data.

In an attempt to improve the transfer of knowledge to practice, Green & Glasgow (2006), proposed some quality criteria for external validity to included in systematic reviews. A copy of these criteria is reproduced in Table 6.2. Influenced by the Re-Aim model (*R*each, *E*ffectiveness, *A*doption, *I*mplementation and *M*aintenance: see www.re-aim.org), which was designed to assist the planning, conduct, and reporting of studies aiming to translate research into practice (Glasgow, Klesges, Dzewaltowski, Estabrooks, & Vogt, 2006), Green and Glasgow's criteria emphasize context as well as program implementation and adaptation processes. The systematic review should also examine the process and implementation data for useful indications concerning intervention adaptation and dissemination (Armstrong et al., 2008). The criteria proposed are also designed to assist in the planning, conduct, and reporting of studies in the aim of translating research into practice, and they suggest that reporting meaningful results to assist in decision-making as well as program maintenance and institutionalization.

Among other criteria to consider when appraising systematic reviews, these should include criteria that assess the potential adverse effects of the type of intervention chosen. The risk that an intervention could increase health inequalities or favor certain types of populations to the detriment of others is an example of such

Table 6.1 Common methodologies according to the type of scientific data sought

Data sought	Methods
Data on health outcomes and their relevance	• Experimental, quasi-experimental • Observational
Implementation data	• Experimental, quasi-experimental • Qualitative • Change theory
Organizational data	• Administrative data • Survey • Comparative, qualitative
Attitudinal data	• Survey, qualitative
Forecasting data	• Time-dependent series • Regression analysis
Economic data	• Cost efficiency, Cost-benefit • Cost-benefit utility • Econometrics
Ethical data	• Distribution analysis • Public consultation
Changing data concerning the general public	• Monitoring • Survey
Social structural data	• Theoretical • Qualitative • Observational

Based on Lomas et al., (2005), and also on Asthana & Halliday (2006), Campostrini, (2007), and Petticrew & Roberts (2003).

adverse effects. Current systematic reviews have little to say on health inequalities or diverse responses across population segments to similar interventions (Asthana & Halliday, 2006; Waters et al., 2006).

The model of Green & Glasgow (2006) helps identify the shortcomings of the evidence on health promotion. Moreover, it has the advantage of drawing attention to the particular priorities and issues of public health, and to balance the study's concerns for internal and external validity. Of course, this would have the effect of increasing the variability of results reported in original studies, but such studies would still be more relevant than if they considered only one type of result (Glasgow & Emmons, 2007).

Up to now, we have proposed criteria for empirical observations to enable the production of systematic reviews that are more relevant in practice. In a field marked by complexity, where empirical observations will always be inadequate to interpret the multiple interactions between the different parts of the system, the use of a deductive process, via the application of theories, could be fruitful. Thus, social science theories could be very useful in clarifying the chaos and complexity involved in the reality of health promotion. Many deplore the underuse of such theories (Potvin & McQueen, 2007) to synthesize research results (McQueen, 2007b; Potvin, 2006). For example, in order to prevent obesity, Summerbell et al. (2005) justifiably underscored the need for multifactorial theoretical approaches that consider the impact of system, setting, and organizational issues together with changes in individual and group behaviors. Researchers are increasingly advancing these

Table 6.2 Proposed quality rating criteria for external validity

---

1. Reach and representativeness

    a. Participation: Are there analyses of the participation rate among potential (a) settings, (b) delivery staff and (c) patients (consumers)?
    b. Target audience: Is the intended target audience stated for adoption (at the intended settings such as worksites, medical offices, etc.) and application (at the individual level)?
    c. Representativeness – Settings: Are comparisons made of the similarity of settings in study to the intended target audience of program settings, or to those settings that decline to participate?
    d. Representativeness – Individuals: Are analyses conducted of the similarity and differences between patients, consumers, or other target subjects who participate versus either those who decline, or the intended target audience?

2. Program or policy implementation and adaptation

    a. Consistent implementation: Are data presented on level and quality of implementation of different program components?
    b. Staff expertise: Are data presented on the level and training or experience required to deliver the program or quality of implementation by different types of staff?
    c. Program adaptation: Is information reported on the extent to which different settings modified or adapted the program to fit their setting?
    d. Mechanisms: Are data reported on the process(es) or mediating variables through which the program or policy achieved its effects?

3. Outcomes for decision-making

    a. Significance: Are outcomes reported in a way that can be compared to either clinical guidelines or public health goals?
    b. Adverse consequences: Do the outcomes reported include quality of life or potential negative outcomes?
    c. Moderators: Are there any analyses of moderator effects – including of different subgroups of participants and types of intervention staff – to assess the robustness versus specificity of effects?
    d. Sensitivity: Are there any sensitivity analyses to assess dose-response effects, threshold level, or point of diminishing returns on the resources expended?
    e. Costs: Are data on the costs presented? If so, are standard economic or accounting methods used to fully account for costs?

4. Maintenance and institutionalization

    a. Long-term effects: Are data reported on longer term effects, at least 12 months following treatment?
    b. Institutionalization: Are data reported on the sustainability (or reinvention or evolution) of program implementation at least 12 months after the formal evaluation?
    c. Attrition: Are data on attrition by condition reported, and are analyses conducted of the representativeness of those who drop out?

From Green & Glasgow, *Evaluation & the Health Professions* (Vol. 29 No.1) p.137, copyright © 2006 by (SAGE Publications). Reprinted by Permission of SAGE Publications, Inc.

social theories, and have proposed innovative applications for health promotion (Dooris et al., 2007; Sterman, 2006).

In order for systematic reviews of complex intervention assessments to reach more compelling conclusions than the all too often "further research is needed," proper use of theory should be included as quality criteria in assessing syntheses of original studies (i.e., how the theoretical mechanisms are explicitly defined and tested), instead of relying solely on empirical results (Greenhalgh, Kristanjsson, & Robinson, 2007; McQueen, 2007b). Too often, very different interventions are considered in the same systematic review, based on superficial similarities such as the setting or targeted behaviors (Armstrong et al., 2008). A theory provides the basics on which to build a model to account for diverse results and complex social relations. By extending the underlying theory that relates program activities to short-, medium-, and long-term outcomes, we can better identify the key elements of complex interventions that could potentially impact outcomes (Asthana & Halliday, 2006; Jackson & Waters, 2005). Jackson and Waters (2005), go even further and propose grouping interventions according to their common theoretical bases, then combining the results to examine the impact of a particular theoretical model on effectiveness. For McQueen (2007b), the evidence makes sense only in light of the theory underlying its construction.

To facilitate translation of research results into practice, systematic reviews should include expert practioner panels in addition to technical and scientific experts. In the long term, this would result in more relevant syntheses (Glasgow & Emmons, 2007; Summerbell et al., 2005). Thus, organizations that produce systematic reviews could develop models for translating community-developed research practices that would emphasize mutual engagement by researchers and users, who would negotiate, create, and share resources to create a more relevant body of knowledge that could be readily applied in practice (McDonald & Viehbeck, 2007). Consensus conferences constitute another way to combine and discuss research results along with other types of information (Callon, Lascoumes, & Barthe, 2001; Lomas et al., 2005). The aim is to clarify decision-making on issues that are clouded in uncertainty. Dialogues are held between scientists and other stakeholders affected by the results, using clear objectives, and following a participatory process that is transparent and inclusive, with the aim of combining the different forms of information (scientific and informal), interpreting them, and yielding "a judgment that is evidence-informed, better matched to the context of application, more efficiently implemented, and more widely acceptable" (Lomas et al., 2005, p. 5).

Toward a Realistic Approach to Producing Systematic Reviews in Health Promotion

A particular difficulty with the empirical and experimental models is the "black box" concept: attention is paid to the input (the intervention) and the outcomes of that intervention in terms of impacts, whereas the mechanisms that transform input into outcomes are ignored. This is a problem with many health promotion interventions, since they are usually implemented with varying degrees of reliability, having adapted to the context and constraints of the setting. It appears that the literature on community health promotion interventions prefers the evidence-based model, with priority given to the possibility of replicating an intervention instead of considering the unique contextual characteristics (McLaren, Ghali, Lorenzetti, & Rock, 2007). Thus, a review of community programs inspired by the North Karelia project revealed that only 19% of the programs considered the importance of context or the need to adapt the intervention (McLaren et al., 2007). In a systematic review on interventions to prevent overweight and obesity in youth, the authors concluded that the best practices also featured the ability to be sustainably integrated into the infrastructure and adapted to the school context (Doak, Visscher, Renders, & Seidell, 2006). Because they expanded their inclusion criteria to consider a wider range of interventions from a large diversity of sociocultural contexts, they were able to support the notion that an appropriate program could be adapted to its context. Documenting aspects of the implementation processes is also important, insofar as they influence the impacts and outcome indicators (Sharma, 2006). Not taking these aspects into account in primary evaluation increases the risks of type III errors, or concluding that the intervention failed to achieve positive results due to poor design, such that it was impossible to make a noticeable difference (Tones & Tilford, 2001). One currently used method is to include an assessment of the intervention delivery process in the research synthesis. Such assessments can help unravel the factors responsible for success or failure of the outcomes of the intervention's application (Armstrong et al., 2008).

As underscored by McQueen (2007a), the debate about evidence has certainly engendered important theoretical advances in the practice and assessment of health promotion. Many have put forward the realist approach as a promising framework for performing assessments and systematic reviews (Dooris et al., 2007; Pawson, Greenhalgh, Harvey, & Walshe, 2005; Poland et al., 2008). The realist investigation enables diverse results on a particular research question to be synthesized, taking into account implementation settings, to shed light on the nuts and bolts of the intervention or program, to the benefit of the individuals running the intervention (Pawson et al., 2005). The realist approach is guided by a theory (Williams, 2003), whose departure point is the distinction between the *real* (the world of objects, whether physical or social), the *actual* (i.e., events and experiences that may or may not be observable), and the *empirical* (what is observed) (Williams, 2003; see also Poland et al., 2008; Potvin, Gendron, & Bilodeau, 2006).

According to the realist approach, the research question is formulated as: "What works in this program, for whom, and in which circumstances?" The first step in a realist synthesis is to make explicit the theoretical presuppositions on how the intervention functions and produces its expected impact. Next, theoretical models are empirically confronted. The results of the synthesis combine the theoretical understanding and empirical data, and explain the relationship between the intervention's application setting, operating mechanisms, and outcomes (Pawson et al., 2005). Synthesizing the evidence requires refining the theory in order to understand how the intervention works.

The realist model of systematic review appears as a promising approach to meet the complexity of health promotion interventions in a number of ways (Pawson et al., 2005; Potvin et al., 2006; see also Tones & Tilford, 2001). First, the realist synthesis is more meaningful for practitioners and decision-makers because it provides a richer and more detailed understanding of complex social interventions. It attempts to grasp what actually takes place, with all its multiple aspects, changes, and uncertainties (instead of using the experimental model to control and restrict). The investigative logic is pluralist and flexible, as it considers the merits of multiple methods (without a hierarchal ranking) to investigate the processes and impacts of the intervention. This approach makes judicious use of all the quality criteria proposed by Green & Glasgow (2006) to document the external validity of original studies, not solely from a standpoint of generalizability of results, but rather to verify their applicability and facilitate their transfer to other, similar settings. The literature review is not limited to studies published in the scientific literature; it may consider publications outside the formal channels, known as *grey literature*. Finally, the production of realist syntheses provides opportunities for non-researchers, practitioners, and policy makers to offer their input on the conclusions, recommendations, and practical applications (Pawson et al., 2005).

Moreover, this approach has begun to be used in parallel with more traditional approaches. A recent systematic review by the Cochrane Collaboration assessed the impact of nutrition programs for disadvantaged school children and concluded that they could have a modest beneficial effect on the children's physical, psychological and social health (Kristanjsson et al., 2007). Of the 18 studies retained, 7 were randomized controlled trials. One objective of this review was to understand the ways in which program delivery impacted outcomes such as children's growth, cognitive development, and performance. Although the retrieval of descriptive data on the setting, the involvement of the various actors, and implementation details helped researchers interpret the quantitative results and generate hypotheses, three of the researchers involved subsequently conducted a realist examination to more precisely identify which particular intervention aspects were associated with effectiveness, and interpreted them in terms of historical and political context (Greenhalgh et al., 2007).

The spread of this method has been limited by the small number of evaluation studies in health promotion in general and realist evaluation designs in particular (Poland et al., 2008). Nevertheless, encouraged by theoretical advances, intervention assessment projects based on the realist approach are underway in France, with the aim of lessening social inequalities in health (Ridde & Guichard, in press). On the other hand, like any relatively novel method, the realist approach needs to be refined and expertise developed by health promotion researchers, including aspects such as the use of theory, which is not common in the field (McQueen & Kickbusch, 2007). We may also expect some resistance from public health researchers to adopte this approach, since it differs substantially from the traditional systematic review. Instead of a replicable method that follows rigid rules, the logic of realist review is guided by principles. Above all, it requires a shift in the dominant public health paradigm away from the ontology of empirical realism and toward the ontology of critical realism (Potvin et al., 2006). Although some believe we should employ a realist ontology rather than the sum of its parts to understand the mechanisms of a complex intervention, they may still be ensnared by positivist certainties when they develop an empirical methodology to operationalize the approach (Hawe, Shiell, & Riley, 2004). More work is required on defining the concepts and operationalizing the elements of the assessment approach in realist syntheses (Pawson et al., 2005; Poland et al., 2008).

Conclusion

The production of systematic reviews that provide a rational basis to guide practices poses a real dilemma for health promotion. Among others, the users of such evidence entertain a broader range of questions than those that are currently prioritized by synthesis projects, and which are related to effectiveness outcomes. In this chapter, we have presented the limitations of synthesis projects currently being produced in relationship with the characteristics of health promotion. First, it is apparent that the answer to these questions is closely connected to the concept of evidence, a concept that must continue to evolve to better respond to issues in the assessment of complex, context-sensitive, and evolving interventions. Second, we explained which aspects of health promotion research syntheses make them more attractive to users. In light of this analysis, we proposed some criteria to include when appraising systematic reviews in order to encourage their translation into practice: the inclusion of original studies according to the principle of methodological pluralism, with a focus on context, the implementation process, and program adaptation. Second, original studies retained in the review should make explicit the theoretical mechanisms underlying the intervention's functioning, and ideally, these theoretical mechanisms would be comparable. The resulting analysis would be primarily useful to verify the responses of various population segments to similar interventions and to identify the potential adverse impacts of population interventions. Finally, systematic reviews should be more meaningful for practitioners and decision-makers, insofar as they can offer their input in the review process. Furthermore, in light of these criteria, it appears that the production of systematic reviews using the critical realist approach offers the potential to better respond to the challenges of producing evidence that is liable to be adopted in practice. It remains to be verified whether this realist approach can in fact respond to the fourth practical dilemma raised in Chapter 3 of this book.

Compared to research in epidemiology and clinical medicine, research in health promotion has been underfunded by the major research granting programs, and cannot produce a sufficient body of evidence to document the effectiveness of interventions (Glasgow et al., 2003; McQueen, 2007b; Mullen & Ramirez, 2006; Potvin, 2006). Investments must be made in evaluative health promotion research in order to generate evidence that would truly advance practices. Moreover, both health promotion researchers and funding organizations should include more theory-based protocols in their assessments (Glasgow et al., 2003; Greenhalgh et al., 2007).

References

Armstrong, R., Waters, E., Moore, L., Riggs, E., Cuervo, L. G., Lumbiganon, P., et al. (2008). Improving the reporting of public health intervention research. Advancing TREND and CONSORT. *Journal of Public Health, 30*, 103–109.

Asthana, S., & Halliday, J. (2006). Developing an evidence base for policies and interventions to address health inequalities: The analysis of "Public Health Regimes". *The Milbank Quarterly, 84*, 577–603.

Balk, E. M., Lau, J., & Bonis, P. A. L. (2005). Reading and critically appraising systematic reviews and meta-analyses: A short primer with a focus on hepatology. *Journal of Hepatology, 43*, 729–726.

Callon, M., Lascoumes, P., & Barthe, Y. (2001). L'organisation des forums hybrides. In M. Callon, P. Lacoumes & Y. Barthe. *Agir dans un monde incertain. Essai sur la démocratie technique* (pp. 209–262). Paris: Seuil.

Campostrini, S. (2007). Measurement and effectiveness: Methodological considerations, issues and possible solutions. In D. V. McQueen & C. M. Jones (Eds.), *Global perspectives on health promotion effectiveness* (pp. 181–200). New-York: Springer.

Contandriopoulos, A. P., Champagne, F., Denis, J. L., & Avargues, M. C. (2000). L'évaluation dans le domaine de la santé. Concepts et méthodes. *Revue d'épidémiologie et de santé publique, 48*, 517–539.

Des Jarlais, D. C., Lyles, C., Crepaz, N., & TREND Group. (2004). Improving the reporting quality of non-randomized evaluations of behavioral and public health interventions: The TREND statement. *American Journal of Public Health, 94*, 361–366.

Doak, C. M., Visscher, T. L. S., Renders, C. M., & Seidell, J. C. (2006). The prevention of overweight and obesity in children and adolescents: A review of interventions and programmes. *Obesity Reviews, 7*, 111–136.

Dooris, M., Poland, B., Kolbe, L., De Leeuw, E., McCall, D. S., & Wharf-Higgins, J. (2007). Healthy settings: Building evidence for the effectiveness of whole system health promotion-Challenges and future directions. In D. V. McQueen & C. M. Jones (Eds.), *Global perspectives on health promotion effectiveness* (pp. 327–352). New York: Springer.

Elm, E. von, Altman, D. G., Egger, M., Pocock, S. J., Gotzsche, P. C., & Vanderbroucke, J. P., for the STROBE initiative (2007). Strengthening the reporting of observational studies in epidemiology (STROBE) statement: Guidelines for reporting observational studies. *British Medical Journal, 335*, 806–808.

Evans, L., Hall, M. Jones, C. M., & Neiman, A. (2007). Did the Ottawa Charter play a role in the push to assess the effectiveness of health promotion? *Promotion & Education, Suppl. 2*, 28–30.

Flay, B. R. (1986). Efficacy and effectiveness trials (and other phases of research) in the development of health promotion programs. *Preventive Medicine, 15*, 451–474.

Fortin, M. F. (2006). *Fondements et étapes du processus de recherche*. Montréal, Québec: Editions de la Chenelière.

Glasgow, R. E., & Emmons, K. M. (2007). How can we increase translation of research into practice? Types of evidence needed. *Annual Review of Public Health, 28*, 413–433.

Glasgow, R. E., Klesges, L. M., Dzewaltowski, D. A., Estabrooks, P. A., & Vogt, T. M. (2006). Evaluating the impact of health promotion programs: Using the RE-AIM framework to form summary measures for decision-making involving complex issues. *Health Education Research, 21*, 688–694.

Glasgow, R. E., Lichtenstein, E., & Marcus, A. C. (2003). Why don't we see more translation of health promotion research to practice? Rethinking the efficacy-to-effectiveness transition. *American Journal of Public Health, 93*, 1261–1267.

Green, L. W. (2006). Public health asks of system science: To advance our evidence-based practice, can you help us get more practice-based evidence? *American Journal of Public Health, 96*, 406–409.

Green, L. W., & Glasgow, R. E. (2006). Evaluating the relevance, generalization, and transferability of research. Issues in external validation and translation methodology. *Evaluation & the Health Professions, 29*, 126–153.

Greenhalgh, T., Kristanjsson, E., & Robinson, V. (2007). Realist review to understand the efficacy of school feeding programmes. *British Medical Journal, 335*, 858–861.

Hawe, P., Shiell, A., & Riley, T. (2004). Complex interventions: how "out of control" can a randomised controlled trial be? *British Medical Journal, 328*, 1561–1563.

Hawkins, N. G., Sanson-Fisher, R. W., Shakeshaft, A., D'Este, C., & Green, L. W. (2007). The multiple baseline design for evaluating population-based research. *American Journal of Preventive Medicine, 33*, 162–168.

International Union for Health Promotion and Education. (1999). *The evidence of health promotion effectiveness: Shaping public health in a New Europe. Part two, evidence book*. Brussels, Belgium: ECSC-EC-EAEC.

Jackson, N., & Waters, E., for the Guidelines for systematic reviews in health promotion and public health taskforce (2005). Criteria for the systematic review of health promotion and public health interventions. *Health Promotion International, 20*, 367–374.

Kristanjsson, E., Robinson, V., Petticrew, M., Macdonald, B., Krasevec, J., Janzen, L., et al. (2007). School feeding for improving the physical and psychosocial health of disadvantaged elementary school children. *Cochrane Database of Systematic Reviews, 1*, CD 004676.

Lobstein, T., & Swinburn, B. (2007). Health promotion to prevent obesity: Evidence and policy needs. In D. V. McQueen & C. M. Jones (Eds.), *Global perspectives on health promotion effectiveness* (pp. 125–150). New York: Springer.

Lohr, K. (2004). Rating the strength of scientific evidence. Relevance for quality improvement programs. *International Journal for Quality in Health Care, 16*, 9–18.

Lomas, J., Culyer, T., McCutcheon, C., & McAuley, L., & Law, S. (2005, May). *Conceptualizing and combining evidence for health system guidance*. Canadian Health Services Research Foundation. http://www.chsrf.ca/other_documents/pdf/evidence_e.pdf

McDonald, P. W., & Viehbeck, S. (2007). From evidence-based practice making to practice-based evidence making: Creating communities of (research) and practice. *Health Promotion Practice, 8*, 140–144.

McLaren, L., Ghali, L. M., Lorenzetti, D., & Rock, M. (2007). Out of context? Translating evidence from the North Karelia project over place and time. *Health Education Research, 22*, 414–424.

McNeil, D. A., & Flynn, M. A. T. (2006). Methods of defining best practice for population health approaches with obesity prevention as an example. *Proceedings of the Nutrition Society, 65*, 403–411.

McQueen, D. V. (2007a). Critical issues in theory for health promotion. In D. V. McQueen, I. Kickbush, L. Potvin, J. M. Pelikan, L. Balbo & T. Abel (Eds.), *Health and Modernity. The role of theory in health promotion* (pp. 21–42). New York: Springer.

McQueen, D. V. (2007b). Evidence and theory: Continuing debates on evidence and effectiveness. In D. V. McQueen & C. M. Jones (Eds.), *Global perspectives on health promotion effectiveness* (pp. 281–304). New York: Springer.

McQueen, D. V., & Anderson, L. M. (2001). What counts as evidence: Issues and debates. In I. Rootman, M. Goodstadt, B. Hyndman, D. V. McQueen, L. Potvin, J. Springett & E. Ziglio (Eds.), *Evaluation in Health Promotion: Principles and Perspectives* (pp. 63–81). Copenhague, Denmark: World Health Organization.

McQueen, D. V., & Jones, C. M. (Eds.) (2007). *Global perspectives on health promotion effectiveness*. New York: Springer.

McQueen, D. V., & Kickbusch, I. (2007). Introduction. Health promotion. The origins of the Third public health revolution leading to a new public health. In D. V. McQueen, I. Kickbush, L. Potvin, J. M. Pelikan, L. Balbo & T. Abel (Eds.), *Health and Modernity. The role of theory in health promotion* (pp. 1–5). New York: Springer.

Mullen, P. D., & Ramirez, G. (2006). The promise and pitfalls of systematic reviews. *Annual Review of Public Health, 27*, 81–102.

Moher, D., Schulz, K. F., & Altman, D. G. (2001). The CONSORT statement: revised recommendations for improving the quality of reports of parallel-group randomised trials. *Lancet, 357,* 1191–1194. http://www.consort-statement.org/

Oxford Centre for Evidence-based Medicine (2001). *Levels of evidence and grades of recommendation.* Oxford (May, 2001). Downloaded in February 2008 from http://www.cebm.net/index.aspx?o=1025.

Pawson, R., Greenhalgh, T., Harvey, G., & Walshe, K. (2005). Realist review. A new method of systematic review designed for complex policy interventions. *Journal of Health Services Research & Policy, 10,* 21–34.

Petticrew, M., & Roberts, H. (2003). Evidence, hierarchies, and typologies: Horses for courses. *Journal of Epidemiology and Community Health, 57,* 527–529.

Poland, B., Frohlich, K., & Cargo, M. (2008). Context as a fundamental dimension of health-promotion program evaluation. In L. Potvin, D. V. McQueen, L. Anderson, Z. Hartz & L. de Salazar (Eds.), *Health promotion evaluation practice in the Americas. Research and values.* New York: Springer.

Potvin, L. (2006). Should we worry about the enthusiasm toward evidence-based health promotion practices? *Promotion & Education, 13,* 228–229.

Potvin, L. (2008). STROBE and the standardization of scientific practice. *International Journal of Public Health, 53,* 9–10.

Potvin, L., Gendron, S., & Bilodeau, A. (2006). Três posturas ontológicas concernentes à natureza dos programas de saúde: Implicações para a avaliação. In M. L. M. Bossi & F. J. Mercado (Eds.), *Avaloação qualitative de programas de saúde. Enforques emergentes* (pp. 65–86). Petropolis, Brazil: Vozes Editorial.

Potvin, L., & Goldberg, C. (2007). Two roles of evaluation in transforming health promotion practice. In M. O'Neill, S. Dupéré, A. Pederson & I. Rootman (Eds.), *Health Promotion in Canada. Critical perspectives.* (pp. 347–360). Toronto: Canadian Scholar's Press.

Potvin, L., & McQueen, D. V. (2007). Modernity, public health and health promotion. A reflexive discourse. In D. V. McQueen, I. Kickbush, L. Potvin, J. M. Pelikan, L. Balbo & T. Abel (Eds.), *Health and Modernity. The role of theory in health promotion* (pp. 12–20). New York: Springer.

Potvin., L., & McQueen, D. V. (2008). Practical dilemmas for health promotion evaluation. In L. Potvin, D. V. McQueen, L. Anderson, Z. Hartz & L. de Salazar (Eds.), *Health promotion evaluation practice in the Americas. Research and values.* New York: Springer.

Raphael, D. (2000). The question of evidence in health promotion. *Health Promotion International, 15,* 355–367.

Ridde, V., & Guichard. A. (In press). Réduire les inégalités sociales de santé. Aporie, épistémologie et défis. In C. Niewiadomski & P. Aïach (Eds.), *Lutter contre les inégalités sociales de santé.* Rennes, France: ENSP Éditions.

Rosen, L., Manor, O., Engelhard, D., & Zucker, D. (2006). In defense of the randomized controlled trial for health promotion research. *American Journal of Public Health, 96,* 1181–1186.

Rychetnik, L., & Wise, M. (2004). Advocating evidence-based health promotion: reflections and a way forward. *Health Promotion International, 19,* 247–257.

Rychetnik, L., Hawe, P., Waters, E., Barratt, A., & Frommer, M. (2004). A glossary for evidence-based public health. *Journal of Epidemiology and Community Health, 58,* 538–545.

Sackett, D. L. Rosenberg, W. M. C., Gray, J. A. M., Brian Haynes, R. B., & Richardson, S. W. (1996). Evidence-based medicine: What it is and what it isn't. *British Medical Journal, 312,* 71–72.

Sanson-Fisher, R. W., Bonevski, B., Green, L. W., & D'Este, C. (2007). Limitations of the randomized controlled trial in evaluating population-based interventions. *American Journal of Preventive Medicine, 33,* 155–161.

Sharma, M. (2006). School-based interventions childhood and adolescent obesity. *Obesity Reviews, 7,* 261–269.

Smith, B. J., Tang, K. C., & Nutbeam, D. (2006). WHO health promotion glossary: New terms. *Health Promotion International, 21,* 340–345.

Sterman, J. D. (2006). Learning from evidence in a complex world. *American Journal of Public Health, 96*, 505–514.

Summerbell, C. D., Waters, E., Edmunds, L. D., Kelly, S., Brown, T., & Campbell, K. J. (2005). Interventions for preventing obesity in children. *Cochrane Database of Systematic Reviews, 3*, CD 001871.

Tones, K., & Tilford, S. (2001). Evaluation research. In K. Tones & S. Tilford (Eds.), *Health promotion. Effectiveness, efficiency and equity. 3rd ed.* (pp. 149–192). Cheltenham, U.K.: Nelson Thornes.

Victora, C. G., Habicht, JP., & Bryce, J. (2004). Evidence-based public health: Moving beyond randomized trials. *American Journal of Public Health, 94*, 400–405.

Waters, E., Doyle, J., Jackson, N., Howes, F., Brunton, G., & Oakley, A. (2006). Evaluating the effectiveness of public health interventions: The role and activities of the Cochrane Collaboration. *Journal of Epidemiology and Community Health, 60*, 285–289.

Wilkinson, R., & Marmot, M. (2003). *Social determinants of health. The solid facts. 2nd ed.* Geneva: WHO.

Williams, S. J. (2003). Beyond meaning, discourse and the empirical world. Critical realist reflections on health. *Social Theory & Health, 1*, 42–71.

World Cancer Research Fund, & American Institute for Cancer Research (2007). Judging the evidence. In World Cancer Research Fund & American Institute for Cancer Research. *Food, Nutrition, Physical Activity, and the Prevention of Cancer: a Global Perspective* (pp. 48–62). Washington DC: AICR.

World Health Organization. (1986). *The Ottawa Charter for health promotion.* Downloaded in February 2008 from: http://www.who.int/hpr/NPH/docs/ottawa_charter_hp.pdf

Chapter 7
From Knowledge to Action: Challenges and Opportunities for Increasing the Use of Evaluation in Health Promotion Policies and Practices

Zulmira M. A. Hartz, Jean-Louis Denis, Elizabeth Moreira, and Alvaro Matida

> *The gap between scientific knowledge and its concrete translation into improvement of people's quality of life is well-known. (Berghmans & Potvin, 2005 p. 19)*

How to make evaluation useful and used are familiar topics that appear to be perennial concerns for evaluators in general. We often talk about the utilization of evaluation research results in policies almost like an inevitable output of evaluation, but we must recognize the challenges that can impede or limit this pursuit. In the health promotion field, for example, these challenges can help us explain the well-known gap between available scientific knowledge, potential effectiveness of social interventions, and improvement in people's quality of life, as quoted above.

Our objective in this chapter is to present some theoretical assumptions and related factors associated with evaluation use as discussed in the literature, and to provide a framework that could increase opportunities to influence health promotion practices and policies with evaluative research. Our main working hypothesis is that although in the health promotion field we do not have an extensive experience with this specific subject, we can learn a lot about it, not only from the lessons of social and health programs evaluation in general, but also from the sociology of innovation, when evaluation is conceived as intervention on programs (Schwandt, 2005) and innovation implemented in the "social space of programs" (Potvin, Gendron, & Bilodeau, 2006).

The first section thus begins with a theoretical overview guided by utilization models. It is followed by a brief discussion of levels and mechanisms of use or influence and complemented by specific comments on a set of health programs guidelines oriented by utilization-focused evaluation. Here we combine the expressions use and influence, following recent positions that we will present later in this chapter. The term influence is broader than use and it refers to the capacity or power

Z.M.A. Hartz
Foundations Oswaldo Cruz, Rio de Janeiro, Brazil

L. Potvin, D. McQueen (eds.), *Health Promotion Evaluation Practices in the Americas,*
DOI: 10.1007/978-0-387-79733-5_7, © Springer Science+Business Media, LLC 2008

of persons or things to produce effects on others by intangible or indirect means (Kirkhart, 2000). Thus, influence is more related to multidirectional, incremental, and unintentional than a merely instrumental use.

The second section constructs an operational framework integrating these and other contributions to innovations studies, applicable to health promotion activities. We conclude by focusing on some initiatives and directives that appear to be good opportunities for increasing the influence of evaluation findings, while offering some watchful advice on the risks associated with eventual misused practices of utility-driven evaluation. The overall goal is to present different approaches, skills, tools, and methods increasing potential utility or usability (Scriven, 2005) of evaluation in health promotion, permitting to design research with visibility to the consequences for public policies.

Knowledge Utilization and Policy Making

There is a consensus in the consulted literature that the evaluation's use theories originate from the United States (Caracelli, 2000; Kirkhart, 2000; Patton, 1997; Preskill & Torres, 2000; Rossman & Rallis, 2000; Sridharan, 2003; Weiss, 1988, 1999; Weiss, Murphy-Graham, & Birkeland, 2005). These studies inspired Canadian and Central and South American authors in the understanding of the theoretical basis for using knowledge evidence in health policy development and services (Borowski, Hanney, Lindquist, & Roger, 2005; CDC, 1999; Champagne, Contandriopoulos, & Tanon, 2004; Denis, Lehoux, & Champagne, 2004; Elias & Patroclo, 2005; Lehoux, Battista, & Lance, 2000; Trostle, Bronfman, & Langer 1999). Their contribution will be summarized according to the four blocks or pillars of our framework: (1) models of and values underlying evaluation use; (2) modes of knowledge production; (3) levels of evaluation influence; and (4) utilization-focused evaluation. All these authors conceive the relationship between science and practice, or decision-makers and researchers, as controversial given the different frames of reference with which these actors approach the situation, leading to unsatisfied expectations. Even if this question is not specific to public health or health promotion, we suggest that we have to deal with it as an issue of research, considering the increasing demand for utility in our work.

Models of and Values Underlying Evaluation Use

Building upon a theoretical review, Weiss et al. (2005) characterize three main types of evaluation use models in policy: instrumental, to give direction to policy and practice; political or symbolic, to justify preexisting preferences and actions; and conceptual, to provide new ideas, or concepts, that are useful for making sense of the policy scene.

The first kind of use, i.e., as direction for decision-making, is often what people have in mind when they think about evaluation and suggests a sense of emergency for making decisions. However, pure instrumental use of evaluation results is not common and, after some time, evaluation results becomes so entangled with other factors contributing to decision that it is almost impossible to discern their specific contribution. The symbolic use refers to situations where evaluation results provide support for policies designed and decided on different bases such as intuition, professional experience, organizational interest, self-interest, or other reasons. If sometimes authors deride the symbolic use of evaluation results, Weiss et al. (2005) argue that it is only in the rare cases where decision-makers distort or omit significant evaluation findings that such a use leads to evaluation being misused. On the other hand, she recognizes that evaluation is often used to buttress an existing point of view by congressional committees, bureaucracies, and organizational administrations, and that the same tendency can be observed in academic reviews. The conceptual use comes when research and evaluation studies are useful, even if decision-makers might not base their decision directly on the evidence they provide, but they find themselves influenced or enlightened by evaluation results. Although some authors consider process use as a distinct category of evaluation results use, Weiss et al. (2005) consider such a use only as a specification about the type of evaluation results that is being used in the first three categories.

As it is the case with most current theoretical models, evaluation use types embody values associated with three different scientific paradigms (classic positivist, constructivist, and neo-positivist) legitimating their orientation (Champagne et al., 2004). The classic positivist set of values associated with the conceptual model of evaluation results use is characterized by a total control of the evaluator over the interpretation of evaluation results, low participation of actors other than researchers in the research endeavor, and a more passive role for researchers in transferring result to decision-makers. The responsibility of researchers stops once results are made available. The constructivist sets of values that support the symbolic or political model, maintains the evaluator's control, but presupposes an intense participation from other actors in the knowledge production process. Finally, the neo-positivist values, which have wide flexibility, can be present in all models characterized by unspecific or targeted use of research findings, mixed control over the evaluation process, and variable degrees of participation by a wide range of actors. In a previous work, Weiss (1999) suggested that other values can produce endarkenment rather than enlightenment when implementing evaluation findings into a policy. She mainly refers to the notion of interests, a paramount in policy-makers' decisions, and to the role played by ideologies, as filters of opportunities that leave out options that are not in accordance with decision-makers' beliefs and preferences.

Modes of Knowledge Production

For Denis et al. (2004), "most knowledge utilization models pay little attention to the production process of knowledge" (p. 30), and they do not agree on either the strategies to increase knowledge use, or the status of scientists and practitioners in such a process. However, all those models imply fine-tuned communication between these domains, to facilitate knowledge use, closely dependent on two knowledge production modes, invoked from the works of Gibbons et al. (1994) and Nowotny, Scott, and Gibbons (2001). Both, Mode 1 and Mode 2, result from the institutionalization of science in modern societies around two archetypes. Mode 1 corresponds to the traditional form of organizing academic and research production, where scientific recognition is achieved mainly through the production of new knowledge inside disciplinary boundaries. The peer-review system works as a safeguard for research quality and a prerequisite for any process of wider dissemination.

In Mode 2, new knowledge is valuable, but insufficient. The emphasis is on the practical outcomes of the knowledge to solve critical problems as implicit in the notion of research and technological development, and on increasing knowledge contextualization. Science must not be constrained, assuming a mutual influence between the University and society, between research groups and organizations. Using the example of Canadian funding agencies, the authors recognize that Mode 2 has been adopted and implemented especially in some areas of health research, thus favoring the emergence of enthusiastic reactions by increasing the use of knowledge, even though it is inquired "whether the emergence of the knowledge-based society might be linked, somewhat paradoxically, to a weakening of science" (Denis et al., 2004, p. 37). Consequently, fearing that some fundamental principles of science could be eroded (e.g., independence, methodological rigor, and organized skepticism), they conclude that Mode 2 "and its explicit valuation of knowledge use and intense relationships between science and practitioners should be a complement to, but not a substitute for, Mode 1" (Denis et al., 2004, p.38).

Echoing the same centrality of practice and scientific communities in the modes of knowledge production, we would like to mention other important contributions, starting with Caracelli (2000), who underlines the evolution of the evaluator's role from a dispassionate outsider to a co-investigator in the program (acting like a facilitator, problem-solver, educator, coach, and critical friend). Such an evaluator can even be called a partner and co-producer of knowledge, from the perspective of a learning inquiry approach and/or learning organizations (Preskill & Torres, 2000; Rossman & Rallis, 2000). In agreement with this perspective, and from a constructivist standpoint where evaluation should serve educational purposes and where success is judged by what others learn, Rossman and Rallis (2000) defend the notion that dialogue replaces discussion. This means dashing to pieces examining arguments, evoking the notions of percussion and concussion – striking or hitting. For them, dialogue means conversation, valuable and constructive communication that situates evaluators and program leaders as co-learners and co-responsible for knowledge use.

Schwandt (2005) analyzes the complex interactions between researchers and practitioners, exposing the material and linguistic activities that people change and develop, and arguing against the "pervasive notion of instrumental rationality" (Schwandt, 2005, p. 97), a narrow view in which evaluators are applied scientists in "a kind of evidence-based mania about all forms of social services and educational practices" (Schwandt, 2005, p. 96) that tends to view the world of concrete and practice dilemmas as an embarrassment. Although recognizing that we must try to lead scientific evidence to deliberations, Schwandt's practice-oriented approach ponders that the notion of transferring knowledge in the form of theory or other prescriptions for practice is questionable, whereby the imperative to evaluate is at the core of practical action of every professional.

Levels of Evaluation Influence

Although those theoretical contributions are of utmost importance for presenting the abstract foundations that sustain the range of evaluation uses-users, they tell us little about how to systematically analyze the evaluation's influence or utility. In an attempt to fill this gap, we will explore the work of Kirkhart (2000), Henry and Mark (2003) and Mark and Henry (2004), examining the complementary levels and mechanisms of influence in order to understand how (and to what extent) evaluation shapes, affects, supports, and changes persons and systems.

Kirkhart's position stems from a historical and critical view of the process use model, but still maintained the narrowness of the results-based construct it was intended to correct: "the terms utilization and use were associated with the data bases influence of evaluation findings . . . The initial response was bringing other forms of influence under the umbrella of use . . . attached to the influence process on persons and systems being evaluated (process use) . . . This has proven to be only a partial solution, one that in some ways has perpetuated the construct under representation" (Kirkhart, 2000, p. 6). According to Kirkhart (2000), the umbrella of influence must both combine and distinguish, in a logical model, three dimensions: the sources of evaluation elements presumed to be able to generate change (process, results or symbolic influence); intentions, defined by the purpose consciously recognized and anticipated (intended) or by unintended findings; and its temporal dimension (immediate, end-of-cycle, or long-term). Therefore, intended and unintended influences may occur separately or in combination at different points in time or sources.

Following Kirkhart (2000), Henry and Mark (2003) go beyond use to understand which mechanisms or mediators (coming from an extensive review of social science literature) explain the evaluation's influence. Evaluation, "viewed in this way . . . is analogous to an intervention or a program . . . that produces consequences that can be good, bad, neutral, mixed or indeterminate . . . A theory of evaluation should focus on the subset of evaluation consequences that could plausibly lead towards or away from social betterment" (Henry & Mark, 2003, pp. 295–296). Their theoretical groundwork fills two gaps: the relative lack of studies involving systematic comparative research in the literature on use, and the lack of attention to the processes, "through which evaluation findings and processes may translate into social betterment" (Henry & Mark, 2003, p. 294). For these authors, there exist different mechanisms corresponding to three levels of influence: individual, interpersonal, and collective. These forms are not mutually exclusive and all these elements of one form can stimulate other elements, either within or across levels. Lehoux et al. (2000), in their work analyzing the pathways of influence on health technology assessment, add incentives or removal of (dis)incentives, as mechanisms of knowledge use in institutional environment, the final decision-making set. These authors distinguish also the micro-macro levels of observed effects or outcomes, from professional practices to health policy.

Utilization-Focused Evaluation

The fourth block to consider in conducting knowledge transfer research or to suggest ways to better integrate evaluation results into the policymaking process is Patton's (1997), structured on the premise that use does not just happen naturally. It needs to be facilitated, and facilitating use is a central part of the evaluator's job. This means incorporating stakeholders and other local protagonists in all steps of evaluation studies, and the same applies when dealing with environment contingencies (Weiss, 1999; Mark & Henry, 2004). Explicitly inspired by Patton (1997, 1988), guidelines produced by the Centers for Diseases Control (CDC, 1999), and already adopted in Community Health Programs (Baker, Davis, Gallerani, Sanchez, & Viadro, 2000; CBPH, 2000), indicate how to manage what are considered the five critical elements for utility in health program evaluations: design, preparation, feedback, follow-up, and dissemination. In the design phase, one should already be organized to achieve intended uses by primary users, "who are in a position to do or decide something regarding the program" (CDC, 1999, p. 7). In the preparation phase, the objective is to rehearse or simulate uses of evaluation, discussing how potential findings or hypothetical results might affect program improvement (positive and negative implications). As for the evaluation progresses, feedback is supposed to create an atmosphere of trust, encouraging stakeholders to participate routinely in the sharing of provisional interpretations of findings and draft reports. An active follow-up to support users, after the final evaluation's report, attempts to prevent misuses or overlooking the lessons learned. Finally, dissemination is defined as "the process of communicating either the procedures or the lessons learned . . . to a relevant audience in a timely, unbiased and consistent fashion" (CDC, 1999, p. 24). Evaluation standard criteria checklists are available for each of these steps, facilitating an (auto) meta-evaluation audit directed to increase potential utility.

Although evaluators' adherence to CDC criteria can minimize some of the obstacles to utilization derived from evaluation itself, evaluators face a difficult undertaking when constrained by environmental contingencies of competing processes or inhibiting conditions (Mark & Henry, 2004). Again, factors impeding changes, particularly between health researchers and policymakers, are considered by Trostle, Bronfman, and Langer (1999) as the most important barriers to overcome. These factors are: the content quality of research and policies, with emphasis on language problems (referred to as mutual intellectual disdain); actor interaction issues, like the role of foreign donors in developing countries, or from different technical backgrounds and political cultures, confronting experience and scientific information;

the communication channel process in political and organizational contexts, reinforcing narrow professional interests.

Lavis, Farrant, and Stoddart (2001) and Lavis et al., (2002), also identified institutional interest-related barriers when analyzing factors associated with using information in Canadian public health policy departments and NGOs. In this sense, Weiss (1999) notes that the institutionalization of channels and procedures to connect evaluation findings to stakeholders, despite conscientious efforts by some nations, is often absent or fails to function well. It seems that nobody has "strong incentives to maintain them (the channels) and improve their functioning", laments the author (Weiss, 1999, p. 479).

To overcome such problems, the creation of networks linking researchers and practitioners has been advocated as a privileged strategy to increase the use or implementation of research evidence into health care and systems (Canadian Health Services Research Foundation – CHSRF, 2005; Fixsen, Naoom, Blase, Friedman, & Wallace, 2005; NIRN, 2005). The knowledge translation strategy of the Canadian Institute of Health Research (CIHR, 2004) supports "networks that bring stakeholders together in order to build and sustain the necessary connection and ongoing interaction among knowledge creators and knowledge users" (p. 7). It takes a position "radically different from the traditional view of 'knowledge transfer' as a unidirectional flow of knowledge from researchers to users … relied mostly on dissemination approach … not proven to be effective in encouraging the adoption and implementation of new research results" (p. 4). In their first statement, Knowledge Translation is a broad concept corresponding to "the exchange, synthesis and ethically-sound application of knowledge … to accelerate the capture of the benefits of research for Canadians through improved health, more effective services and products, and a strengthened health care system." (p. 4).

Here we must distinguish between two main network modalities. On the one hand, knowledge networks refer to a more formal category consisting of experts working together, whereas communities of practice include individuals or groups with a common interest of improving their practice or professional development. Both types of network differ from soft networks such as electronic list discussions that can integrate, as a content resource of the area, other modalities or can be mere catalyst tools or "match-making" (CHSRF, 2005). To summarize, evaluation's influence arises from multiple pathways counteracting or creating a hospitable environment, where networks attempt to address persistent problems. Low success uptake is mainly attributed to differences in world view, language and culture between the communities of researchers and policy makers.

Evaluation Use Framework

"Though the problems of translating or applying research in policy-making are legion, solutions are rare … bridges should be built between research and policy … But knowledge is often lacking about where … how, or by whom" (Trostle et al. 1999, p. 103 and p. 112).

Trostle's puzzle with regard to the challenge of building bridges between scientific and political cultures was the motivation for Latour's clamor for help (2001). For him, this is a paradoxical challenge, because whenever lay people begin to build this bridge, scientists react as if talking about science is their exclusive domain, which further deepens the abyss. The first stage to overcome this barrier must be to understand when this war in science was invented. This is what he has investigated in his science studies that emphasized local, material, and mundane sites where sciences are practiced.

Findings from those studies demonstrate that the divorce between science and politics cannot be resolved without overcoming the old philosophical opposition, strengthened by modernists, between object-subject, scientific content and context, and social and technical productions. Although these distinctions have been used for decades, they have been totally dismantled by the science studies' evidence of the multiple translations between them. Therefore, through the study of laboratory practice as part of their social studies of innovation, Callon and Latour (1986) developed the sociology of translation, that explains and eventually supports the operational transformation of political questions into technical questions, and vice-versa (Callon, 1986; Latour, 2001, p. 117).

Translation takes the position left empty by the obsolete dichotomy between the object and the subject, the external world and the mind, in the familiar dispute of internal versus external explanations in science. This is also referred to as the Actor-Network Theory, which conceives the network as a socio-technical entity emerging and increasingly stabilized in connections and associations between material and non-material elements (artifacts, humans, texts, symbols, concepts), stressing the mutual constitution and transformation of elements in the process and generation of knowledge as effects of network-building (Russel & Williams, 2002). Callon and Latour's (1986) Translation Theory presupposes that all process and research findings (potentially useful innovations) are modified by "acting" interests (human and nonhuman actors) in the process of building an actor-network by multifaceted interactions, where only the trajectory of negotiations describes the final implemented product. In contrast to the metaphor of physical diffusion of research findings, where artifacts and ideas are transported unchanged from one context to another, translation indicates that these artifacts and findings are, and must be transformed by, the actors involved in the process with a realignment, allocation, and definition of attributes or roles of actors.

It is important to justify briefly why the sociology of translation could be an appropriate approach to improve the use or influence of health promotion evaluative research, articulating its contribution with the theoretical basis of evaluation use models previously shown, in an operational framework. Three basic principles guided this choice, all of which related to the socio-technical nature of health promotion programs. (1) Akin to programs they seek to study and evaluate, health promotion evaluation projects constitute social organizations or living systems, and as such should be characterized by their objectives, components or activities (teleological, structural, and functional dimensions), but also by their life cycle (evolutionary dimension) and the dialectical relationship with the environment (contextual dimension), where the "program aims to modify some aspects of the environment - the target of change - and is in turn modified by contextual elements" (Potvin, Haddad, & Frohlich, 2001, p. 47). (2) Distinctiveness in health promotion research, making explicit efforts to reflect the core values of equity, participation, and empowerment in decisions about how the research is conducted (Lahtinen, Koskinene-Ollonqvist, Rouvinene-Wilenius, Tuominen, & Mittelmark, 2005), compels us to summon the requirement of representing and respecting these specificities. This involves contextualizing study process and results as well as lay people participation in health promotion evaluations. Those people are almost always excluded from professional networks. (3) The work of Bilodeau, Chamberland, and White (2002) demonstrates quite clearly that public health programs or health promotion actions are collaborative and multi-partner interventions, operating in open systems where different actors negotiate the structure and realization in their social relationships, in iterative and interactive ways. Understanding and operating in such systems require a theory of innovation that replaces diffusion with translation logic of action, in order to foster program implementation, quality, and effectiveness. The sociology of translation allows analyzing transformations and mutual adaptation of the actors, context, and project in the development of an innovation, conceiving the situations as networks linking participant actors and resources (Callon, 1986).

Translation therefore refers to the continuous re-interpretations operated by the actors about their roles as innovation producers in programmed action, and that can only emerge if carried out by a network. This theory contends that controversies always precede the emergence of an innovation project, because actors have different points of view (Latour, 2001). To solve the controversies, actors are oriented toward a compromise solution to cooperate, while at least partially responding to their own interests (Bilodeau et al., 2002).

In the operational analysis of translation, the core of our framework (Fig. 7.1), four moments (not necessarily following a pre-determined sequence) are distinguished in the development of networks and innovations (Bilodeau et al., 2002; Potvin, 2007; Russel & Williams, 2002; Spinuzzi, 2005). Problematization is the first step, in which a focal actor conducts a provisional definition of the problem or project, beginning to identify the interests of other relevant actors in the situation, consistent with his own, as well as the main controversies. This allows to map the social space of programs. Interestment is made of the actions deployed to convince other actors to accept their roles in the alliance to reach a common objective with the obligatory passage by the focal actor or main translator. An interpretative flexibility is requested with the attribution by the groups of different meanings to an artifact, according to their backgrounds, purposes, and commitments. Enrollment is the process of network-building in which the actors' support is obtained for the development of a socio-technical entity. It is a successful interestment of other actors in order to strengthen the network in the pursuit of a common objective. Finally, mobilization is the set of methods or negotiations to ensure that spokespersons from relevant communities or collectives have the legitimacy to lead actions and displace the network.

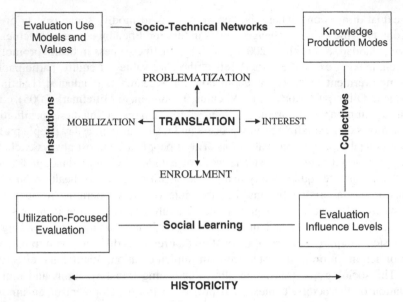

Fig. 7.1 Integrated framework for evaluation use studies

In program evaluation, these moments form a social learning process in which researchers, implementers, and users learn from experience and interactions. Learning cannot be framed only in individual and cognitive terms. Framed as social and political institutional transformations it involves the combined action of understanding, analyzing, and giving new meaning to routines (Russel & Williams, 2002). A few principles and conceptual complements of scientific studies and the translation theory, in the paragraphs below, appear as essential for a better understanding of the other framework's elements, links or bridges in their mutual and continuous dynamics.

In common usage, institution refers to a site and laws, people, and customs that are continuous in time. In traditional sociology, institutionalized is used as a critique of the poor quality of overly routine science. Here, the meaning is positive, considering institutions as providers of the necessary mediations for maintaining actors. The word actant is often used to evoke the inclusion of nonhumans in the actor's definition, frequently restricted to humans, while the term collective refers to the associations of humans and nonhumans. This representation of reality surpasses the usual division between subject and object, society and nature that renders invisible the political process by which the cosmos is one living whole. In the history of science, these terms refer to a largely obsolete dispute between those who claim to be more interested in the content of science and those who focus on its social context (internal and external explanations of validity).

Finally, Latours's glossary reiterates that 'translation', in its linguistic and material connotations, refers to displacements of actors whose mediation is indispensable for any action to occur. Instead of a rigid opposition between context and content, chains of translations refer to the work through which actors modify, displace, and translate their various and often contradictory interests. The term mediation, in contrast with intermediary, which is fully defined by its input and output, always exceeds its predictable conditions. This makes a sound difference between those who recognize in the entanglements of practice mere intermediaries and those who recognize mediations as real actors or 'events'. Later on, it replaces the discovery notion and can be defined as any experiment or action having consequences for the historicity of all elements of the network meaning, not merely the passage of time, but the fact that something has been transformed, in a continuous space and time network.

Returning to the Fig. 7.1, we can see that the four blocks or pillars, reviewed in the Chapter's first section, are integrated in the framework as a changing assemblage of technical and social components (expertise, tools, interest groups, people and their values). They interact and shape each other in a dynamic ensemble of the collective, building socio-technical networks of institutionalized practices in the creation and production of new events (innovations). They keep continually being translated in their implementation and use, leading political commitments and technical objectives into scientific knowledge (Russel & Williams, 2002).

If we now explore the similarities and possibilities of health promotion appropriation in the whole framework, we may begin with Rootman, Goodstadt, Potvin, & Springett, (2001), in their work on the use of knowledge from health promotion evaluations. For these authors, all three models proposed in Weiss' typology (2005), and discussed previously, are implicit in the first block of Fig. 7.1 and are seen as legitimate. These authors also recall that addressing theoretical assumptions embedded in programs (as it was done here with translation theory) can have more influence on policy and public opinion ("nothing is as practical as a good theory"–p. 21). It is also possible to apply the levels and mechanisms of evaluation's influence (Henry & Mark, 2003; Mark & Henry, 2004), and even amend them, by focusing choice and key concepts from health promotion theories and models for change (Bryant, 2002; HPA, 2005).

Health promotion evaluators could improve their work process by adapting lessons learned from a utilization-focused evaluation perspective, in community interventions, being aware that each step affects the potential usefulness of tools and results (CBPH 2000; De Leeuw & Skovgaard, 2005; Raphael, 2000). Gardner (2003) highlights the importance of a shared understanding by the evaluator(s) and potential users of epistemological foundations, shaping science production and the relationship between the roles of evaluators and stakeholders. From this perspective, utilization-focused evaluation, also means a "user-friendly evaluation approach". In short, it is supposed that translation operations must be recognized as an integral part of health promotion interventions and evaluations, equally driving the evaluation capacity and institutional innovations.

Shifting the attention from the theoretical perspectives of the framework to evaluators' practice, the challenge to translate research to decision, and vice-versa, rises one question at once: How to teach/learn translation skills? In an attempt to give some clues to answer this question, Box 1 gives an example of the evaluation capacity-building process focusing on evaluation's usefulness or influence in socio-technical networks of AIDS prevention and control programs. It is also an opportunity to observe that some aspects of translation that could seem disconnected, at first, prove to be intertwined in this training project. Freire's problematization approach, described therein, joins translation as a complementary tool (Freire, 1967). This experience fills also a frequent omission in evaluation capacity projects, because "training often focuses on the scientific and technical aspects of conducting research, rather than how to develop and influence health public policy and practice" (Rychetnik & Wise, 2004, p. 253).

Box 1 Evaluation capacity-building and sociotechnical networks: A practical example of the Brazilian national aids program The Brazilian National Aids Program is situated under the Ministry of Health, and in 2002 its National Coordinating Office called for the development of a National Evaluation Plan with a strong commitment to institutionalize evaluation at all levels of the Program. Therefore, in 2003 a monitoring & evaluation (M&E) unit was created with technical and financial cooperation from the Centers for Disease Control (CDC), a partnership to foster training of the necessary human resources, including the Program, the National School of Public Health and the Tulane University School of Public Health, in the scope of the Evaluation Plan (Ministerio da Saude, 2004; Santos, 2005). The initiative was tailored according to specific needs of the program, and at least two major premises supporting this experience appear completely in keeping with our framework: the proposed pedagogical approach and the socio-network of internal evaluators as an interface for technology transfer.

Proposed Pedagogical Approach

The pedagogical approach was based on Freire's concept of problematization to empower students with their own experiences, developing an understanding of new concepts. The three stages of Freire's approach were developed through five key processes described in Freire's approach: 1) experiential connections with a problem, (generative contents), in this case evaluation and ethical issues related to the provision of public health services; 2) systematizing these experiences through adult learning techniques, such as role-playing and small group work; 3) locating experiences within a theoretical framework; 4) discussion of possible alternatives and options for solving problems and improving reality; and 5) application of this process to the original reality.

Freire's theory, despite the fact that he denied having developed a theory, encompasses three stages: investigative, thematization, and problematization (Freire, 1967). The first – investigative – is a period of disturbance, lively discussion and discovery. Small group discussions and challenging situations pose to the participants' generative contents, which are chosen for cognitive value and social meaning. Generative contents work as a key to build a topic, in convergence/divergence to the participant's own thoughts an values. Freire's second stage is thematization, when the generative contents are highlighted, codified and decodified, taking into account the participant's experience and the available theory (giving a meaning and revising this meaning). The last stage – problematization –, which for Freire is a process of appropriation of your own thoughts, reflection and values, and contrasting them with reality for concrete action (Gadotti, 1994). According to the author, problematization is not a mere utilization of newly acquired knowledge, but a conscious effort to transform reality for social betterment. Problematization, Freire says, is "hominization", that is, a process of becoming a new man, directly linked to the ability to mobilize knowledge not only for technical responses, but for social betterment above of all. In Freire's words, "the starting point for organizing the program content of educational or political action must be the present, existential, concrete, reflecting aspirations of the people. Utilizing certain basic contradictions, we must pose this existential, concrete, present situation to the people as a problem which challenges them and requires a response –not just at the intellectual level, but at the level of action" (Freire, 1987 p. 85).

Therefore, problematization goes beyond problem-posing, since conception encompasses not only an instrumental response, but also a reflexive and interactive response necessarily committed to social change. This approach engages professionals in a dialogue with experts (there are no teachers and students) as learning subjects (sujeitos aprendentes), encouraging both to draw on their existing experience and synthesize this experience into a new understanding of the problem and solutions that could be put into action (praxis). The center of the educational process is shifted from contents for creative mobilization to sympathetic interaction. That is, the mechanical sharing of a fixed reality is replaced by an ever-accelerating coming to be. This approach relies heavily on small group activities, internalization of key issues through constant dialogue, and an inductive process of learning, drawing on prior experience, relearning, and synthesis. However, some issues arose regarding the development of the course methodology. One was the extent to which the methodology could or should be delivered in a pure form, that is, excluding traditional, didactic, expert-driven presentations. These issues arose for several reasons: 1) some instructors were unable to adapt to the methodology; 2) students requested some didactic presentations; and 3) some materials lend themselves to didactic approaches (e.g., sampling methodology, presentation of existing instruments, etc.).

The resolution of a controversy among the curriculum committee members was an agreement to disagree: The course coordinators moved forward with a mixed methodology that used both problematization and a more didactic or traditional approach. Thus, the curriculum development committee continued development of course modules with the understanding that the methodology would be delivered in a mixed form. The committee members maintained their commitment to the course and its completion, and continued to work as a collegiate group to carry out this process (CDC, 2005).

The Network of Internal Evaluators as an Interface for Technology Transfer

The Network for Monitoring and Evaluation (ReM&A – Rede de Monitoramento e Avaliação) is a subcomponent of the capacity-building in evaluation. The network's main objective is to contribute to the institutionalization of the M&E in the Brazilian STD/Aids Program through a virtual forum that encourages an integrated and multidisciplinary practice of M&E, addressing program implementation and improvement (UNAIDS, 2000). Their specific objectives are to disseminate and strengthen the evaluation culture in the Program; to share experiences and best practices ; to create and spread a database of M&E consultants; to encourage meta-evaluation practices; to support evaluation teaching; and to develop M&E actions in the different areas of the Program.

Implementation of ReM&A began in 2005, although its planning and negotiation started nearly a year earlier. The network's creation has been a process of discussion among several actors and involving interests of the program staff, national and international donors to the program, and other areas. Students saw the network as a way to continue the learning process and continue to engage in exchanges as a community. Those who came from the areas of the country with few resources saw the network as a critical tool for responding to training needs. Sharing experiences with countries having different levels of responses to the epidemic has been a good experience for the Brazilian Program. This is relevant not only in terms of capacity-building or for making M&E a sustainable activity, but also to legitimate the Brazilian M&E response and the participant's professional identity.

The network has two levels of access. The first is open to every professional interested in M&E and to specialists working in the M&E field. Its primary challenge is to facilitate circulation of technologies and knowledge for the benefit of context. Technology and knowledge circulate without being accompanied by everything they owe to the social space within they were generated. Thus, a false perception of participation may emerge, denying cultural disjuncture or improving gaps between historical, economic, and cultural differences (Bourdieu, 1997), especially considering the technological gap among different social groups, particularly in Brazil. Moreover, one should account for the instability of evaluation as a field of knowledge and practice, and the necessity of a strong polemical level to prevent the network's active moderators from dictating what should be done or discussed (Latour, 1991, 1997). The second level concerns eventual arrangements aimed at solving specific problems in the Program. This second level refers to a community of practices directly oriented toward the resolution of focused questions related to the Program's priorities. It is strictly related to utilization and mobilization of available knowledge and technology to obtain better solutions to M&E problems in the Program. In terms of the local level, it is necessary to put M&E into practice in daily work and everyday life (Edmundo, Guimarães, Vasconcelos, Baptista, & Becker, 2005). In addition, the network aims to provide an environment to analyze and negotiate (translate) the incorporation of new technologies.

Negotiations (translation) to start ReM&A lead to a consensus that the issue capable of stimulating the initial interactions (enrollment) is the development of an evaluation proposal. This specific issue would problematize very practical and theoretical questions in M&E. The active moderators have to provide challenges and space for consequential debates (translation) for each step in the development of the proposal, such as evaluability (evaluation needs assessment, the evaluation question, evaluation approach, and design); implementation of the evaluation process; dissemination of the evaluation results; and meta-evaluation, including the influence of the evaluation processes. Considering the complexity of the Brazilian AIDS epidemic, actions involve a wide range of dimensions and components. This provides the network an enormous amount of issues, such as M&E of health promotion and protection, of information and communication, of epidemiological surveillance systems, of human rights and society's response, and so on. Therefore, the priority of this network is to support the National Program in these several possible subjects for M&E in an articulated exercise of reflection and practice, capable of obtaining an integrated flow of mobilized knowledge.

Concluding Remarks

If the importance of research influence in health policy and key utilization issues has been described for at least 20 years, this chapter is consistent with the general picture of under-utilization recognized by Hanney, Gonzalez-Block, Buxton, and Kogan, (2003) or Almeida and Bascolo (2006). Notwithstanding, we must highlight, or reiterate at least, three promising opportunities for more influential evaluations of health actions that seem good examples for the promotion field.

First, the Brazilian politics for institutionalizing evaluative practices in AIDS program, with the support of the evaluation capacity-building project (Box 1), is being expanded into the national strategy of family health, involving a formal partnership between universities and state secretariats in the evaluation of primary health care, including health promotion actions. In this sense, it is important to underline that institutionalizing evaluation and/or the increment of evaluation capacity are referred by all consulted authors as factors that can improve the evaluation's use and, per se, be an inductive mechanism in relevant outcomes for social betterment (Mark & Henry, 2004).

Second, the previously mentioned networks for health innovation, launched by the Canadian Institutes of Health Research (CIHR, 2004), whose characteristics include co-governance by users and researchers, constitute a good model for communities of practice. This kind of initiative is recognized by Borowski et al. (2005) as being potentially able to bridge the gap between researchers and policymakers that has arisen from the "producer-push and user-pull modes" of knowledge transfer (p. 9). Even if the main currency of change remains the classical research influence, it is much more flexible and democratic, in a shared improvement of researchers and practitioners, than the evidence-based models defended by the National Implementation Research Network (NIRN, 2005).

Third, the notion of translation, an integrative concept based on a multidirectional understanding of research and medical practice, in a back-and-forth movement, has been incorporated by scientific and clinical networks supported by medical and scientific societies, and also by healthcare and academic institutions, particularly in North America (Sontag, 2005). It is also a good example of a partnership strategy developed to improve research utilization, based on the need for multi-level analysis involving ethical, technological, political, and social issues, in a feedback loop to provide crucial information for improving human health.

Despite these positive signs, in a simulation of the evaluation's influence published by Christie (2007) recently, the author states that "if evaluation utilization is arguably the most widely researched area, receiving substantial attention in their theoretical basis, the empirical literature on evaluation's influence is sparse and there is only limited research that disaggregates the influence of evaluation on programs, policies, and participant improvement" (p. 9). Once more, it is necessary to invoke Latour (2001), with his metaphor of a circulatory system of scientific facts, to understand how to improve socio-technical events that can promote the evaluation's influence at the public level. He recognizes that it is impossible to provide a general description of all heterogeneous and surprising loops and ties that keep scientific events alive in the circulatory system. The chain of translations is the conceptual and operational hard core of the framework. Only such a network is capable, by its knots and ties of well-articulated propositions, to maintain an adequate flow between the vital circuits of the circulatory system of scientific facts or innovations.

These propositions do not mean statements of truth or falsehood, but a good articulation between what is said and the common world of the different realities progressively unified in the translation process, reminding us that scientific and political contexts are indissoluble. In the socio-technical perspective, the evaluation's usefulness becomes inherent to the translation process. The circulating or internal reference produced with objective actors' displacements qualifies the chain of transformations in such a way that when problems or controversies enter the scene, improving its descriptive capacity, the result is already a better and broader understanding for programs of action and minimization of anti-program reactions. It is thus indispensable to invest much more time learning to actively follow up this circulatory system's historicity, overcoming its immediate and intrinsic usefulness to indicate its influence on the social betterment objectives of health promotion actions.

Finally, we give two recommendations for vigilance concerning the possible risks associated with a kind of utility-driven evaluation that can jeopardize the efforts to defend investments for investigating its influence. The first is from Scriven (2005), advising that we should not forget that the evaluation impact may occur years after its submission, often after being rejected when submitted and, most important, if a valuable outcome is an effect of the evaluation, it cannot compensate for low validity or external credibility, since it is not a primary criterion for merit. The second refers to the demand for cost-effectiveness estimates as part of the evaluation influence analysis, especially in developing countries (World Bank, 2004), which can be understood as a dangerous persuasion tool caused by a prescriptive reading of utilization-focused evaluation. If the use is to be the central outcome of any evaluation, because without it the evaluation cannot contribute to social betterment (Christie, 2007 p. 8), it can become a Holy Grail merely if we forget that evaluation, as social practice itself, needs to define first an appropriate common specification of the social betterment to which health-related or other social interventions are supposed to contribute (Henry, 2000).

References

Almeida, C., & Bascolo, E. (2006). Use of research results in policy decision-making: A review of the literature. *Cadernos de Saude Publica, 22*, S7–S33.

Baker, Q. E., Davis, D. A., Gallerani, R., Sanchez, V., & Viadro, C. (2000). *An evaluation framework of community health programs*. Durham NC: The Center for Advancement of Community Based Public Health. Downloaded in November 2007 from: www.cdc.gov/eval/evalcbph.pdf

Berghmans, L., & Potvin, L. (2005). Health promotion and local and regional actors: Lessons from the conference. *Promotion & Education, Supplement 3*, 71–74.

Bilodeau, A., Chamberland, C. & White, D. (2002). L'innovation sociale, une condition pour accroître la qualité de l'action en partenariat dans le champ de la santé publique. *Revue Canadienne d'évaluation de Programme*, 17, 59–88.

Borowski, H., Hanney, S., Lindquist, E., & Roger, R. (2005). *Bridging the gap: The use of research evidence in policy development*. Edmonton: Health Technology Assessment, Alberta Heritage Foundation for Medical Research. Downloaded in November 2007 from: www2.eastwestcenter.org/research/popcomm/pdf/2_Selected_Readings/Use%20of%20 Research%20in%20Policy.pdf

Bourdieu, P. (1997). For a sociogenetic understanding of intellectual works. In C. Calhoun, E. LiPuma, & M. Postone (Eds.), *Bourdieu: Critical perspectives* (pp. 264–275). Chicago: The Chicago University Press.

Bryant, T. (2002) Role of knowledge in public health and health promotion policy change. *Health Promotion International*, 17, 89–98.

Callon, M. (1986) Éléments pour une sociologie de la traduction. La domestication des coquilles de St-Jacques. *L'année sociologique, 36*, 169–208.

Callon, M., & Latour, B. (1986). Les paradoxes de la modernité. Comment concevoir les innovations? Clés pour l'analyse sociotechnique. *Prospective et santé, 36*(hiver), 13–29.
Canadian Health Services Research Foundation. (CHSRF, 2005). A spotlight on networks. *Links,
8*(1), 9.
Canadian Institutes of Health Research. (CIHR, 2004). Innovation in action: Knowledge translation
strategies 2004–2009. Downloaded in November 2007 from: www.cihr-irsc.gc.ca/e/26574.htlm
Caracelli, V. J. (2000). Evaluation use at the threshold of the twenty-first century. *New Directions
for Evaluation, 88*, 99–112.
Community Based Public Health (CBPH, 2000). An evaluation framework of community health
programs. Downloaded in November 2005 from www.cbph.org
Centers for Diseases Control. (CDC, 1999). Framework for program evaluation in public health.
Mortality and Morbidity Weekly Report, 48(RR-11), 1–40.
Center for Diseases Control (CDC, 2005). Annual report global aids program – CDC: reporting
period: September 2003 – Octobrt 2004. Brady W; Westman S; Moore J (Org). Brasília DF:
CDC/GAP.
Champagne, F., Contandriopoulos, A. -P., & Tanon, A. (2004). A program-evaluation perspective
on processes, practices, and decision-makers. In L. Lemieux-Charles, & F. Champagne (Eds.),
Using knowledge and evidence in health care: Multidisciplinary perspectives (pp. 139–171).
Toronto: University of Toronto Press.
Christie, A. C. (2007). Reported influence of evaluation data on decision-makers' actions: An
empirical examination. *The American Journal of Evaluation, 28*, 8–25.
De Leeuw, E., & Skovgaard, T. (2005). Utility-driven evidence for healthy cities: Problems with
evidence generation and application. *Social Science & Medicine, 61*, 1331–1341.
Denis, J. -L., Lehoux, P., & Champagne, F. (2004). A knowledge-utilization perspective
on fine-tuning dissemination and contextualizing knowledge. In L. Lemieux-Charles, &
F. Champagne (Eds.), *Using knowledge and evidence in health care: Multidisciplinary perspectives* (pp. 11–41). Toronto: University of Toronto Press.
Edmundo, K., Guimarães, W., Vasconcelos, M. S., Baptista, A. P., & Becker, D. (2005). Network
of communities in fight against AIDS: Local action to address health inequities and promote
health in Rio de Janeiro, Brazil. *Promotion & Education Supplement*, 3, 15–19.
Elias, F. T. S., & Patroclo, M. A. A. (2005). Research use: How to build a theoretical model of
evaluation? *Ciência & Saude Coletiva*, 10, 215–227.
Fixsen, D. L., Naoom, S. F., Blase K. A., Friedman, R. M., & Wallace, F. (2005). *Implementation
research: A synthesis of the literature*. Tampa, FL: University of South Florida, Louis de la
Parte Florida Mental Health Institute, The National Implementation Research Network (FMHI
Publication #231).
Freire, P. (1967). *Educação como prática de liberdade* Rio de Janeiro: Jorge Zahar.
Freire, P. (1987) *Pedagogy of the oppressed*. New York: Continuum Publishing Corporation.
Gadotti M. (1994) *Reading Paulo Freire: His Life and Work*, Albany: Sunny Press.
Gardner, F. (2003). User friendly evaluation in community-based projects. *The Canadian Journal
of Program Evaluation, 18*, 71–89.
Gibbons, M., Limoges C, Nowotny, H. Schwartzman, S., Scott, P., & Trow, M. (1994). Intro-
duction. In M. Gibbons, C. Limoges, H. Nowotny, S. Schwartzman, & P. Scott (Eds.), *The
new production of knowledge: The dynamics of science and research in contemporary society*
(pp. 1–16). London: Sage.
Hanney, S. R., Gonzalez-Block, M., Buxton, M. J., & Kogan, M. (2003). The utilisation of health
research in policy-making: concepts, examples and methods of assessment. *Health Research
Policy and System, 1*, 2.
Health Promotion Agency. (HPA, 2005). Health Promotion theories and models. Downloaded in November 2007 from: www.healthpromotionagency.org.uk/Healthpromotion/Health/
section5.htm
Henry, G. T. (2000). Why not use? *New Directions in Evaluation, 88*, 85–98.
Henry, G. T. & Mark, M. M. (2003). Beyond use: Understanding evaluation's influence on attitudes
and actions. *The American Journal of Evaluation, 24*, 293–314.

Kirkhart, K. E. (2000). Reconceptualizing evaluation use: An integrated theory of influence. *New Directions for Evaluation, 88*, 5–23.

Lahtinen, E., Koskinene-Ollonqvist, P., Rouvinene-Wilenius, P., Tuominen, P., & Mittelmark, M. B. (2005) The development of quality criteria for research: A Finnish approach. *Health Promotion International, 20*, 306–315.

Latour, B. (1991). Technology is society made durable. In J. Law (Ed.), *A Sociology of monsters. Essays on power, technology and domination* (pp. 103–131). London: Routledge.

Latour, B. (1997) On actor-network theory: A few clarifications. Downloaded in November 2007 from: www.nettime.org/Lists-Archives/nettime-l-9801/msg00019.html

Latour, B. (2001). *A esperança de pandora*. São Paulo: Edusc.

Lavis, J. N., Farrant, M. S. R., & Stoddart, G. L. (2001). Barriers to employment-related healthy public policy in Canada. *Health Promotion International, 16*, 9–19.

Lavis, J. N., Ross, S. E., Hurley, J. E., Hohenadel, J. M., Stoddart G. L., Woodward, C. A., & Abelson, J. (2002) Examining the role of health services research in public policymaking. *Milbank Quarterly, 80*, 125–154.

Lehoux, P., Battista, R. N., & Lance, J-M. (2000). Monitoring health technology assessment agencies. *Canadian Journal of Program Evaluation, 15*, 1–33.

Mark, M. M., & Henr, G. T. (2004). The mechanisms and outcomes of evaluation influence. *Evaluation, 10*, 35–57.

Ministerio da Saude (2004). *Programa Nacional de DST e Aids. Monitor Aids.* Brasilia: Centers for Disease Control and Prevention.

Nowotny, H., Scott, P., & Gibbons, M. (2001). *Re-thinking science: Knowledge and the publica in an age of uncertainty.* Cambridge: Polity press

Patton, M. Q. (1997) *Utilization-focused evaluation: The new century text.* (3 ed.) California: Sage.

Patton, M. Q. (1988). The evaluator responsibility for utilizationé. *Evaluation Practice, 9*, 5–24.

Potvin, L. (2007). Managing uncertainty through participation. In D. V. McQueen, I. Kickbusch, L. Potvin, J. M Pelikan, L. Balbo, & T. Abel (Eds.), *Health & modernity. The role of theory in health promotion* (pp. 103–128). New York: Springer.

Potvin, L., Gendron, S., & Bilodeau, A. (2006). Três Posturas Ontológicas Concernentes à Natureza dos Programas de saúde: implicações para a avaliação. In M. Bosi, & F. J. Mercado (Eds.), *Avaliação qualitativa de programas de saúde. Enfoques emergentes* (pp.65–86). Sao Paulo: Editora Vozes.

Potvin, L., Haddad, S., & Frohlich, K. L. (2001). Beyond process and outcome evaluation: a comprehensive approach for evaluating health promotion programmes. In I. Rootman, M. Goodstadt, B. Hyndman, D. V. McQueen, L. Potvin, & J. Springett (Eds.), *Evaluation in health promotion. Principles and perspectives* (pp. 45–62). WHO Regional Publications, European Series no. 92.

Preskill, H., & Torres, R. T. (2000). The learning dimensions of evaluation use. *New Directions for Evaluation, 88*, 25–38

Raphael, D. (2000). The question of evidence in health promotion. *Health Promotion International, 15*, 355–367.

Rootman, I., Goodstadt, M., Potvin, L., & Springett, J. (2001). A framework for Health Promotion Evaluation. In I. Rootman, M. Goodstadt, B. Hyndman, D. V. McQueen, L. Potvin, & J. Springett (Eds.), *Evaluation in health promotion. Principles and perspectives* (pp. 7–38). WHO Regional Publications, European Series no 92.

Rossman, G. B., & Rallis, S. F. (2000). Critical inquiry and use as action. *New Directions for Evaluation, 88*, 55–69.

Russel, S., & Williams, R. (2002). Social shaping of technology: frameworks. Findings and implications for policy with glossary of social shaping concepts . In K. Serensen & R. Williams (Eds.), *Shaping technology, guiding policy: Concepts, spaces & tools* (pp. 37–131). Cheltenham: Edward Elgar Publishing Limited.

Rychetnik, L., & Wise, M. (2004). Advocating evidence-based health promotion: reflections and a way forward. *Health Promotion International, 19*, 247–257.

Santos, E. M. (2005) Plano Nacional de Monitoramento e Avaliação Downloaded in December 2007 from: http://www.aids.gov.br/data/documents/storedDocuments/%7BB8EF5DAF-23AE -4891-AD36-1903553A3174%7D/%7B4CA2F147-2C19-4C45-B964-3C0C441835EA%7D/ PNM&A_site%20.pdf

Schwandt, T. A. (2005). The centrality of practice in evaluation. *The American Journal of Evaluation, 26*, 95–105.

Scriven, M. (2005). *Key evaluation checklist.* Downloaded in November 2007 from: www.wmich.edu/evalctr/checklists/kec.pdf

Sontag, K. -C. (2005). Implementation of translational medicine. *Journal of Translational Medicine, 3*, 1–5.

Spinuzzi, C. (2005). Reading roundup: Callon on translation. Downloaded in December 2007 from www.spinuzzi.blogspot.com/2005_05_22_archive.html

Sridharan, S. (2003). Introduction to special section on "What is a useful evaluation". *The American Journal of Evaluation, 24*, 483–487.

The National Implementation Research Network) (NIRN, 2005). Implementation Research: a synthesis of the literature. Downloaded in December 2007from: http://nirn.fmhi.usf.edu/ resources/publications/monograph

Trostle, J., Bronfman, M., & Langer, A. (1999). How does research influence decision-makers? *Health Policy and Planning, 14*, 103–114.

UNAIDS (2000). *Putting knowledge to work: Technical resource networks for effective responses to HIV/AIDS.* Downloaded in November 2007 from: http://data.unaids.org/Publications/ IRC-pub05/JC483-PuttingKnowledge_en.pdf

Weiss, C. H. (1988). Evaluation for decision : is anybody there ? Does anybody care? *Evaluation Practice, 9*, 5–19.

Weiss, C. H. (1999). The interface between evaluation and public policy. *Evaluation, 5*, 468–486.

Weiss, C. H., Murphy-Graham, E., & Birkeland, S. (2005). An alternate route to policy influence. How evaluation affects DARE. *The American Journal of evaluation, 26*, 12–30.

World Bank. (2004). *Influential evaluations. Evaluations that improved performance and impacts of development programs.* Washington DC: The World Bank

Part III
Aligning Evaluation with Health Promotion Principles: Experiences from the Americas

Chapter 8
Figurative Thinking and Models: Tools for Participatory Evaluation

Denis Allard, Angèle Bilodeau, and Sylvie Gendron

In sociological terms, an evaluation can be considered as a collective decision to step back, take a second look, and formulate a judgement on a public program. This collective decision is usually borne by a limited number of actors who elaborate their thinking with the advice and support of an evaluator. In the past two decades, major developments in the field of evaluation have emerged through the practice of "participatory evaluation." This approach requires an expansion of the number of actors beyond the initial proponents and the evaluator so as to expand as much as possible the scope of the reflection. A public program involves many actors, all of whom have interests at stake, some of which are liable to be divergent. When judgements are made without somehow including the diverse stakeholders or their spokespersons, issues concerning the results and their utilization are more likely to surface (Weiss, 1983a). Over the years, evaluators have become increasingly aware of the relevance of being inclusive. Hence the proliferation of participatory forms of evaluation to account, to various degrees, for stakeholders' concerns (Weiss, 1983b; Monnier, 1992), grant them control over the evaluation process (Chinman, Imm, & Wandersman, 2004; Fetterman, 2001), and enable them to transcend their respective positions and work together to elaborate descriptions, judgements and future directions (Abma, 2006; Guba & Lincoln, 1989; Niemi & Kemmis, 1999; Van der Meer & Edelenbos, 2006).

The process of developing shared knowledge poses a number of methodological challenges for the evaluator. Partners must work together to create new knowledge (Ryan, 2004; Ryan & De Stefano, 2001), and they must be able to monitor progress along the way. The work is usually conducted within a limited timeframe during which a vast amount of information must be managed and competing ideas reconciled as much as possible. Moreover, evaluators and partners must make a concerted effort to synthesize all viewpoints into a collective endeavour. In our experience, the discursive toolbox for written, linear accounts, albeit necessary, benefits from the addition of an inclusive toolbox of figurative images that includes metaphors, schemas and matrices. These are simple to present, discuss, modify and use as touchstones as the evaluation process unfolds. Indeed, figurative thinking can do

D. Allard
Université de Montréal, Montreal, QC, Canada

L. Potvin, D. McQueen (eds.), *Health Promotion Evaluation Practices in the Americas*,
DOI: 10.1007/978-0-387-79733-5_8, © Springer Science+Business Media, LLC 2008   123

more than just illustrate a waypoint in the discussions. Models can be at the forefront of the evaluation when they are used as tools for collective reflection.

Based on our field experience with figurative thinking, we propose a working hypothesis for the integration of analogies, schemas, models, and matrices as essential tools for participatory evaluation. The modelling process is core to this proposition. In the first section, we formulate and refine our proposition. The second section presents a detailed illustration of the use of figurative tools at various stages in the work process of a steering committee for a participatory evaluation project. In the third section, we discuss the development of figurative thinking and modelling to further contribute to participatory forms of evaluation.

Integrating Figurative Thinking Tools

To cite Morin (1986), human thinking is dialogical. It opposes and combines analysis and synthesis, or digital and analogical ways of thinking. The digital mode separates what is connected whereas the analogical mode connects what is separated (Morin, 2001). The first reduces reality into categories; the second relates images across realities. In the social sciences, thinking is expressed mainly as linear discourse. Even analogies, which are primarily based on images, are used most often in their written or spoken forms. Occasionally, images may be introduced as complements to the text, or they may serve to synthesize, summarize or illustrate the text. In any case, the discursive mode remains dominant. However, the inverse situation is equally possible; the discourse becomes the outcome or complement of the figurative language (Radnofsky, 1996) to express thoughts under construction. Exchanging ideas in teamwork situations and via the Internet often employs figurative modes of expression whereas thinking is often initiated and developed through images and graphs. Figurative representation is therefore an appropriate choice for the collective construction process because it expresses concepts in a more compact, readily shared form. However, figurative approaches and techniques have not yet been well defined, particularly in the field of program evaluation, and there is a need to develop a methodological landscape of figurative thinking tools.

Based on a review of our evaluation work (Allard & Adrien, 2007; Allard & Ferron, 2000; Allard, Audet, St-Laurent, & Chevalier, 2003; Allard, Kimpton, Papineau, & Audet, 2006; Allard & Adrien, 2007; Bilodeau, Allard, & Chamberland, 1998), we propose an integration of basic figurative thinking tools (Fig. 8.1). First, this thinking can be expressed with two main tools: the schema and the matrix. Walliser (1977) agrees when he says that the graph and the matrix are the primary elements in the modelling syntax. The schema provides a spatial framework where images and concepts are connected, generally with arrows, according to certain organizing principles such as time, hierarchy levels and interaction modalities. The matrix is a table that facilitates the intersection of concepts, essentially via their dimensions (D1, D2) and attributes (A1, A2, A3). The resulting matrix cells refer to the specific content of the associations or, more synthetically, new categories

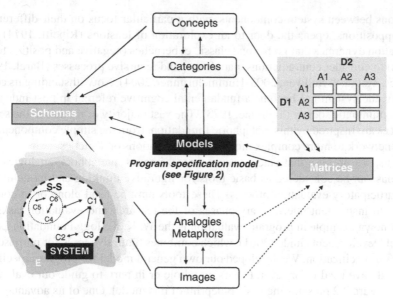

Fig. 8.1 Working hypothesis for the integration of figurative thinking components

(Barton, 1965). The matrix is often used to complement the schema because it helps to develop the meanings of the arrows and allows new relations between concepts and categories to be explored.

At a first level, these two main figure types are based on concepts and images. At a second level, the concepts are transformed into categories (Juan, 1999; Mark, Henry, & Julnes, 2000) and images into analogies. The analogy is a form of metaphor (Ascher, 2005; De Coster, 1978) where the use of one object to represent another goes beyond general characterization (e.g., likening a public program to a journey) to feature specific parallelisms (e.g., the program is a journey that must be prepared, provided with a clear plan, and adjusted when unexpected events occur). An analogy may also be isomorphic when it is used to conceptualize different realities along similar terms. General System Theory is an example of isomorphic thinking (Bertalanffy, 1968; Le Moigne, 1977). It was developed to account for concrete systems – from the cell to society – using a transtheoretical model. This isomorphic image of a system is represented summarily in Fig. 8.1. Basically, it is a set of relations (arrows) between components (C). These relations form structures (C1-C2-C3) that are contained within a frontier (dotted line) that identifies the system. In open systems, exchanges with the environment (E) are necessary. Within the system, an assemblage of specific, marked-off relations (C4-C5-C6) may be considered a subsystem (S-S). Thus, a system may be conceived as part of a nested hierarchy of systems, and transformation over time (T) may be defined as system genesis.

This brief outline is based on first-generation systems theory. Recent research on systems theory has introduced more complexity (Lapierre, 1992). The analysis of relations between system components, with a particular focus on their differences and oppositions, opens the door to an exploration of tensions (Ribeill, 1974) and regulation dynamics that go beyond classic cybernetics (negative and positive feedbacks) to consider contradictions, paradoxes, and recursive processes (Barel, 1989; Barnes, Matka, & Sullivan, 2003, Hummelbrunner, 2004). Notwithstanding its complexity, the system has become a fundamental cognitive referent in post-industrial or programmatic society (Touraine, 1973). The vast majority of models in the social sciences are inspired by this metaphoric foundation, from the simple components or ideas network to more complex models of organizations or societies.

Thus, we propose that categories, matrices, images, metaphors, analogies and schemas can be considered as basic tools for figurative thinking and modelling in the participatory evaluation process. These tools may be used alone or in combination to instrument intermediary phases of the research and evaluation tasks. A well-known example in program evaluation is the W. K. Kellogg Foundation Logic Model Development Guide (2001), which combines figurative tools for purposes of program specification. We developed our own general model for program specification and have used it for several years, in whole or in part, to guide our evaluation work. Figure 8.2 presents the basic blueprint of this model. One of its advantages is that various aspects of program theory, as described in the evaluation literature, are clearly differentiated in this model.

The first distinction is derived from Chambers, Wedel, & Rodwell (1992), who marks the difference between problem theory and program theory. In the field of public health, we usually define our problem theory in terms of the underlying determinants of health. A schema can represent this theory very well. The transition

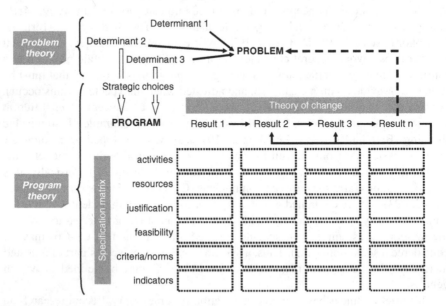

Fig. 8.2 General model for program specification

from a problem theory to a program theory is done by strategically selecting one or several determinants that would contribute to the solution of the problem and then identifying the attendant program interventions to address these determinants (Renger & Titcomb, 2003). This strategic conversion is generally implicit in program theory. Once the strategic choices are made, the program can be schematically developed along a logical path of results (Gottfredson, 1986). This is most often associated with stakeholder use of the theory of change. The process must follow certain operational steps, including (1) the creation of implementation conditions, (2) the implementation process itself and (3) the intermediate and long-term outcomes that should, in principle, resolve the problem.

Besides schematically representing the theory of change, a matrix structure can be used to specify the different dimensions of each program result and, in turn, help monitor program progress. First, and most traditionally, the activities and resources required to achieve the results can be described in detail. The next two dimensions relate more specifically to the bases underlying the planned action and its feasibility. On the one hand, actors are invited to reflect on the justifications for each step of the program, that is, the rationales (including those supported by scientific studies and theories) that suggest that the proposed activities will produce the desired outputs, which are in turn required to produce the end results. On the other hand, issues surrounding feasibility and context are addressed. Thus, for each result, we can explore realistic middle-range theories (Pawson & Tilley, 1997) to explain how the expected results will vary with underlying causal mechanisms triggered or not by the program activities/resources in their practical circumstances. Program specification therefore becomes an evaluative reflection on the program's plausibility (Smith, 1989). Finally, the matrix allows us to foresee some of the criteria, norms, and guiding indicators for program implementation and performance.

Applied Example of Figurative Thinking in Participatory Evaluation

The objective of our project was to evaluate an Intervention Assistance Committee (IAC) that had experienced particular difficulties contacting persons that could not, or would not, take precautions to prevent HIV transmission or inform their partner(s) that they were seropositive (Allard & Adrien, 2007). These persons were referred to as risk behaviour clients (hereinafter RB). An Evaluation Steering Committee (ESC) was responsible for formulating a judgement on the relevance and utility of the IAC. Figurative tools and models were developed for the ESC to use in three key phases of the evaluation. The first phase involved constructing a shared understanding of the ESC's evaluation mandate. The second phase focused on the use of the research results and their translation into judgements with respect to the IAC. The third phase examined the implications of these evaluation results for future IAC directions. The following sections present some of the tools used in each of the three phases, illustrated by specific project contexts.

Situating Partners in the Evaluation Process

The IAC arose out of the Montreal Public Health Department's concern to manage RB cases within a prevention and health promotion framework as a first step before bringing in the legal system. A committee made up of representatives from the community of front-line workers dealing with persons living with HIV was formed and a flexible policy for RB case management was developed to support practitioners in their efforts to educate and persuade RB clients rather than use more coercive methods. The main support mechanism proposed was a multidisciplinary committee of experts to coordinate the interventions of diverse professionals and institutions involved with the more problematic cases. Due to administrative constraints that hindered the coordination and delegation of responsibilities among the institutions, the initial IAC prototype eventually settled for more modest objectives. The IAC was limited to an advisory role, and practitioners could request consultations on ethical, preventive and legal aspects of RB cases.

The IAC evaluation project was initiated by the IAC itself when members realized that, despite efforts to promote its services, only a very small number of practitioners had requested consultations. This raised doubts about the utility and relevance of the IAC. The IAC chair therefore suggested that experts be invited to undertake an evaluation. He then enlisted external researchers, submitted an application and obtained research funding for the evaluation. Since some members of the funded research team were closely tied to the IAC, the external researchers requested that the evaluation project be directed by an Evaluation Steering Committee (ESC) who would be responsible for the evaluation report. The ESC was made up of ten persons, five of whom were members of the research team. Three of these five were, and still are, members of the IAC. The other two researchers were external and had never been connected with the IAC. Of the five remaining ESC members, four were past or potential IAC users. Two were recruited from HIV/AIDS community organizations, one from a specialized medical clinic and the fourth from a community clinic. The final member was a bioethics specialist. As a member external to both the IAC and the Public Health Department, he chaired the ESC. The ESC meeting agendas were prepared jointly by the chair and an evaluation specialist external to the IAC. This external specialist led ESC meetings and also acted as an independent knowledge broker (Ryan, 2004) for knowledge produced by, and for, the evaluation. The idea to facilitate ESC discussions using figurative depictions was inspired from his work. Although the ESC members were not the primary producers of the figurative language, they used and transformed it to initiate, support and illustrate their co-constructions.

Since the funding application had already set forth the evaluation goals as well as the ESC composition and responsibilities, the first ESC meetings were spent drawing up a clear and shared vision of its mandate. Several members, including some of the researchers, had only limited experience in evaluation, and more importantly, with evaluation steering committees. It was important for the ESC to understand the difference between a research and evaluation process and to clearly grasp that judgement construction would be the essential function involved. Although several

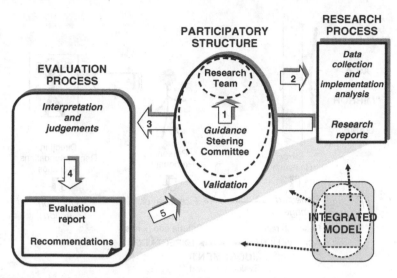

Fig. 8.3 Integrated participatory evaluation model

tools were developed to guide the discussions, two simple models were used in particular. The first presented in Fig. 8.3, provides an overview of the participatory evaluation process. The participatory structure, primarily consisting of the ESC, but open to other stakeholders that could be mobilized to validate the committee's work, acted as a mediator to integrate data collection and analysis on the one hand, and to facilitate interpretation and judgement formulation according to the selected criteria on the other. The ESC oversaw the research team, whose reports were used to produce the concluding evaluation report containing the final judgements and recommendations. This model clarifies the role of ESC members as knowledge integrators and defines as their primary responsibility to produce an evaluation report comprised of judgements and their justifications.

To shed light on this essential but not necessarily familiar notion of judgement process that underlies all evaluation, we have used a metaphor (House, 1993; Kaminsky, 2000) to portray judgement as the result of a comparison between an expectation (criterion, norm, benchmark, desired outcome, ideal, etc.) and an achievement (e.g., research report on program process and observed outcomes). The metaphor depicts evaluation as a mirror game. When a person looks in a mirror, an image is created, a reflection of reality generated by the image-producing mechanisms of the mirror. Data analysis and the research report are the image-producing mechanisms in the evaluation process. In addition, the person facing the mirror incorporates a personal combination of intentions and interests into the judgement of what is reflected. In our example, presented in Fig. 8.4, the person examines his appearance and considers his body too frail. If the desired ideal (i.e. the standard, norm or benchmark) is a more muscular appearance and the mirror (the observation mechanism) is of sufficient quality, a thin person might make this judgement. This reasoning is akin to what Fournier (1995) names the general logic of evaluation, or

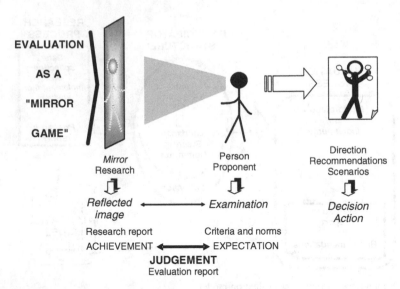

Fig. 8.4 Metaphor used to explore the judgement process

what Scriven (1998) refers to as minimal theory, i.e. establishing evaluation criteria and standards, measuring performance, comparing with the standards, and integrating all the information into a judgment. Furthermore, the mirror game leads directly to a course of action, or scenarios and recommendations in the evaluation process, to fill the gap between the judgement and the ideal. In this case, a bodybuilding program might be considered the solution.

This metaphor can be extended to describe a participatory evaluation process. In other mechanisms (not illustrated here, but imaginable), we might add other actors to the person looking in the mirror. A friend, for example, could change the person's viewing angle or position of the person, use the mirror in another setting, question the criteria that inform the examination, and consequently transform the final judgement. A professional evaluator usually plays this reflexive role. Our friend looking in the mirror might also be joined by family members, with their varying degrees of interest in participating in the judgment and in the formulation of subsequent recommendations or action scenarios. This would necessitate discussion of the mirror-produced image, the criteria, the judgment and the ensuing course of action. The person might initially decide on a bodybuilding program, based on a judgement of thinness, but he might also change his plan to outdoor activities with the family, based on a judgement of pallor, lack of flexibility and insufficient recreational time spent with the family. The role of the family in our metaphor parallels the involvement of the ESC in the judgement process and demonstrates the very concreteness of the dialogue and discussion framework through which the ESC members elaborated their judgment. They were able to work analogically by imagining new situations and transposing them to comparable contexts, and in a pinch, they could review the metaphor's capacity to address the different aspects of a judgement. In the words of De Coster (1978), the use of this metaphor exceeds the potential of a discursive analogy tool in rhetorical-didactic relations (research or evaluation is often associated with the production of a mirror that reflects the actor's reality, but goes no further) and attains that of methodological analogy (as in our mirror analogy where "a" in reality "X" corresponds to "b" in image "Y"), which gives rise to unexpected associations and new hypotheses.

Securing the Transition from Research Results to Judgement

Essentially, the proposed evaluation of the implementation and functioning of the IAC was meant to judge its utility for practitioners confronted with RBs, and more broadly, its relevance. This was initially accepted by the ESC members with the understanding that the project goal could be adjusted over time to better respond to issues as they arose. This was the case at the third meeting when, in light of initial results on the number and nature of RB cases analyzed by the IAC, members raised the issue of coverage, or the IAC's capacity to reach targeted practitioner groups. This shifting locus of control, as Themessl-Huber & Grutsch (2003) named it, led to the addition of a coverage criterion to those of utility and relevance. Thus, from its inception, the ESC decided to examine the IAC through the filter of three criteria. They also knew from the mirror game metaphor that the definitions of the criteria could vary between individuals, leading to differing requests for information as well as diverse or even dissenting judgements. In addition, they were aware that the criteria were not independent from each other, and that the resultant judgements would be interrelated. Therefore, their challenge was to orient the evaluation with an attempt to integrate the three criteria and use the results in order to progressively structure their judgements.

The ESC kept track of its judgements by monitoring the work with a matrix that ultimately helped represent the final judgement. Figure 8.5 presents the end version, which was included in the evaluation report. The matrix intersects the three evaluation criteria with the two dimensions: orientation and action. These dimensions were identified during ESC discussions on the available coverage data, in which two separate questions were addressed: (1) did the IAC meet the expectations articulated in its main orientations and those expressed by each member? and (2) was the IAC sufficiently well known and exempt from access barriers to achieve the desired coverage? These two dimensions were then considered in the discussion on utility, which focused on two questions: (1) was the IAC useful in providing accurate ethical and legal information to support decision-making in RB cases? (2) was the IAC demonstrably useful in identifying precise intervention modes and their application in practice? Finally, the examination of relevance, which took on greater importance when the ESC began to consider future directions in light of the coverage and utility criteria, was also split into two questions: (1) what is the relative importance of IAC activities among all the possible actions to manage problematic RB cases? (2) how suitable are the current IAC mechanisms for meeting priority

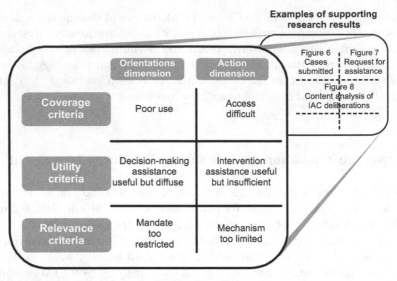

Fig. 8.5 Integrated judgement matrix: Working hypothesis

needs that have apparently not obtained an adequate response? The cells in this matrix contain brief descriptions of the judgements that, taken together, set the tone for the evaluation report conclusions. In the final report, however, each judgement is qualified and supported with data, analyses and other relevant information. This detailed presentation highlights the fact that the matrix represents only majority viewpoints on each criterion. Accordingly, we have retained a working hypothesis subtitle for the matrix, since it corresponds to the state of discussions, based on available research data, at the time of the final account of the judgements.

The ESC's work was marked by continuous transitions between data analyses, discussions and judgement formulation. To facilitate rapid assimilation of this evolving information within a limited timeframe, syntheses were depicted as figures and models. Three examples of figurative techniques used to support judgement formulation are presented below (identified in the background of Fig. 8.5), combining the metaphor, the matrix and the schematic diagram.

The first two figures depict the coverage criteria for the IAC's capacity to reach practitioners that needed support to manage RB cases. Depending on the circumstances, the IAC included between five and ten members with expertise in HIV/AIDS and ethical and legal matters. The IAC was available to assist all practitioners that submitted a request and were willing to discuss the RB case. The IAC designers had stressed the importance of the practitioners' participation in the discussion. There was also a more or less explicit expectation that the majority of practitioners referring cases to the IAC would be those who dealt with a large number of cases. However, the data indicated that practitioner participation did not correspond to these expectations. About 70 RB cases were submitted to the Public Health Department, and among those, less than half (26) were discussed by the

IAC, and of these 26 cases, it was noteworthy that only four were RB cases from the gay community, which is by far the most affected by the AIDS epidemic. In addition, of the 26 cases, only six were discussed in the presence of the concerned practitioners. Based on these observations, the ESC pursued two series of activities. First, it decided to obtain a more accurate picture of the RB cases examined by the IAC over time before drawing any conclusions. Second, it wanted to take stock of the interview data collected from former and potential IAC users as part of the evaluation project to better understand the underlying reasons for poor practitioner participation in the IAC discussions. In light of this, the ESC formulated several hypotheses that were deemed essential to explore via the interviews.

Figure 8.6 provides an example of the time distribution of RB cases handled by the IAC. This chronological matrix (Miles & Huberman, 2003) reports specific types of RB cases submitted by time period, along with some relevant characteristics. The particularity of this matrix lies in the use of different figurative elements to illustrate case characteristics and convey their complexity. Figure 8.6 shows only one possible use of this matrix. Based on information concerning the origin of requests for consultation, gender of RB cases and practitioner presence at IAC case discussions, the ESC drew two conclusions.

Firstly, the average number of cases analyzed by the IAC was slightly over three per year. However, if we exclude cases handled or notified by the IAC members themselves during the Committee's pilot testing years, the average falls to almost two cases per year. The matrix also differentiates cases that were directly notified to the IAC by a victim (oval) or indirectly by a third party (T), parent or friend of

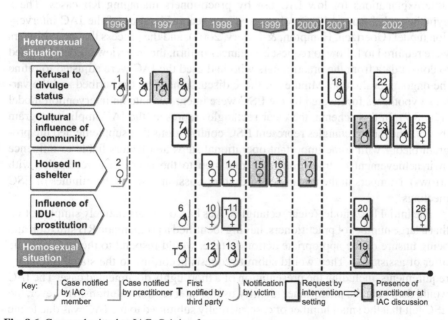

Fig. 8.6 Cases submitted to IAC: Origin of request

a victim. These requests were eventually refused by the IAC due to the possibility of false declarations and the ethical implications of unwarranted investigations. The higher number of cases in the last year was the result of IAC promotional efforts, most likely in response to the evaluation project that required an analysis of IAC discussions. A closer examination of these cases showed that some could have been dealt with more rapidly in contexts other than the IAC, such as consultations with partner notification counsellors. The 2002 increase was thus partly due to marketing efforts combined with the evaluation apparatus. In addition, Fig. 8.6 clearly underscores the small number of cases that involved practitioner participation in IAC discussions.

Secondly, cases analyzed by the IAC were primarily heterosexual RBs. Four major categories were identified. The first comprises almost exclusively HIV-infected men that refused to divulge their status to their partners. The second contains men having a concept of personal responsibility that was largely shaped by the image of HIV/AIDS in their ethnic community. A third category refers to women who, due to serious physical or mental health handicaps, lived in shelters and threatened the health of the people around them by their sexual behaviours. A fourth category includes RB cases that reported injection drug use and prostitution.

Presentation of the coverage data generated opposing views within the ESC. On the one hand, some members questioned the relevance of the IAC based on the resources that were mobilized for such a small number of cases. Other members cited the potential consequences of unmanaged cases, be it just one case, and argued that the interview data on utility should be closely examined before reaching a conclusion. Discussions within the ESC also gave rise to several possible explanations for low IAC use by practitioners managing RB cases. These hypotheses led, somewhat involuntarily, to a reconsideration of the IAC intervention model (Goertzen, Hampton, & Jeffery, 2003), and the process that practitioners were required to follow to request assistance. In turn, the interview guides designed to collect data from the practitioners who had used the IAC were adjusted to refine the ongoing evaluation. Minutes of these discussions were transcribed and the various hypotheses formulated by the ESC were integrated into an intervention model (Fig. 8.7). In this schema, the clear rectangles represent the IAC implicit program theory. The dark rectangles represent ESC contributions that supplemented the program theory with some important operational steps and factors liable to influence their achievement or transition from one step to the next (clear rectangles with arrows). Numbers in the rectangles refer to discussion items in the minutes of ESC meetings.

The initial IAC model (clear rectangles) was based on the relatively simple notion that a large number of practitioners, having identified a problematic RB situation and being unsure of the appropriate action to take, would respond to the IAC's public offer of assistance. They would submit requests according to the stated eligibility requirements, including the presentation of a thoroughly documented case. The IAC would then help the practitioner identify useful intervention solutions. However, the ESC felt that the small number of cases actually submitted to the IAC was due to the absence of certain influent factors, identified in the model by dark rectangles, which

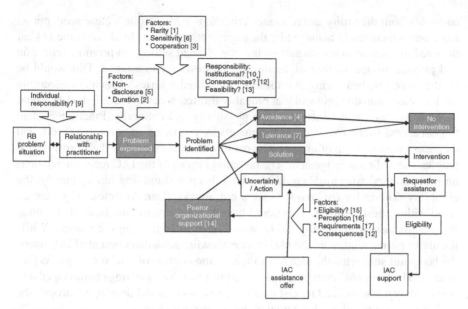

Fig. 8.7 Practitioner request for IAC assistance process: Representation of ESC

therefore gained further consideration. For instance, for a problem to be identified, it must be somehow expressed. This constitutes a challenge, particularly for gay men, where responsibility for HIV transmission is a community as well as an individual issue. Thus, for many practitioners, each person in this community should be alert to the danger and has the responsibility to protect oneself. RBs may then become a non-issue.

At the same time, clinical factors may play a role in problem identification. Problematic situations are not always clearly apparent; clients may be reluctant to speak out and the short duration of clinical consultations may leave many cases undetected. Various organizational factors also come into play. The type of clientele served by a clinic may mean that RB cases are rare, thus requiring greater sensitivity and cooperation on the part of practitioners to identify them. Even when a problematic case is identified, an adequate organizational structure is still required to support appropriate action. Not all organizations have clearly defined roles and responsibilities for dealing with RB cases, nor do they necessarily have a clear vision of the consequences or feasibility of different types of interventions, whether preventive or coercive. Thus, practitioners reacting to a RB situation might take a different approach than making a request for assistance to relieve their uncertainty. Some might avoid such situations in the first place, while others might tolerate them, and in a best-case scenario, some might find solutions on their own or with the help of colleagues or supervisors. Nonetheless, a small number of the detected cases ended up receiving no intervention at all, which led to two important observations by the ESC members. The first is that the IAC evaluation should be combined with research on the institutional and professional practices concerning RB cases. The second, which addresses both the utility and relevance criteria, is that, despite a clear need, not all RB cases are currently managed by the organizations. This should alert the IAC of the need to do more outreach and go into the clinical settings to promote reflection and provide advice, instead of waiting for requests for assistance. This would be all the more justified seeing that the ESC identified a series of factors concerning the IAC case selection protocol that probably limited access. Overall, the IAC could be perceived as a remote service, both physically and culturally. Practitioners had to gain access to the IAC, fulfil requirements by preparing an extensive report, and then meet with a group of experts who could ultimately question their professional practices and clinical judgement. The potential impact of the IAC recommendations on practitioners' workloads could also have been a stumbling block. Finally, the eligibility criteria for IAC requests were not always clear. At times, they were an issue within the IAC itself. This could have caused unease and hesitation among the practitioners who actually did or would have liked to submit a request. While the above points reinforced the idea of interviewing actual and potential IAC users, the last point supported the idea of examining the content of IAC meetings. As part of the evaluation, IAC members had agreed to have their meetings audio taped and observed by a researcher. Our last example presents a model developed through the analysis of four meetings, for a total of eight case discussions.

The analysis aimed to determine how discussions between Committee members oriented the solutions proposed to the practitioners, as well as which factors influenced the exchange of ideas. A first reading of the meetings verbatim showed that, overall, discussions were marked by divergent positions that sometimes cast doubt on the very bases for establishing the IAC. Moreover, these oppositions hindered the formulation of clearly shared recommendations. A content analysis was conducted, based on the idea that human discourse is structured by contradictions and oppositions (Léger & Florand, 1985). The analysis revealed a particular structure in the IAC deliberations, as schematically illustrated in Fig. 8.8.

From the outset, the structure emerges as an oscillation between two poles on a single axis of opposition, for both the practitioner submitting the request and IAC members. The cases discussed at meetings are characterized by a pressing need for action. Practitioners seek solutions to problems involving ethical issues, legal responsibilities and intervention approaches for cases with which they are likely to lose contact, such as patients transferring to other healthcare services, talking about leaving, or dying. Thus, there is an emergency situation and the hope is that the IAC will rapidly provide a solution. However, this sense of urgency is countered by IAC members who assert the need for caution, which may be largely justified by a lack of accurate information, including high-risk sexual behaviours, or unreliable supporting evidence. Such incomplete information is reflected in the IAC deliberations on potential solutions that tend to be phrased in conditional terms (if such and such is verified, you could do this or that). This cautionary stance gives rise to requests for verification, which place everyone in what is known as the investigation dilemma.

This dilemma was central to the discussions. Since its inception, the IAC has been guided by two ethical issues and has continually debated their relative importance. On the one hand, an RB case puts past, present, and future victims at risk, and on the

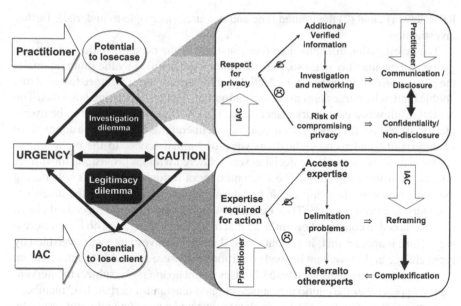

Fig. 8.8 Opposing relationships model: Content analysis of IAC deliberations (4 meetings)

other hand, this person's privacy and rights must be respected. Thus, we observed a balancing mechanism at work in IAC discussions. When the balance tipped too far in favour of actions designed to protect the victims – the usual ethical trigger for practitioner consultation – an IAC member would raise caution about acting precipitously and prejudicing the basic rights of the RB. The problem was that the IAC did not usually have complete or reliable information on the RB's high-risk activities. Practitioners often reported unsubstantiated evidence, and definitive proof of conscious, voluntary HIV transmission was rare. Hence, the IAC's requirement for more specific facts as well as additional, confirmed information before identifying further appropriate action. Meanwhile, the RB situations presented to the IAC were characterized by three features: instability, both psychological and geographic for some of the concerned parties; hostile relations that could result in violence; and social contexts of secrecy and concealment. Investigating a case under such conditions meant going outside the initial network of the practitioner that appealed to the IAC. Practitioners were then required to expand their investigation to other clinicians and individuals that had been in contact with the RB to corroborate certain facts. Consequently, the problem of divulging personal information arose, assuming that these other individuals had relevant information, as well as the possibility that they could use any information that they received, however minimal, to harm the RB. In short, the expanded scope of the investigation in itself carries the threat of negative consequences, since the RB's confidentiality would be compromised. This pressure would then shift the balance towards confidentiality, which speaks to two practitioners' issues: (1) the right to disclose personal information contained in the client's file to another organization, and more importantly to an individual in the

RB's network; and (2) the limited time and resources available to undertake further investigation.

The investigation dilemma therefore consisted of the need to conduct an investigation and the inability to do so, both of which were justified by the same rationale: the protection of privacy and confidentiality. IAC discussions therefore featured this double bind, which translates as an oscillation between two opposing positions. The overall result was a cautionary stance, since the IAC had no choice but to be exemplary in its respect for privacy. Consequently, deliberations evolved in an atmosphere of uncertainty, and recommendations were of limited scope. In the eight above-mentioned cases, not a single decision was rendered without provisions for further investigation and verification. The small number of follow-up meetings held during the study period made it impossible to determine the extent to which the investigative work had been pursued. They essentially highlighted changes (deceased client, client returned to country of origin, etc.) that made the investigation no longer necessary. Thus, it appears that, in certain cases, the need to investigate was overruled by rapid change and movement beyond conditions that were amenable to intervention.

In opposition to situations where RB cases might no longer be subject to intervention, it appears that the cautionary stance created tension for certain IAC members. The practitioner, who was the IAC's client, expected a specific and rapid response. When such responses were not provided, practitioners were likely to become disenchanted, end the consultation process, and influence their colleagues who may in turn have become reluctant to seek advice in the future. Because the very survival of the IAC rested upon a minimal amount of requests, there was a perceived need to provide responses, even for incompletely documented cases or when IAC members felt they did not have all the necessary information or knowledge. To offset this limitation, the IAC had to refer to other experts, which placed it in another quandary known as the legitimacy dilemma.

The practitioner or intervention team that requested support from the IAC did so to obtain expert advice in order to take appropriate action to manage a problematic situation. This meant access to solutions on how to proceed. In five of the eight RB cases, the initial request concerned partner notification procedures, and for two additional cases, advice was sought on supporting high-risk behaviour change. In only one case was the issue of an organization's legal responsibility raised. However, the IAC initiated its intervention with a general review of problem situations brought to its attention. This reframing occurred spontaneously and, in the heat of discussion, raised several points: the ethical principles that must be safeguarded by the IAC; individual versus collective responsibility for HIV transmission; comparable cases and past recommendations; legal and organizational constraints; and resources for action. Throughout the discussion, IAC members of various affiliations voiced diverse, if not dissenting, opinions. This only made the problem, as well as potential solution avenues, more complex, thereby confronting the IAC with the limits of its expertise. One way to offset these limitations was to expand the network of expertise by referring to other resources. This process was itself complex, since it could involve practitioners returning to their team to reformulate the problem or define their own solutions, or they might be instructed to appeal to a public health authority with a legal mandate to enforce health protection measures on persons who are impervious to supportive change general (psychiatrist, psychologist) or specific (probation officer, community organization) resources, including those with which certain of its members might be associated. The legitimacy dilemma therefore resides in the IAC case management. Practitioners drew attention to this dilemma. Those who participated in IAC meetings expressed their appreciation of the IAC's capacity to reveal the complexity of the situations confronting them. However, they also expressed their disappointment at having to leave those meetings without a more definite answer, and at having to pursue further consultations when they felt there was an urgent need to take action. Additional referrals only exacerbated practitioners' time and resource constraints, especially when they felt there was a need for a quick response to a situation. The problem has thus come full circle.

This model illustrates the structural features of the IAC deliberations, and reveals the limitations of the challenges inherent in formulating practical advice for dealing with complex situations. Utility is also restricted by the IAC's role as a consulting body that must await solicitation. Nevertheless, instead of questioning the IAC's role, the ESC identified the need to revise both the mandate and the scope of its support apparatus in order to extend its operation.

Translating Judgements into Action

Having recognized the need for change, the IAC agreed to put together a transition scheme to become a more functional device. In accordance with their mandate, the ESC submitted their judgements and recommendations for discussion to a wider network of actors to obtain feedback on the feasibility of their change scenario. At the outset, the ESC proposed an expanded version of the IAC. Instead of responding to requests as they arise, the IAC could adopt a broader advisory role that would be more connected to intervention settings. For instance, the IAC could become more active in raising awareness of RB issues and supporting more reflexive practices. It could also document ongoing practices in the field and facilitate knowledge sharing of best practices. The IAC would still be part of the regional public health authority. However, in addition to the current advice providers (a nurse and a physician) to practitioners, the new IAC would have access to a permanent team that would conduct research, develop position papers and disseminate pertinent information to the intervention community. The ESC developed an organizational model and presented it for validation (Brandon, 1999). Two validation groups were identified: a group of actors from state and regional institutions, who could either support or sit on the new IAC, and the actual IAC. Each group was provided with a brief presentation of the resultant judgements and supporting data. The change scenario, in the form of a schematic diagram, was then presented for discussion.

This consultation phase led to an essential modification in the ESC proposal. The new organizational apparatus (see Fig. 8.9 for the revised model) more clearly delineates two distinct functions. First, a regional mechanism is designed to reinforce

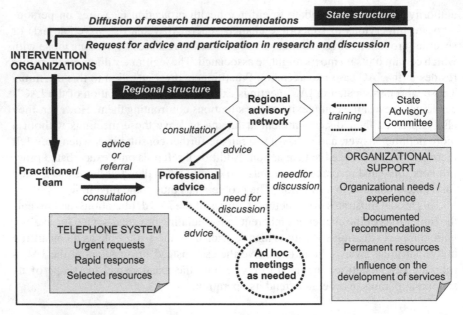

Fig. 8.9 Organization proposed by ESC after validation

the existing telephone answering system for urgent practitioner requests. Both the public health nurse and physician would continue to handle urgent requests, and would also have access to a network of resource persons for consultation as needed, and, in the rare cases that necessitate further deliberation, ad hoc meetings. Thus, the standing committee would be abolished. Instead, there would be a space where practitioners could access a solution bank built from previous similar cases. The experience acquired over time by the designated public health professionals, within and beyond the IAC, coupled with ongoing reflection and knowledge development, would provide for an excellent response capacity.

Second, it was suggested that a State Advisory Committee with ready access to academic and government resources be established to work more systematically with intervention settings and provide tools for coping with RB issues. This new Sate Advisory Committee would have permanent paid staff to document ongoing practices, conduct research and disseminate position papers to practitioners. The proximity of this Advisory Committee to government decision-makers would also facilitate the development of dedicated resources (e.g., psychologists to help RBs change their behaviours). This higher level (state) structure could also work with regional agencies to ensure ongoing information exchange and training. To ensure a smooth transition period, the current IAC was designated to propose the establishment of the State Advisory Committee and eventually to be a part of it. Moreover, IAC members could pursue their actions at regional level by joining the network of resource persons available to the public health authority nurse and physician, who would continue providing telephone assistance upon request. Therefore, after consultation, the proposed model aims to radically change a structure that was no longer viable. On the one hand, the new structure ensures that practitioners would always have access to timely advice. On the other hand, it demonstrates the government's willingness to support RB case management. Given the complexity of the issues at stake and the limitations of the evaluation process itself, the final recommendation of the ESC was to review the implementation progress of the proposed changes two years onwards.

Development of Figurative Thinking and Models for Participatory Evaluation

The examples presented here testify to the ways in which figurative thinking and models can contribute, at different points in time, to a participatory evaluation. In particular, models can help specify the respective participant positions / interests in the evaluation process, and establish significant links between research data, judgements, and action scenarios. To say that these figures were determinant would be presumptuous. We have not directly verified the extent to which the ESC members integrated these figures into their ongoing reflections, nor how the course of their deliberations was influenced by the various syntheses provided. Nevertheless, our experience suggests that figurative thinking can contribute to the participatory evaluation process in several pertinent ways. That said, the above-presented case underscores how figurative thinking and models can facilitate, limit, or ultimately improve and enhance the participatory process. Figure 8.10 presents the functions of different models and specifies how they facilitated and limited the progress of the evaluation, and how they could have improved it. According to Walliser's typology (1977), we differentiated the models by whether they described a current reality (descriptive model), specified an expected situation (normative model), or simulated a future situation (prospective model).

The five functions models can play are: identification, illustration, revelation, simulation, and finalization. Identification is particularly apparent in Figs. 8.3 and 8.4, which are designed to provide a shared representation of the evaluation mandate. The "Integrated participatory evaluation model" presented in Fig. 8.3 has an official feel to it, since it was part of the funding application and establishes the ESC's boundaries and leeway with respect to the research team. Moreover, it clearly outlines the evaluation mandate and responsibilities. Figure 8.4 further clarifies the mandate and signals that the purpose of the evaluation is to produce a judgement. The mirror game provides an appropriate metaphor for steering the ESC's work on the basis of a shared understanding. Presentation and discussion of these two figures helped clarify the group's identity for the entire project. Both representations were referred to at subsequent meetings, particularly when co-constructing judgements and considering IAC change scenarios. This proved very helpful in a limited timeframe where energy was supposed to be spent on debating results and not the nature of an evaluation. However, these models had the negative effect of

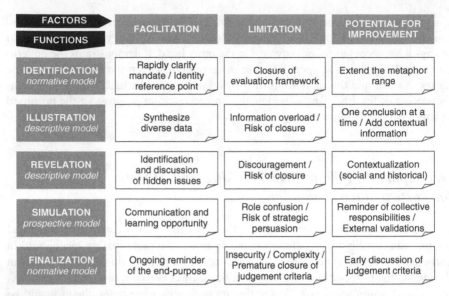

FACTORS / FUNCTIONS	FACILITATION	LIMITATION	POTENTIAL FOR IMPROVEMENT
IDENTIFICATION *normative model*	Rapidly clarify mandate / Identity reference point	Closure of evaluation framework	Extend the metaphor range
ILLUSTRATION *descriptive model*	Synthesize diverse data	Information overload / Risk of closure	One conclusion at a time / Add contextual information
REVELATION *descriptive model*	Identification and discussion of hidden issues	Discouragement / Risk of closure	Contextualization (social and historical)
SIMULATION *prospective model*	Communication and learning opportunity	Role confusion / Risk of strategic persuasion	Reminder of collective responsibilities / External validations
FINALIZATION *normative model*	Ongoing reminder of the end-purpose	Insecurity / Complexity / Premature closure of judgement criteria	Early discussion of judgement criteria

Fig. 8.10 Functions of figurative thinking in participatory evaluation

rapidly overruling any possible challenges to the evaluation's general framework. To enhance the participatory process, an ESC could also be given opportunities to express views and positions on the evaluation and learn about the various tools available to achieve its mandate. In this case, metaphors could have been useful, particularly in the way Patton (1997) employed them. He places small everyday items at the centre of a table (pencil, magnifying glass, ruler, knife, etc.) and asks committee members to choose one that readily represents their personal vision of evaluation, then explain why (slides may be shown instead of using real items). This exercise helps uncover the issues that bring together or divide committee members so that consensus around a shared vision may be built. Should consensus be reached around one particular item, the group could move on to develop the metaphor, as illustrated by the mirror game.

The second function, illustration, is exemplified in Fig. 8.6. The ESC members had already reviewed the data in order to get an overview of the cases submitted to the IAC. Their subsequent questions led to the chronological matrix presented here, in terms of both content and outline, providing a synthesis and portrayal of what was more or less implied, and perhaps even obscured, by the IAC. In a sense, Fig. 8.6 dovetails with the next function, revelation. Another advantage of this matrix is that it serves as a background on which to superpose additional information. As a counterpoint, the main limitation is the danger of information overload, which could result in losing sight of the very observations the figure is meant to illustrate. This synthetic representation also poses the risk of premature closure. For the ESC, it could have created an illusion of firm conclusions that obviated further exploration of the data in light of other criteria. For the IAC members, it could have been rather discouraging when considered out of context. Therefore, we offer two suggestions:

illustrate one conclusion at a time so as to limit the quantity of information; and soften the impact of a potentially discouraging picture by adding contextual information or providing results on other program dimensions that suggest alternative explanations. The latter recommendation is borrowed from Patton (1997).

As mentioned above, Fig. 8.6 also illustrates the third function, revelation. Beyond an illustration of the group's resultant analysis, the matrix reveals some important aspects of the IAC's history. Figure 8.8 clearly demonstrates this function as well. By synthesizing the deliberations of four IAC meetings, this figure had a particularly revelatory effect on the IAC members. They were able to identify a certain malaise that inspired them to engage in open discussion. The above-mentioned risks of closure and discouragement remained, however. For some, such an elegant synthetic portrayal of a complex situation might have implied that there were no further avenues for action or exploration. Here again, it is important to present the model in its social and historical perspective.

The fourth function is simulation. In this case, ESC members generally modified the models presented to them. Figure 8.7 depicting the practitioner request process for assistance and Fig. 8.9 presenting the final scenario endorsed by the ESC went through numerous versions as discussions progressed. In this way, simulation provided an opportunity for group communication and learning. Figure 8.7 allowed the intervention theory to be reformulated, while Fig. 8.9 led to a further refinement of the further organizational structure. According to the distinction made by Michel (1994), Figure 8.9 is a transductive schema that translates a final synthesis into an image. However, it was initially an inductive schema that guided and was transformed by the production, comparison and discussion of several representations. That said, when a simulation exercise opened the door to what should have been, or what should be done, ESC members openly expressed their intentions and were in a position to influence the process. Care therefore had to be taken to ensure that the collective responsibilities of the ESC were not obscured by power struggles and individual persuasion tactics. When ESC members alternated between research, evaluation and planning activities, there was also a strong potential for role confusion. Simulation work should therefore proceed cautiously, with periodical reminders of the group's collective responsibilities and recourse to additional actors to examine and validate the emergent proposals.

The issue of collective responsibilities brings us back to the purpose of the ESC's work, which was to produce an evaluative judgement. Throughout our project, Fig. 8.5 had this finalization function, underscoring the end-purpose of our work. The integrated judgement matrix presented the criteria that were used for judgement making and brought attention to their potential interrelations. The matrix underscores an important limitation as well. It reveals the complexity and imperfection of a judgement. It can therefore create a feeling of insecurity. At the same time, it can help identify program areas that require consolidation or modification. It is therefore not surprising that the ESC members frequently referred to this matrix as they discussed future scenarios and drew up their recommendations. They were fully aware that deficiencies in coverage and utility could be mitigated by reconfigurations to ensure relevance. Still, this type of matrix would be much more useful if its content were discussed early on in the process, while being mindful of the danger of premature closure on the judgement criteria. By and large, all the figures presented here can fulfil several of the functions that we have briefly outlined above. Substantial work is still required, however, to develop a more complete classification and functional framework.

Conclusion

Our extensive experience with figurative tools in participatory evaluation has convinced us that they are more than illustrative extensions of stakeholder discussions. At different stages of an evaluation, they can provide valuable material for evaluative thinking and processes.

In this chapter, we have exposed a working hypothesis, with an emphasis on the central role of models that combine schemas and matrices, images and analogies, concepts and categories. We have also provided an example of an evaluation project where figurative tools were voluntarily used in a steering committee to clarify its mandate, support data synthesis and interpretation, and formulate a judgement as well as recommendations. Our models worked in synergy to stimulate both figurative and discursive thinking throughout the evaluation partnership. In the end, we set out the diverse functions these tools can have in participatory evaluation, how they can facilitate, limit or even threaten the process, and where there is room for methodological development.

However, several issues ought to be addressed to further develop a sound and structured figurative thinking practice. First, there is the balance between discursive and figurative thinking tools in a participatory evaluation project, as well as the degree to which they ought to be used in relation to other types of tools. We have shown that there certainly is space for both these complementary processes. However, what could be optimal combinations, in what circumstances, and with which stakeholders is still open for discuss. Furthermore, to what extent should discursive and figurative methods be pursued to enhance and express the evaluation processes experienced by each stakeholder? Simons & McCormack (2007) have endorsed the integration of creative arts in evaluation. Participatory evaluators in developing countries (Case, Grove, & Apted, 1990) have also used innovative approaches in their methodology, using familiar oral traditions, such as storytelling and drama, or common objects (e.g. drawing in the sand).

As we seek to enhance participation in evaluation, a second issue arises with respect to participants' capacities to engage with these tools. For instance, how do we prepare, guide and assist stakeholders unfamiliar with such tools to enhance their understanding and fully participate in the evaluation project? Moreover, different forms of representation may elicit different meanings from different actors, as well as require differing modes of communication that are not necessarily familiar to all stakeholders. In fact, there is room for confusion that could be a deterrent to participation. Because it is familiar to most people, the metaphor could have a definitive advantage over other forms of representation. Still, even such familiarity should not obviate the need to clearly explain the potential rules and dangers of a metaphoric stance. Therefore, the evaluator must make provision for time and resources to ensure participant capacity development with respect to the tools presented herein. In this vein, diverse categorization and classification methods (Mark et al., 2000) can be explored with participants to produce useful matrices.

A related issue refers to the production of schemas: how could we ensure their management to facilitate ongoing discussion, collective productions and linkages with additional documents judged pertinent by participants, while also keeping track of the processes? Although schemas can be produced with basic slide or paint software like Microsoft® Powerpoint®, which we used in our example, more specialized software ought to be considered. For instance, Mindjet® MindManager® Pro6 is one example where a mindmap (a schematized ideas network) is an integrating mechanism for multiple documents and complex exchanges throughout a group project. Therefore, different types of software should be tried out in concrete evaluation situations to further develop figurative thinking methods.

A third issue pertains to the data synthesis and interpretation functions of figurative thinking tools. In particular, how can they facilitate cross-linkage of different forms of data, most notably integration of quantitative measures and qualitative observations generated through our complex evaluation projects? A number of software products, such as those used for content analysis and statistical analysis, provide various options for representations of data and analysis; charts, causal pathway models and factorial analysis figures are good examples. These are all part of the figurative artillery of quantitative data and could benefit from interaction with qualitative figures. For instance, a chart could be integrated into a schema where images or categories give an overview of potential interpretations; or several charts could be combined into an image which becomes a metaphor for an evaluation object (e.g. a human body made of charts to synthesize the characteristics of program participants). The objective should always be to involve stakeholders in a more penetrating and comprehensive view of the data.

Other issues will certainly arise as various actors who engage in participatory evaluation processes require that results be useful and utilized. Although evaluators have quickly become aware of the need to create rhetorical spaces (McKie, 2003) that enable all actors to have equal access to discussions and decisions, efforts to create these spaces have largely remained within a discursive mode of communication. However, the road is now mapped out. We must systematically continue to expand the modes of communication to include figurative thinking tools in participatory evaluation.

References

Abma, T. A. (2006). The practice and politics of responsive evaluation. *American Journal of Evaluation, 27*, 31–43.

Allard, D., & Adrien A. (2007). *Infection au VIH et personnes ne prenant pas les précautions nécessaires afin d'éviter la transmission du virus - Évaluation d'implantation du Comité d'aide aux intervenants*. Montréal: Direction de santé publique.

Allard, D., Audet, C., St-Laurent, D., & Chevalier, S. (2003). *Évaluation du programme expérimental québécois de traitement des joueurs pathologiques – Rapport 6 – Monitorage évaluatif – Entrevues initiales auprès des décideurs et des coordonnateurs.* Québec: Institut national de santé publique du Québec.

Allard, D., Bilodeau, A., & Lefebvre, C. (2007). Le travail du planificateur public en situation de partenariat, In M.- J. Fleury, M. Tremblay, H. Nguyen & L. Bordeleau (Eds.), *Le système sociosanitaire au Québec – Gouvernance, régulation et participation* (pp. 479–494). Montréal: Gaëtan Morin.

Allard, D., & Ferron, M. (2000). *Évaluation du programme PAD-PRAT – Vie et reproduction d'un programme.* Montréal: Institut de recherche en santé et sécurité du travail.

Allard, D., Kimpton, M. A., Papineau, É., & Audet, C. (2006). *Évaluation du programme expérimental sur le jeu pathologique – Monitorage évaluatif – Entrevues avec les directions et les coordonnateurs sur l'organisation des services et leur évolution.* Québec: Institut national de santé publique du Québec.

Ascher, F. (2005). La métaphore est un transport. Des idées sur le mouvement au mouvement des idées. *Cahiers internationaux de Sociologie, CXVIII,* 37–54.

Barel, Y. (1989). *Le paradoxe et le système – Essai sur le fantastique social.* Grenoble: Presses universitaires de Grenoble.

Barnes, M., Matka, E., & Sullivan, H. (2003). Evidence, understanding and complexity – Evaluation in non-linear systems. *Evaluation, 9,* 265–284.

Barton, A. (1965). Le concept d'espace d'attributs en sociologie. In R. Boudon & P. Lazarsfeld (Eds.), *Le vocabulaire des sciences sociales* (pp. 140–170). Paris: Mouton.

Bertalanffy, L. von (1968). *General system theory.* New York: George Braziller.

Bilodeau, A., Allard, D., & Chamberland, C. (1998). *L'évaluation participative des priorités régionales de prévention-promotion de la santé et du bien-être.* Montréal: Direction de santé publique.

Brandon, P. R. (1999). Involving program stakeholders in reviews of evaluators' recommendations for program revisions. *Evaluation and Program Planning, 22,* 363–372.

Case, D. D., Grove, T., & Apted, C. (1990). *The community's toolbox: The idea, methods and tools for participatory assessment, monitoring and evaluation in community forestry.* Bangkok: Regional Wood Energy Development Program in Asia (May 8, 2002); http://www.fao.org/docrep/x5307e/x5307e00.htm

Chambers, D. E., Wedel, K. R., & Rodwell, M. K. (1992). *Evaluating Social Programs.* Boston: Allyn and Bacon.

Chinman, M., Imm, P., & Wandersman, A. (2004). *Getting to outcomes 2004 – Promoting accountability through methods and tools for planning, implementation and evaluation.* Santa Monica: Rand Corporation.

De Coster, M. (1978). *L'analogie en sciences humaines.* Paris: Presses universitaires de France.

Fetterman, D. M. (2001). *Foundations of empowerment evaluation.* Thousand Oaks: Sage.

Fournier, D. M. (1995), Establishing evaluative conclusions: A distinction between general and working logic. *New Directions for Evaluation, 68,* 15–31.

Goertzen, J. R., Hampton, M.R., & Jeffery, B. L. (2003). Creating logic models using grounded theory: A case example demonstrating a unique approach to logic model development. *Canadian Journal of Program Evaluation, 18,* 115–138.

Gottfredson, G. G. (1986). A theory-ridden approach to program evaluation – A method for stimulating researcher-implementer collaboration. *Evaluation Studies Review Annual, 11,* 522–533.

Guba E. G., & Lincoln Y. S. (1989). *Fourth generation evaluation.* Newbury Park: Sage.

House, E. R. (1983). How we think about evaluation. *New Directions for Program Evaluation, 19,* 5–25.

Hummelbrunner, R. (2004). *A systems approach to evaluation – Applications of systems theory and systems thinking in evaluations.* Lausanne: Fourth European Evaluation Society Conference.

Juan, S. (1999). *Méthodes de recherche en sciences sociohumaines – Exploration critique des techniques.* Paris: Presses universitaires de France.

Kaminsky, A. (2000). Beyond the literal: Metaphors and why they matter. *New Directions for Evaluation. 86*, 69–80.

Lapierre, J. W. (1992). *L'analyse des systèmes – L'application aux sciences sociales*. Paris: Syros.

Léger, J. M., & Florand, M. F. (1985). L'analyse de contenu: deux méthodes, deux résultats?". In A. Blanchet & R. Ghiglione (Eds.), *L'entretien dans les sciences sociales* (pp. 237–273). Paris: Dunod.

Le Moigne, J. L. (1977). La *théorie du système général – Théorie de la modélisation*. Paris: Presses universitaires de France.

McKie, L. (2003). Rhetorical spaces : Participation and pragmatism in the evaluation of community health work. *Evaluation, 9*, 307–324

Mark, M. M., Henry, G. T., & Julnes, G. (2000). *Evaluation – An integrated framework for understanding, guiding, and improving policies and programs*. San Francisco: Jossey-Bass.

Michel, J. L. (1994). La schématisation de l'avenir – Autour des travaux de Robert Estivals. *Revue de bibliologie, schéma et schématisation, 4*, 35–58.

Miles, M. B., & Huberman, A. M. (2003). *Analyse des données qualitatives*. Bruxelles : De Boeck.

Monnier, É. (1992). *Évaluations de l'action des pouvoirs publics*. Paris: Economica.

Morin, E. (1986). *La méthode – 3. La connaissance de la connaissance /1*. Paris: Seuil.

Morin, E. (2001). La *méthode – 5. L'humanité de l'humanité – L'identité humaine*. Paris: Seuil.

Niemi, H., & Kemmis, S. (1999). Communicative evaluation – Evaluation at the crossroads. *Lifelong Learning in Europe, 1*, 55–64.

Patton, M. Q. (1997). *Utilization-focused evaluation – The new century text*. Thousand Oaks: Sage.

Pawson, R., & Tilley, N. (1997). *Realistic evaluation*. London: Sage.

Radnofsky, M. L. (1996). Qualitative models: Visually representing complex data in an image/text balance. *Qualitative Inquiry, 2*, 385–410.

Renger, R., & Titcomb, A. (2002). A three-step approach to teaching logic models. *American Journal of Evaluation, 23*, 493–503.

Ribeill, G. (1974). *Tensions et mutations sociales*. Paris: Presses universitaires de France.

Ryan, K. (2004). Serving public interests in educational accountability: Alternative approaches to democratic evaluation. *American Journal of Evaluation, 25*, 443–460.

Ryan, K., & De Stefano, L. (2001). Dialogue as a democratizing evaluation method. *Evaluation, 7*, 188–203.

Scriven, M. (1998). Minimalist theory: The least theory that practice requires. *American Journal of Evaluation, 19*, 57–70.

Simons, H., & McCormack, B. (2007). Integrating arts-based inquiry in evaluation methodology: Opportunities and challenges. *Qualitative Inquiry, 13*, 292–311.

Smith, M. F. (1989). *Evaluability assessment – A practical approach*. Boston: Kluwer.

Themessl-Huber, M. T., & Grutsch, M. A. (2003). The shifting locus of control in participatory evaluations. *Evaluation, 9*, 92–111.

Touraine, A. (1973). *Production de la société*. Paris: Seuil.

Van der Meer, F. B., & Edelenbos, J. (2006). Evaluation in multi-actor policy processes. *Evaluation, 12*, 201–218.

Walliser, B. (1977). Systèmes et *modèles – Introduction critique à l'analyse des systèmes*. Paris : Seuil.

Weiss. C. H. (1983a). The stakeholder approach in evaluation: Origins and promise. *New Directions for Program Evaluation, 17*, 3–12.

Weiss. C. H. (1983b). Toward the future of stakeholder approach in evaluation. *New Directions for Program Evaluation, 17*, 83–96.

W. K. Kellogg Foundation. (2001). *Using logic models to bring together planning, evaluation, & action – Logic model development guide*. Michigan.

Chapter 9
Dilemmas in Health Promotion Evaluation: Participation and Empowerment

Marjorie MacDonald and Jennifer Mullett

Over the past few years, there has been dialogue and debate in the health promotion literature on appropriate approaches to health promotion evaluation (Labonte & Laverack, 2001; Springett, 2001). A basic premise of this book is that evaluation must be sensitive of the principles of health promotion to be able to contribute to the overall objectives of health promotion. In this chapter, we take up the challenge inherent in this premise and hope to contribute to the dialogue on appropriate approaches to health promotion evaluation. We do this by retrospectively comparing two unique cases in which we experienced challenges in enacting the principles of participation and empowerment in our evaluations. In a cross-case analysis, we identify and elaborate on the themes that emerged in the comparison and draw some conclusions about the application of these principles in evaluating health promotion.

Health Promotion Principles: Participation and Empowerment

We selected the principles of participation and empowerment for two reasons. First, we believe they are foundational to the health promotion process. Second, the two principles are inextricably related, both practically and theoretically (Becker, Israel, Schultz, Parker, & Klem, 2002; Laverack Wallerstein, 2001; Speer, Jackson, & Peterson, 2001). Wallerstein (2006), for example, emphasizes that there is a reciprocal relationship between empowerment and participation, in that community participation is facilitated by an existing sense of community and psychological empowerment while these, in turn, are promoted by participation. "The most effective empowerment strategies are those that build on and reinforce authentic participation. . . ." (Wallerstein, 2006, p. 5).

Arnstein (1969), in her classic ladder of citizen participation presented a typology of eight levels of participation ranging on a continuum from no participation at all through token participation to citizen control. Others have used the terms authentic participation (Laverack Wallerstein, 2001), genuine participation (Simovska, 2004),

M. MacDonald
University of Victoria, Victoria, British Columbia, Canada

L. Potvin, D. McQueen (eds.), *Health Promotion Evaluation Practices in the Americas*,
DOI: 10.1007/978-0-387-79733-5_9, © Springer Science+Business Media, LLC 2008   149

or deep participation (Butterfoss, 2006) to refer to levels of participation that generally correspond to the highest levels on Arnstein's ladder. The meanings of these terms vary slightly with the context and circumstances, but in general, no participation means that research or program participants are not involved in any way in planning, implementing, or evaluating health promotion initiatives, other than as subjects in an evaluation, or as recipients of the services offered in the program. In token participation, a person or group may be consulted but have no control over decision-making. Or, an individual may be selected on the basis of sharing characteristics of that group although that person may not have communication with or receive input from the group he or she is supposed to be representing (e.g., an aboriginal person is selected to represent the interests of all aboriginal persons). Authentic participation is more difficult to define, but Rebein (1996) has argued that an evaluation is truly participatory when individuals who are the focus of an evaluation or a program are involved at all levels and stages of the processes from planning through to evaluation and use of the data. This means that participants are full and equal members of the research or program planning team, have opportunities to make a significant contribution to the process, and are involved in decision-making.

Wallerstein (2006) has argued that it is through authentic participation that individual and collective capacity is developed, transformational learning takes place, and empowerment occurs. This type of participation is an ideal to strive for, but can be very difficult to achieve despite the best intentions. We make a case here for the benefits of a variety of degrees of participation, arguing that they are no less important than forms of authentic participation as described above, in that participants themselves are satisfied with their participation, view it as genuine, and realize benefits.

The editors initially defined empowerment as enabling individuals and communities to assume more power and control over the personal, socioeconomic, and environmental factors that affect their health. This aligns closely with the definition of health promotion in the Ottawa Charter (World Health Organization, 1986), and so, to distinguish empowerment from health promotion, we prefer a blend of the definitions identified by Butterfoss (2006, p. 326) and Wallerstein (2006, p. 17). Empowerment is a multilevel construct that describes a social action process by which individuals gain mastery over their lives, their organizations, and their communities, in the context of changing their social and political environment, to improve equity and quality of life.

Method: Within Case and Cross-Case Analysis

We used a case-oriented approach to examine our individual health promotion evaluation projects and conduct a comparative analysis of our two cases (Miles & Huberman, 1994; Stake, 1995). Our projects were distinct cases, each involving health promotion interventions, but had different funders, purposes, participants, time frames, approaches, and methods.

In our analysis, we moved back and forth between inductive derivation of concepts or themes from the data, and a more deductive review of data to support those themes. In the first stage of analysis, we met to discuss our cases together, and based on that preliminary discussion we inductively derived a tentative framework that specified potential similarities and differences across projects. This provided a basic outline for us to reflect critically on our individual evaluations. In the second stage, we determined separately how our respective data could illustrate this framework. Each of us developed detailed narratives about the application of the principles of participation and empowerment and the issues associated with each application.

In stage 3, we met to review and discuss each other's narratives. We analyzed similarities and differences across cases and again inductively identified themes that appeared to be emerging from our cases and revised our framework accordingly. We then separately organized our own narratives in relation to the themes. Although this entire process was a retrospective secondary analysis, this iterative process of moving between data and analysis both inductively and deductively is consistent with many approaches to primary qualitative data analysis (Flick, 2006; Glaser & Strauss, 1967; Miles & Huberman, 1994; Schwandt, 2001; Strauss & Corbin, 1997).

In the final stage, we analyzed our narratives together and identified six themes in the data on which the successes and challenges of enacting participatory and empowering evaluation appeared to hinge. These were: the nature of the intervention and evaluation, power, evaluation methods, vulnerability, evaluation as intervention, and researcher/practitioner way of being.

Case Descriptions

Case 1: Supporting the Evaluation of Community Development Initiatives

The Queen Alexandra Foundation for Children in Victoria, British Columbia (BC), Canada was one of the recipients of the Strategic Investment Initiative Fund (SIIF), funded by the British Columbia Ministry for Children and Families. The purpose was to strengthen the capacity of communities to support families and children, reduce the number of children brought into protective care, and demonstrate innovative child welfare practices (Queen Alexandra Foundation, 2004). The Foundation put out a call for proposals for innovative projects and subsequently funded twenty-one. The funding criteria required that, if appropriate, those affected by the initiative should be involved in its development, implementation, and evaluation.

The discussions about participation and empowerment in Case 1 draw primarily from six community-based health promotion evaluations; three youth projects and three projects aimed at supporting parents (mostly mothers) of young children. The first youth project engaged at-risk youth in ecological restoration activities (Kotilla, 2005) with volunteer members of non-profit community environmental groups. Some of the youth participants were doing mandatory community service hours while others enrolled voluntarily in the program. The second youth project focussed on youth aged 6–12 in an isolated, socio-economically disadvantaged community with no industry, a high proportion of single parent families, and few resources to support families experiencing hardship. The aim was to increase youth resilience and developmental assets in their lives. Crime Prevention Canada funded the third project, an evaluation of projects in four communities aimed at positive youth development (Miller, Mullett, & VanSant, 2006). The three parent projects assisted mothers to provide a safe environment for their children, some of whom the Ministry of Children and Family Development had deemed to be at "high risk" of abusing their children, or having them apprehended. The purpose was to assist in reuniting families whose children had been in care, prevent others from going into care, and to enable or empower parents to provide safe care for their children. The mothers in these programs experienced a range of problems (e.g., learning disabilities, mental illness, substance abuse, and dysfunctional extended families) that presented concerns for their children's safety.

Case 2: The School-Based Prevention Project

The provincial government in British Columbia (BC), Canada requested proposals from community-based alcohol and drug agencies, in collaboration with school districts, to implement locally developed substance misuse prevention programs in secondary schools (Grades 8–12). Program developers conceptualized prevention from a health promotion perspective. The School-Based Prevention Project introduced Prevention Coordinators into selected schools to guide program development at the community/school level. The coordinator's role was to facilitate a collaborative, participatory, community development process with schools to identify their own substance misuse issues and to develop, implement, and evaluate strategies to address these concerns (MacDonald & Green, 2001).

We conducted a provincial level, multi-site evaluation to examine the effectiveness of the overall project in achieving desired outcomes. A significant challenge to systems-level evaluation, however, is local autonomy, which usually results in major differences among communities in both the intervention and its evaluation. Such differences make evaluative comparisons across communities difficult. Within the larger Project evaluation, one focus was to evaluate program development and implementation within and across sites. We incorporated local level evaluation to address the uniqueness of programs in each community. The Prevention Coordinator at each school facilitated program development and evaluation at that site.

Cross-Case Comparison of Participation

In this section, we compare the enactment of participation in the two cases. First, we present a summary table that outlines three main themes for comparison in both cases, and then we elaborate on these themes as they apply in each case. These themes are: the nature of participation, power dynamics, and evaluation methods to promote participation. We chose these themes because they were relevant in some way to both cases, although their relative importance to each case varied. For this reason, we are not able to rank them in order of importance or against any general set of criteria. We expect that, although the themes may be generalizable to other situations, their importance and relevance will be dependent on the specific health promotion program and its context. Each health promotion program is unique, even when comprising standard elements, because "the boundary between the intervention and the social process or context in which it occurs is often blurred" (Springett, 2001, p. 140). Thus, although this framework and its categories may provide a useful heuristic for other health promotion evaluators to consider in planning and carrying out their evaluations, we do not claim that this represents any sort of comprehensive planning model or "toolbox" of methods to facilitate participation (Table 9.1).

The Nature of Participation

The nature of participation in health promotion evaluation is determined by a variety of factors, but in our cases four factors stood out. These were: the level of the evaluation, who participates in the process, who or what determines the issue in the intervention, and participant engagement.

Level of Evaluation

The nature of participation and the influences on participation in health promotion evaluation depend on the level at which the intervention and evaluation take place. Participation looks quite different when the intervention takes place at a local community level than when it takes place at a larger system level. In Case 1, all the projects were local level community projects situated primarily within community organizations. In Case 2, the intervention took place at both the local and provincial levels. At the local level, it may be that there is greater potential for authentic participation, for building trust, and for developing empowering relationships. This is because the scale of both the intervention and the evaluation is smaller and the number of participants is relatively fewer than at the system level, where the intervention might incorporate multiple sites, multiple levels, and thousands of people. Smaller projects may also provide greater opportunities for building trust and establishing empowering relationships.

Who Participates?

Our case studies identified three issues with regard to who participates. These are: initial versus subsequent groups of participants, the issue of representation, and nonvoluntary participation.

Rarely discussed in the literature is the issue of differing degrees of participation between initial and subsequent groups. Involving youth participants in designing

Table 9.1 Case comparison of participation

Challenges and issues	Case 1: Queen Alexandra community projects	Case 2: School-based prevention project
Nature of Participation		
Levels of analysis	• Local level – community project	• Provincial level, multisite • Local level, community/school project
Who participates?	• Initial versus subsequent groups of participants • Sometimes non-voluntary participation • Issue of vulnerability	• Initial versus subsequent groups of participants • Issue of representation
Who/what determines the issue?	• Funding requirements • Issue pre-defined by program staff	• Funding requirements • Lack of interest in defined issue
Participant engagement	• Participating in intervention vs. evaluation • Avoiding appearance of testing • Challenges of vulnerability	• Participating in intervention vs. evaluation • Survey interpretation
Power Dynamics	• Agency as authority	• Researchers and participants as equal or not-so equal partners • Control over outcomes
Evaluation methods to promote participation	• Relationships vs. rigour • Managing role conflict • Evaluation as intervention • Not all participatory methods are created equal (focus groups, photovoice, asset focused tools)	• Use of student survey to promote participation • Health promotion planning model • Steering committee

an evaluation raises the issue that, although this activity may be participatory for the first group, subsequent groups of participants are, in effect, subjects because they are responding to questions or surveys that others have developed. Even in the Case 1 youth ecological restoration project, in which the coordinator maintained a painstaking and vigilant attitude towards participation throughout, the first youth participants were more involved in the design of the evaluation than later participants. They edited the questions, eliminated some and rewrote others in more kid friendly language. The subsequent youth participants did not have this same opportunity. Nonetheless, as the program gained a reputation in the community and referrals increased, the information provided by each youth at all stages of the project became important for the continued refinement of the project. In this way, all youth participants, not just the initial group, were co-investigators, helping to continuously revise and refine the project so that it would be of benefit to future participants.

In a similar attempt to involve youth in the school-based project evaluation, we initiated a collaborative process to develop the provincial level survey instrument. Students in two schools participated in developing the survey content and format. Then, classes in those schools participated in pilot testing the survey and assisted with revisions to the instrument. As with Case 1, students who subsequently completed the questionnaire were subjects in the survey. Thus, the number of students who were able to participate in an active, decision-making way in planning the evaluation was small. As in the first case, however, some students not involved initially did participate later in the survey's interpretation and application. Thus, the nature of participation varies depending on the stage of the project. A broad conceptualization of participation is necessary to capture the variations throughout the life of any project. As argued by Gregory (2000), there is an inevitable lack of comprehensiveness in participation because we are not able to include, at any given stage of a project, all those who came before, and those who will follow.

The issue of representation was of less concern in the much smaller scale Case 1 projects, in which participants were essentially representing themselves. It was more of an issue in the school-based project where one of the challenges was in establishing a representative advisory group to guide the project. A provincial advisory committee was created, comprising representatives of various constituencies. The project involved many schools from across the province, with thousands of students, parents, teachers, school administrators, and community agency staff. Rebein (1996) has argued that because it is practically impossible to include all stakeholders in active roles, evaluators should, at the very least, include representatives of various stakeholder groups to participate. Although the school-based project advisory group represented many stakeholder groups, it was difficult to ensure adequate representation. One or two students cannot possibly represent the diverse groups that comprise the provincial student population. In fact, the type of student that is most likely to function well in this type of adult group may not reflect the characteristics of students mostly at risk for drug use. Similarly, a single administrator, parent, or teacher representative may not reflect the interests of the diverse membership of their stakeholder groups.

Arnstein (1969) and others might argue that assuming a single individual can represent the interests of a broad constituency reflects tokenism. Gregory (2000) further suggests that the views of the few selected representatives may be overemphasized, and because they are considered to represent faithfully the views of the larger group, could be used to justify evaluation findings. Others have argued (Jayaratna, 1994) that representation can only be participatory with elected representatives and if there is a process of involvement extended to members by the representative (i.e., input sought, information reported back, and decisions discussed with the larger group being represented). This type of democratic representation did not characterize the school-based project advisory group. The size and scale of the provincial level evaluation made any kind of democratic process unwieldy and unworkable.

Nonetheless, when a project covers many sites and geographic locations, this level of participation may be all that can be achieved with some representatives better than none. Perhaps including representatives who are able to put forward diverse perspectives, concerns, and interests of multiple groups for consideration in planning is the only realistic alternative. But, this should also be coupled with a critical reflexivity on the part of evaluators about what the lack of comprehensive participation might mean for the evaluation results. In particular, consideration must be given to what might have been found had we included those whose voices were not heard (Gregory, 2000).

At the local level, even in schools in which there was a high level of student participation, only certain segments of the school population participated. Some Prevention Coordinators focussed their activity on students identified as being at high risk for drug use whereas in others they focussed on a whole school approach and involved a much more diverse group of youth. The approach taken by a Prevention Coordinator was both a theoretical and a philosophical choice, but that decision had implications for the nature of participation in a particular school.

For the most part, parents involved in the school-based Project tended to be those already involved in Parent Advisory Council activities and generally reflective of a more privileged parent population. Involved teachers most often taught health and physical education, and occasionally science or social studies. Most other teachers were not interested in participating because they viewed drug use prevention as outside their areas of expertise and interest. They supported the Prevention Coordinator doing the work, but they were not interested in participating directly because, as they said, "We have our own jobs to do." What all this means is that participation needs to be appropriate to the context, the scale of the intervention and evaluation, and fit with the needs and wishes of stakeholders who may not want, or be able, to be involved at every stage of the evaluation.

Finally there is the issue of non-voluntary participation. What was more an issue in the Case 1 projects was the fact that for some participants their choices were limited. They were required to participate with some community agency, either in the case of the youth to do community service, or in the case of the mothers to learn parenting skills to retain custody of their children. These participants were particularly vulnerable, and when participation is not voluntary, it is a significant challenge to engage participants in evaluation activities no matter how participatory the methodology. We discuss below the strategies to engage participants and encourage their active involvement under Participant Engagement, and the issue of empowering those who are not voluntary participants in the section on Empowerment. What is critical in this situation, however, is the quality of the coordinator's interactions with participants.

Who Determines the Issue?

There is often a tension between funding agency requirements and local needs. In the school-based project, school districts, schools, and community-based alcohol and drug agencies were involved at the local level in preparing the project proposal.

Thus, the program was driven by the local community, although the extent and nature of participation varied by community. In communities in which participants did not identify substance use as an important issue, it was a challenge to obtain voluntary participation. Health promotion dictates that issue identification should come from the community. Although the project in Case 2 was intended to promote a participatory community development process, the problem definition was restricted by the funding requirements. This issue was not a priority for some schools. Many health promotion programs begin with a focussed issue, often because the funding organization has a mandate to deal with that particular health issue and not others. This is actually the norm in health promotion. True bottom-up community organizing around a specific community-wide concern seems to occur much less often than issue-specific health promotion funded by a particular agency with a mandate to deal with that issue and led by an outsider. In itself, this tendency can create problems for subsequent participation, not just in the program, but in the evaluation. At the same time, Reason has argued that many projects "…would not occur without the initiative of someone with time, skill and commitment, someone who will almost inevitably be a member of a privileged and educated group" (Reason, 1994, p. 334). Prevention coordinators who were successful in facilitating participation, even when the issue of drug use was not a high priority, began the process by dealing with issues that were of concern to the schools, thus following the classic health promotion principle of starting where the community is at (Nyswander, 1955).

In the Case 1 projects, although the mandatory aspect of enrolment caused some difficulties, the evaluation itself had fewer restrictions from the funding agency. It was only required that the evaluation be participatory. At the same time, there was an expectation that staff define project goals and activities prior to participant enrolment, so there was limited opportunity for participant involvement in the development of the programs. There was also an expectation in the proposals to project some outcomes. This was further complicated by the range of participants that might, in fact, constitute the group for the projects. One coordinator expressed the dilemma in this way: "We won't know what can be achieved until we see the first group – who will come and what level of cognitive or mental health functioning they will be at."

The issues discussed above with respect to who participates and who determines the issue are illustrative of a larger set of power relations that inevitably present themselves in community-based health promotion intervention and evaluation. These issues are discussed further in the section below on Power Dynamics.

Participant Engagement

Successful youth engagement in a health promotion initiative is one of the most difficult elements in implementation and the key to positive outcomes. Engaging youth is even more challenging in an evaluation, as the evaluators in both cases discovered. Youth in the Case 1 projects said that the project must be meaningful and fun to warrant their participation (Miller et al., 2006). Similarly, in Case 2, despite high levels of participation in some project schools, participation usually meant taking part in planning and implementing prevention activities rather than in their evaluation. Involved students and teachers often reported that they were not as interested in evaluation as they were in planning and implementation.

There were, however, a few exceptions. In a small number of schools, charismatic and innovative Prevention Coordinators got students very involved in interpreting the results of the survey conducted in their school. Inspired and trained by the coordinator, students took the lead in preparing presentations of the data for other students, parents, and teachers and then used the data to advocate for school change. For example, in one school, the data demonstrated that the school climate was very negative. The students used that information to lobby the school administration for resources and programs that would enhance the school climate. Students in another school used the data to support a student's appointment to the selection committee for hiring a new vice-principal. Comments made by students reflect the satisfaction of involvement: "I feel like I have some say in what goes on in the school," or "I never realized that things I do can actually make a difference." This demonstrates a link between active participation and the experience of empowerment for these students.

In the schools where students were actively involved in the survey, the Prevention Coordinator's role was central and perhaps the most important factor. Effective prevention coordinators played a strong leadership role in facilitating participation, not just by capitalizing on opportunities to support youth involvement, but in recognizing and creating opportunities in situations that might otherwise not be obviously conducive to participatory processes. More than that, however, the most effective coordinators were liked, respected, even revered by the youth in their schools because they were seen as trustworthy, respectful, and real. Students enjoyed spending time with these coordinators and working with them to create meaningful activities for themselves and their peers in the school. Wallerstein (2006) has suggested that effective leadership that promotes participatory decision-making is one of the most important factors in a participatory empowerment process. She also noted that participatory strategies based on group dialogue, collective action, advocacy and leadership training, and transfer of power to participants were essential. All of these were elements in the work of Prevention Coordinators who got students involved in the student survey in their schools. They were also evident in the work of program coordinators in several of the Case 1 projects.

In Case 1, coordinators and the evaluators dealt with the challenge of engaging youth in the evaluation with some innovative strategies to facilitate youth engagement. In the ecological restoration project, the coordinator was eager to take a participatory approach to the evaluation and discussions began with exploring how to involve the youth in designing the evaluation. The first issue was how to establish what the youth knew about ecological restoration so that we could make comparisons at the end of the project. Because the youth were vulnerable (i.e., experiencing behavioral problems, substance abuse, and mental health difficulties), any questions that had the appearance of testing them could risk affecting the relationship between the youth and the coordinator.

To address this problem, a simple technique developed by Kurt Lewin, the originator of action research, was used to facilitate freedom of discussion. By talking about youth like themselves rather than about themselves "it minimized resistance to considering the problems and possibilities" (Lewin, 1952, p.50) and removed the burden of having to apply it to their own lives. Instead of asking the youth at the start of the project: What do you know about watersheds and the environment in this valley? -a question that might cause them embarrassment if they knew very little about the subject – they were asked the following: What do you think kids would like to know about watersheds and the environment in this valley? By removing the personal aspect from the question any reluctance to respond was overcome and the youth were engaged in designing the program curriculum for others by identifying appropriate content.

Power Dynamics

Researchers and Participants as Equal Partners

Although health promotion principles would suggest that researchers, program staff, and program participants should be equal collaborators in the evaluation, this presents considerable challenges. In a study that explored a participatory implementation and research project for diabetes prevention in Kahnawake (Potvin, Cargo, McComber, Delormier, & Macaulay, 2003), the authors identified four key principles that facilitated the success of the participatory intervention and research. The first of these, integration of community members as equal partners, assumes that researchers and health promotion practitioners are in a more powerful position than community members because expert knowledge is often viewed as being of higher importance and value than lay or community knowledge. This assumption is well justified, given the absence of community participation and involvement in so many community health evaluations and given the negative experience with research of many marginalized communities.

In the school-based project, however, the power differential tipped in the opposite direction. At both the local and provincial levels, people in some sites viewed the external researchers and the Prevention Coordinators as outsiders and their very presence in the schools was at the discretion of principals and school districts. In some situations, Prevention Coordinators did not have the power to establish themselves as equal partners let alone take control of either the intervention or the evaluation, at least initially. They had to establish their own credibility before those in the school could begin to view them as an equal partner, and in several sites, they were never fully integrated in this way. Educational researchers have found that in the school system, every day knowledge (or what is referred to as community knowledge) is often valued over knowledge generated from data and research (Clark, 1981; Hargreaves, 1994).

Control over and Reporting on Outcomes

Another manifestation of the Prevention Coordinators' lack of power was evident in the nature of the outcomes that emerged in the evaluation. Overall, most of the local level evaluations were quite positive. This finding is consistent with reports by others of a tendency for internal process-oriented evaluations to focus on positive experiences (Pavis, Constable, & Masters, 2003). There was a strong incentive for positive results to come out of each of the site-specific school-based projects and the reports tended to focus on what was successful. Even when Prevention Coordinators wanted to include the implementation problems and discuss what was not so successful, there was tremendous pressure from some schools and districts to be positive, either to ensure continued funding or that the school would not get a bad name. Prevention Coordinators felt vulnerable in reporting negative results.

In the overall provincial level evaluation, however, it was possible for us to talk about successes and challenges. Several Prevention Coordinators confessed their relief that there was a provincial level evaluation to name some of the problems because the coordinators did not feel they had the power to identify those directly. Given the challenges that coordinators had in garnering the power to facilitate change on behalf of students, one can only imagine what little power the students had to influence changes in the factors that affected their life and work in the school.

The Agency as Authority

In Case 1, power dynamics influenced the level of change in two ways. First, vulnerable mothers could not completely dismiss the fact that although they were engaged in a project that attempted to be very egalitarian, it was still a project within the larger program of the agency that received money from the Ministry. Thus, no matter how well staff handled the processes of empowerment, the project still symbolically represented an authority. In fact, the issues and activities for the project had been decided prior to participants engaging with the project and they were aligned with Ministry goals. Second, extremely vulnerable community members, youth or mothers, often view all agencies with scepticism due to their prior history of being powerless in interactions with agency representatives. It takes time for this perception to dissipate and for participants to be able to discriminate between empowering and disempowering practices. As in other situations, however, the importance of the coordinator or evaluator's way of being was centrally important.

Evaluation Challenges and Methods to Promote Participation

Because the projects in both case studies were quite different, operating at different levels on very different scales, the kinds of evaluation methods used to promote participation differed considerably between cases. The issues encountered in each case were also different. For this reason, it is not possible to present a practical set of strategies or a toolbox that the health promotion evaluator can use in every situation. Below we present first some methods and issues from Case 1 followed by methods and issues from Case 2.

Relationships Versus Rigor in a Field Setting

A lot of health promotion work is done in the field, sometimes one-on-one, with participants. The success of the project and its evaluation is largely related to the ability of the coordinator to develop strong relationships with community members, particularly youth. Coordinators worried about how to balance a rigorous approach to evaluation with the flexibility to respond on a personal level to spontaneous participant comments about their experiences in the project because these comments could provide valuable data. For example, youth often disclose significant changes they have made because of the program, in intimate moments when recording is not possible. The most profound discussions sometimes occur in the car, in the dark. By focusing on the needs of the evaluation (i.e., rigor) instead of the youth, the coordinator can jeopardize the developing relationship.

To address this challenge, the coordinator created a field diary to document what she was able to remember of the discussion. Although the youth were aware that these discussions constituted part of the evaluation, the opportunity to discuss their experiences in their own way and at their own time contributed to the development of the relationship between the coordinator and the youth. Preserving the integrity of the developing personal relationships is important because the success of the project is dependent on them.

An evaluator of health promotion makes use of tools from other disciplines, particularly where field work is conducted. Field diaries are a common tool for example, in disciplines like ecology, ethology and ethnography. Tjora (2006) suggested that in field diaries the researcher reproduces dialogue as close to verbatim as possible because such situated vocabularies may provide clues about the observed person's perception of his or her world. The quality of a method, as defined by the adequacy of the approach to capture the essence of the change that has occurred, may be more important than rigor, or a concern with strict exactness. In fact one could argue that an insistence on rigor in this example would not only interfere with the relationship of the coordinator and the youth but may, disrupting the momentum of the dialogue create an unnatural and self conscious interaction that would be therefore less rigorous. To exaggerate this point the dialogue in that scenario might sound like this: the youth says "I want to tell you how I felt about the work we did today"; the coordinator replies "Please wait until I can record it in detail." Had the coordinator waited until the youth was interviewed at a scheduled time to elicit the same remarks retrospectively it is possible that the comments would not be as rich as those offered in situ. By responding in the moment she preserved the relationship she had developed with the youth and the integrity of the evaluation by reproducing the dialogue as closely as possible in her field diary as soon as she was alone. She was also able to note the circumstances of the dialogue and the events of the day, in other words the contextual frame.

Evaluation as Intervention

Although strong relationships are essential for the success of health promotion projects, they can also present challenges for evaluation. Once a trusting relationship is developed, youth often regard the adults involved as role models.

In one of the youth projects, a participant cited this as the most significant aspect of the intervention project. She said that she learned from the community worker "how to have a life". If this same role model, however, is also the evaluator, the relationship can be very confusing and the evaluator must take extra care to assure the youth participants that the evaluation is about the project and not about them or their ability to learn and change. Failure to make this message clear could undo all the earlier work of relationship and trust building. The coordinator must juggle the roles of confidante and evaluator; even though, if taken literally, these roles are the antitheses of each other.

Active participation by youth in the evaluation is a creative way to address this concern about role conflict. In one case, the youth were trained to do evaluation interviews, with each successive group interviewing the next group. Thus, all participants were both evaluators and participants. In another project, the youth were trained to do focus groups in which the questions were decided collaboratively with the coordinator, the researcher, and the youth.

In the project designed to develop sustainable independent housing, the youth were trained in the photo voice method (Wang & Burris, 1997). They took photos of their idea of a home with a disposable camera and, in discussions with the coordinator, set goals for achieving that home. As the project progressed the photos were reviewed, barriers discussed and new goals set based on the progress to date. The youth created a collage throughout the project that was a pictorial record of the progression towards independent living. This method is important because it was engaging, it gave the coordinator insights into what would constitute success for the youth, the youth and coordinator could see the progression towards a goal (or lack thereof) and both could discuss together the remaining barriers. Not only did all of the above methods reduce role conflict for the coordinator, thereby addressing issues of bias, but the photo voice strategy is another example of evaluation as intervention; that is, a strategy that provides important evaluation data while also being part of the intervention. The photo voice method can be empowering for youth in a variety of contexts (Wang & Burris, 1997).

Not All Participatory Methods Are Created Equal

Community practitioners are often not experienced with evaluation (hence the need for support) and sometimes, to allay their anxiety about conducting evaluation research, they choose to rely on standardized or published tools believing that funding agencies are more likely to approve an evaluation using such instruments. Unfortunately, a published tool is not necessarily a good tool, and even good tools are not appropriate in all contexts. Critically assessing what appears to be a tried and true approach, however, requires confidence and knowledge of methodology. Consequently, to be assured of conducting a good evaluation, some practitioners presented tools they had obtained (or bought) that appeared to them to be relatively simple to administer, yet scientific.

This issue arose recently in the context of the youth project that took place in a socio-economically disadvantaged community and was aimed at increasing the number of developmental assets within their lives. On receipt of funding, the coordinators reviewed their evaluation materials with the evaluator. One of these tools was a Checklist of Assets, a test to be used pre- and post-program to measure improvement in youth assets. Given the aim of the project, it would seem a reasonable instrument to use in the evaluation. However, there are two assumptions implicit in the use of this kind of a tool: (a) it is participatory, and (b) it measures something positive (assets) rather than negative (deficits) and thus would not have a negative effect on the respondent. Unfortunately, neither of these assumptions held up. The coordinator and evaluator reviewed the checklist together and the evaluator suggested that completing the checklist could affect vulnerable youths negatively, particularly if they did not have many of the assets listed. With vulnerable youth one cannot risk making them feel worse about themselves. Rewording a needs assessment so that it is phrased in terms of assets rather than problems may be a wolf in sheep's clothing. In addition, this view of the test as a positive experience for youth also leads to a kind of halo effect for the test in which it is seen as engaging and therefore participatory, which it clearly is not.

In Case 2, as discussed previously, our evaluation demonstrated that a survey instrument was effective in facilitating participation in strategies that serve the goals of health promotion (including empowerment) but it was not the method itself that enhanced participation. Rather, it was a group of motivated and innovative students who wanted to create organizational change in their schools, facilitated by a creative and empowering Prevention Coordinator who encouraged students to make use of this information, got them excited about the possibilities, and then supported them in using the data for their own purposes, resulting in a group of students who felt empowered by the process.

Similarly, in another school, school administrators and teachers used the survey as a benchmark to judge their progress in achieving improvements in their school in preparation for accreditation. The disappointing scores on the first survey stimulated them to engage members of the school community in making specific changes related to student engagement in school processes, school climate, and drug prevention strategies. Thus, they felt empowered to use the survey data effectively to make changes in their school.

A Health Promotion Planning Model

Program funding agencies expected the School-Based Prevention Model to be the foundation for the process in which students, teachers, school administrators, parents, and community agency representatives would participate and be involved in defining the issues, identifying and implementing strategies/programs, and evaluating the outcomes. In fact, Laverack Wallerstein (2001) suggest that a logical framework system of program planning is a tool that can help stakeholders recognize their potential for action and change. This is not always the case, unfortunately, and the extent to which this actually occurred in the Project varied considerably across schools. The model assumes an existing interest in the issue and the willingness of schools for Prevention Coordinators to facilitate a community development and evaluation process around that issue. For many Prevention Coordinators this was not the case. Teachers had often not been involved in the initial decisions to adopt the project. Thus, Prevention Coordinators had to begin by building relationships and enhancing the readiness of the school to take on the issue.

The School-Based Prevention Model (based on the PRECEDE-PROCEED Model) (Green & Kreuter, 1991) was intended to facilitate the process of local issue definition but within the constraints of a pre-defined problem, thus creating a dilemma for the Prevention Coordinators. Some of the schools did not see alcohol and drug use as a major focus for their schools, even though the school had been involved in writing a proposal for funding to do just that. The Prevention Coordinators therefore had to sell the issue before they could begin to work collaboratively with the school community to address the issue of drug use prevention. This was uncomfortable for many of them.

In addition, the model did not fit with the way planning is often done in schools. The model is a systematic planning process in which information is gathered and used to set priorities for action. This rational planning process was foreign to many schools continually dealing with crises that required action in the moment. In fact, some educational researchers have suggested that an evolutionary planning process is more common than rational planning in schools. In such a process, action occurs before planning and plans emerge on the basis of early action (Clark, 1981; Hargreaves, 1994; Louis & Miles, 1990). Most Prevention Coordinators found that proactive planning did not occur and often schools actively resisted it. It was a constant struggle for them not to be drawn into a reactive stance (MacDonald & Green, 2001).

A Steering Committee

The establishment of a steering committee was the second recommended mechanism for facilitating participation and involvement of key stakeholder groups in implementing and evaluating the project. The committee was to steer the process at the local school level and be responsible for securing commitment and participation by members of all the constituencies. In reality, it was very difficult for most Prevention Coordinators to establish steering committees because they first needed to gain entry to the schools, overcome opposition to their roles, put into place the infrastructure to do their work, and sell the issue. Some felt a lot of pressure from the funding agencies to get the steering committee established and thus moved too quickly to invite participation before they had established good working relationships with potential members and identified appropriate participants. Participation floundered.

Overall, most Prevention Coordinators had to work very hard to initiate and maintain a steering committee, and they felt they had to play a very directive role in the process. In the end they were steering the steering committee. In some schools, teachers and administrators argued that they had their own jobs to do and the Prevention Coordinator was being paid to coordinate and implement the program. They did not feel that they should be involved to the extent expected by the funding agencies and the PRECEDE-PROCEED planning model. Some Prevention Coordinators found other ways to work collaboratively and facilitate participation that did not involve having a steering committee. So, mechanisms used to facilitate participation have to be sensitive to the context and fit with the ways of working familiar to the school, at least in the beginning.

In some instances, steering committee members wanted to do things that went against the principles of health promotion espoused by the planning model, creating yet another dilemma for the coordinators. The members were more interested in operating in a top-down way and taking control of the decision-making, rather than facilitating participation and empowerment. What should the Prevention Coordinator have done in this case –defend health promotion principles? If so, which of the principles are most important? If they defended school control of the process, then some other health promotion principles like student participation and empowerment might be lost. If they defended participation and empowerment, then they went against the wishes of the steering committee and the vested interests of the more powerful people in the school thereby risking their ability to implement any successful prevention strategies. This left some of them feeling powerless to influence change.

In this evaluation, it was clear that the mechanisms that were intended to facilitate participation in program development and evaluation were not always effective in achieving that goal, in part because the funders had imposed the goals and the process. The irony of those at the top imposing a bottom-up community development process was not lost on some Prevention Coordinators and schools. At the same time, some Prevention Coordinators were able to make these strategies work for them in engaging participation of community members in both implementation and evaluation of their projects.

Cross-Case Comparison of Empowerment

In this section, we compare the enactment of empowerment in the two cases. First, we present a summary table that outlines the main themes for comparison with respect to the principle of empowerment across both cases, and then we elaborate on these themes as they apply in each case. As with the cross-case comparison of participation above, we chose the themes because they were relevant to both cases, and again, their relative importance in each case varied. The exception is the first category, the way of being of the practitioner, which was the most important factor in both cases (Table 9.2).

Practitioner's Empowering Orientation or Way of Being

Participation is a major factor influencing the development of empowerment at the individual and the community level. It is theorized that in participating, individuals

Table 9.2 Case comparison of empowerment

Themes	Case 1: Queen Alexandra Community Projects	Case 2: School-Based Prevention Project
Way of Being	• Creating a comfortable environment • Building trust and relationships	• Power with vs. power over • Empowering orientation
Empowering Strategies	• Disempowering nature of measurement instruments • Issue of vulnerability • The subtlety of empowerment • Group format • Evaluation as intervention	• Measurement can be empowering • Evaluation as intervention

and communities learn to take control over the influences on their health. Although participation was an important factor in the experiences of empowerment in the projects in both Cases 1 and 2, the main mechanism to promote empowerment was actually the way of being demonstrated by project coordinators, program staff, Prevention Coordinators, and school administrators.

In Case 1, the practitioners were fully aware that some participants had negative experiences with institutions in the past. As part of their plans to build rapport they also concentrated on the physical environment, trying as much as possible to simulate a casual home-like environment. Throughout all their interactions the coordinators used their skills to make participants feel recognized, competent, and part of the group. As participants developed trust for the motivations and the honesty of the coordinators, they in turn came to trust the project. In all of the projects in Case 1, the projects largely succeeded due to the competence and way of being of the coordinators. The significance of this aspect was not fully revealed in the evaluations (probably because the coordinators would have been reluctant to ask about it when conducting the evaluations).

In Case 2, those individuals who worked in collaborative and egalitarian ways, adopting a *power with* approach, had quite different outcomes in their schools than those who tended to take control and work in hierarchical and '*power over*' ways (Labonte, 1993). When both the Prevention Coordinator and the school administrators demonstrated a highly empowering orientation, the level of participation in all aspects of the project was much higher than in schools in which either the Prevention Coordinator or the school administrators did not demonstrate an empowering way of being. Furthermore, student experiences of having a say in school governance were stronger in those schools in which both Prevention Coordinators and administrators demonstrated a highly empowering orientation. Even in schools in which the administration did not demonstrate an empowering orientation, the strength of the Prevention Coordinators' orientation facilitated a significant degree of participation and change. It was in such a school that the students used the survey data to lobby for changes in student involvement in school governance, and the initiation of programs and policies to enhance school climate.

Evaluation Methods That Promote Empowerment

In the Case 1, community action projects coordinators are accountable for producing some kind of change to justify the investment of funds. Without the time or the experience to explore creative research methods that are congruent with the intent of the program, there is often an over reliance on pre and post tests. With a vulnerable population, however, such as the mothers in these programs, the issues are more serious than achieving methodological congruence. These mothers are in a situation in which some one is looking over their shoulder (often a social worker) to ensure that they are doing a good job of keeping their children safe. If they are not, the evaluation could have negative consequences for the mothers. This has important implications for participation.

Any evaluation that appears to be testing a program participant's ability as a parent is disempowering and regarded with distrust. In addition, these mothers have not written a test for many years and find them intimidating. Anything involving paper and pencil looks like a test. In some cases, low literacy is also a limiting factor. We had to carefully design the evaluation questions for interviews or discussions so that they did not imply a previous failure in parenting but rather they contributed to positive reinforcement of their current abilities. In other words, the evaluation had to serve as part of the intervention.

In a project for mothers with learning difficulties, the coordinator and evaluator looked at two assessment forms. It was clear that one of the tests would likely make the mothers feel scrutinized and they could feel inadequate after completing it, whereas the other test was a list of things that a parent might do to make sure that a child is physically safe in and out of the house. We determined that the list of safety issues was quite extensive, and the coordinator knew through her interactions with the mothers that they had already made some of these changes in their homes to ensure safety. If a mother was able to circle some of the items, this could be positive reinforcement and allow her to show what she had accomplished toward making the home environment safer. The other items on the list would be a good reminder of what remained to be done and thus a part of the intervention. Because the list was extensive and there was no timeline for doing them, there need not be a feeling of failure since participants could do these items in the future. While this was not participatory, it was empowering in that the mothers could identify their own progress. Others have also observed that active participation is not always necessary to empower or emancipate participants (Themessl-Huber & Grutsch, 2003; Wallerstein, 2006).

In another project designed to enhance parenting skills, the coordinators and their staff were very experienced in empowering clients, but this type of work, when done well, is extremely subtle, almost invisible work. This is the very quality that makes it empowering – program participants feel they are achieving goals through their own hard work since parenting skills were not specifically taught in a formal structure. Rather, by interacting with the parents while they engaged in routine activities with their children, the coordinators observed teachable moments and engaged parents in discussions about options for dealing with their child's behavior. To the parents it would appear, not as teaching, but as talking with the coordinator. Given this subtlety, how then do you evaluate meeting the objectives of the program?

Standard program evaluation questions such as, "What was the most important thing that you learned in this program?" would get the response: "I didn't learn anything, I just had lunch with my child at the program." Given the context of this program and the nature of the issues experienced by the women, the evaluation was designed so that, (a) it would act as a further intervention for learning, and (b) that it would bring into consciousness (the process Freire (1970) called conscientization) what they had gained in the program while maintaining their power and reinforcing their learning.

We decided to use a group format so that the synergistic dynamics of the group created a kind of collective memory for what had been learned without any one individual having to take particular ownership of learning anything new and therefore acknowledging to the authorities that they didn't know what they were doing previously. It also solved the problem of low literacy experienced by some women. The evaluation consultant, the coordinator and the staff generated the questions.

At the beginning of the group sessions, staff asked participants the evaluation questions and documented participant feedback on flipchart paper. Each question was on a separate piece of paper. After each question was asked, discussed, and documented, participants taped it to the wall in the group room. When discussion of each question was completed, we taped all of the flipchart paper around the room while the group took a break for food. Participants were urged to add any thoughts to the posted questions at any time during the rest of the session. This allowed for processing and discussion time so that those who may not have had an opportunity to get their opinions and thoughts on paper had that chance. This process worked well because (a) it allows parents to demonstrate what they know and therefore continues the empowerment process, (b) it eliminates the pressure individuals might feel to demonstrate a change in knowledge and/or behavior, (c) the group process helps individuals who may have difficulty articulating what they have learned, and (d) it builds on and summarizes what participants have learned and thus provides an opportunity for reinforcing key ideas as a closing exercise.

The approaches used with the mothers were not fully participatory but they did contribute to their sense of accomplishment and therefore were congruent with an empowering approach. An important learning in the Case 1 projects was that top-down projects in which participants did not necessarily engage voluntarily or participate in early planning could still be empowering through participatory dialogue and other processes that allowed for personal meaning making.

In Case 2, we previously discussed several of the strategies used to facilitate participation in the implementation and evaluation of the projects, including the student survey interpretation, the steering committee, and the planning model. Of these, involving students and teachers in interpreting and using the data to facilitate changes in the school environment was the most empowering of the methods used. The others might well have resulted in empowerment if greater participation in the early program decisions had been facilitated. Other than the survey, however, none of these was as effective in facilitating empowerment among participants as the way of being of the prevention coordinator.

Marrying Health Promotion Principles and Evaluation: Lessons from the Field

Throughout this discussion, we have resisted taking a toolbox approach to categorizing the lessons of our work, despite our desire to be very practical about health promotion. It has been a challenge to synthesize our lessons in a systematic way, in part, because the complexity of health promotion processes often defies the imposition of an organizing framework. Nonetheless, we have learned some lessons about facilitating participation and empowerment in evaluation and have found some strategies that work better than others. However, these take the form of generalized principles rather than concrete tools and they are not rocket science. To many health promoters and evaluators, they will seem very basic.

As a result of our analysis, we conclude that the nature of participation and the potential for empowerment in health promotion evaluation, hinge on at least seven factors that emerged as key themes in our cross-case analysis. In Table 9.3, we present these seven cross-cutting themes and the elements of those themes for each of our cases, and following that, we elaborate on those themes.

Nature of the Health Promotion Intervention and Evaluation

Developmental Stage

What is possible in terms of participation, and the potential for empowerment is contingent on the nature of the health promotion intervention and its evaluation as well as on the context within which it occurs. A number of key features of the intervention provide both opportunities and constraints for implementing and evaluating in ways that are sensitive to health promotion principles.

The developmental stage of the intervention is an important consideration. Some health promotion interventions are already established with clear goals and objectives, best practices identified, and resources in place. In Case 1, project proposals prescribed the activities and funding was awarded on the assumption that these activities would be conducted as described. Within the project, participants may have been treated in a participatory way, nonetheless the course is preset. The reason we do evaluation, in fact, is to identify effective programs and practices that can be used in other settings with other populations. The potential for participation in planning and developing the intervention is limited in these circumstances, although

Table 9.3 Thematic analysis

Cross-Cutting Themes	Case 1: Queen Alexandra Community Projects	Case 2: School Based Prevention Project
Nature of the Intervention and Evaluation		
Developmental Stage	• Project previously established with already defined goals and objectives limits participation in the entire planning process • Best practices already defined • Ongoing programming	• New project going through a developmental process provides more scope for participation throughout
Scale	• Early participants more likely to participate in designing evaluation but nature of participation can be re-conceptualized depending on stage • Small scale projects at the community level • Small groups of participants • Capacity for authentic participation may be greater in some ways at the community level	• Early participants more likely to participate in designing evaluation but nature of participation can be re-conceptualized depending on stage • Provincial level – large scale • Multiple sites, thousands of participants • Less potential for authentic participation • Community level – smaller scale, fewer participants • Capacity for authentic participation may be greater in some ways at community level
Power	• Mothers at risk for losing children • Researchers and staff power vs. mothers' power • Nature of participation depends on power dynamics	• Researchers vs. community members as having more power • Pressure on coordinators for positive outcomes • Nature of participation depends on power dynamics
Evaluation Methods	• Some methods appear participatory but are not	• Some methods do not seem participatory but may be
Vulnerability	• Participation can have negative consequences • Issue of voluntary vs. non-voluntary participation • Participation requires painstaking care, trust, and relationship building • Testing perceived as negative and risky	• A different kind of vulnerability than in Case 1 • Different participants vulnerable in different ways • Testing perceived as the norm
Evaluation as Intervention	• Evaluation strategies deliberately designed to reinforce particular effects and to contribute to further learning	• Evaluation strategies sometimes produce incidental vs deliberate intervention effects
Way of Being	• Key factor in aligning health promotion and evaluation	• Key factor in aligning health promotion and evaluation

participation in planning and implementing the evaluation remains a possibility. In other interventions, such as the school-based project, the process is developmental and not specified in advance. In this situation, there is considerably more scope for participating in the entire process.

The developmental stage of the evaluation is also an important factor in defining what kind of participation is possible. In both cases, early participants had more opportunities to participate in designing the evaluation than later participants. It is important to recognize, however, that participation is not static and differs at each stage. Participation occurs along a continuum such that not all people can participate in all stages of a project, but all can participate in some stages. Not all participation can meet the ideals of authentic participation, but many less intensive forms of participation can have important benefits. Thus, participation needs to be concep-tualized broadly, but every opportunity must be taken to encourage participation within the constraints of the intervention and its context.

Scale

The scale of the intervention and evaluation is another factor that influences the quality and nature of participation and empowerment. In Case 1, the interventions were small scale community level projects, with small groups of participants. The potential for participation of a majority of participants and the achievement of empowerment among those participants is therefore considerable. In Case 2, how-ever, the project took place at two levels: local and provincial. Multiple sites were involved with thousands of participants. The potential for a high level of participa-tion throughout the process is greatly constrained in such circumstances; the nature of participation and the methods to facilitate it will necessarily look quite different at the larger system level than they do at the local level.

When it is not possible to involve everyone, we need to find ways to maximize representativeness of participants and build in mechanisms to ensure input and feed-back to stakeholders. Representatives must be selected carefully for their ability to be open, honest, and respectful of diversity. Evaluators should reflect critically on their own processes and draw on the learning from those reflections to feed it back into the evaluation. In large scale projects in which full participation is not possible, decisions about who to focus on for participation can be facilitated first and foremost by consultation with diverse community members, but also by considering project goals, values, and theories guiding both the project and its evaluation. Finally, in sit-uations of non-voluntary participation, careful attention to building trust, developing supportive, respectful, and honest relationships is paramount.

In health promotion, we are concerned not only about individual health and well-being, but also about population health. It is therefore important that we use multiple strategies at multiple levels across multiple sectors in a "whole systems or ecologi-cal approach" (Springett, 2001, p. 140). This complexity requires interventions that take place at both local and systems levels and thus present considerable challenges for achieving effective and authentic participation and engaging in processes that are truly empowering. In fact, other health promotion principles (i.e., intersectoral collaboration and multiple strategies) themselves present constraints to the type of participation that can occur in any given health promotion program. The premise of this book, however, is not that evaluation should demonstrate defined types of participation or empowering strategies, but that evaluators must be sensitive to the principles. What is meant by being sensitive, likely varies. In both cases, we used a number of very simple strategies to facilitate participation and empowerment within the context of these programs. These may not work elsewhere because they may not fit the situation. What is important is that program staff and evaluators need to be responsive to the situation. At the same time, the following personal characteristics are important: leadership, an empowering orientation, respectful and caring relationships, creativity and the ability to be an "animator" (Rahman, 1993). In addition, it is important to create opportunities for group dialogue, collective action, advocacy and leadership training (Wallerstein, 2006). Readers who are looking for creative ways to engage youth can find a number of excellent engagement strategies in a variety of resources (e.g., Paul & Lefkovitz, 2006), but we believe that we were indeed sensitive to these principles even though neither participation nor empowerment was enacted perfectly in our cases.

Power

Power is a central feature in community work of any kind. The word empowerment itself is about power. The nature and type of participation in health promotion evaluation is contingent on the power dynamics in the situation. The influence of power on participation and empowerment was evident in so many ways in both our cases. In Case 1, the projects were smaller, local and scheduled as a series of small groups. In these cases it was easier for the coordinators to develop relationships that approximated if not wholly achieving equality. The coordinators by virtue of their expertise in community development work were skilled in facilitation and education that was participatory. But even their skills could not eliminate the influence of the greater context of the power of government agencies over some of the participants, such as the justice system in the case of the youth or the Ministry for Children and Families in the case of the mothers.

In Case 2, the Prevention Coordinators were actually vulnerable and powerless in several situations. They often were unable to name issues or speak the truth about those issues because school administrators did not want to put themselves or their schools in a bad light. Foucault's notion of power (Foucault, 1980) is relevant here; that is, "power relations permeate all levels of social existence and are therefore to be found operating at every site of social life" (Hall, 2001, p. 77). Everyone is caught up in the circulation of power and any person may be both an oppressor and oppressed. The Prevention Coordinators were in a powerful position relative to students but were themselves vulnerable to the exercise of power by those in authority in the schools.

One issue of power that emerged related to the question of who defines the focus for health promotion. Ideally, the community should decide on the issue of focus for health promotion and its evaluation. When this is not possible because of funding requirements, for example, health promoters and evaluators can begin where the community is at (Nyswander, 1955), working with community-defined issues, building trust, and through critical dialogue and questioning may ultimately be able to mobilize the community around the defined issue, but only if this is a concern that the community agrees is relevant. Without that agreement, the goals of the project will inevitably be co-opted by the status quo.

There are no simple tools for dealing with power relations. They are complex and often unacknowledged. We discuss this issue in more detail in the discussion below, but the most important lesson we learned in our projects was that it is critical to acknowledge the power differentials, and to work collaboratively to find ways to minimize inequities arising out of these differences. Again, we do not have an easy answer, but it boils down to the evaluator or health practitioner's way of being and ability to build trust and establish caring and respectful relationships. It is all about relationships.

Evaluation Methods

Springett (2001) has implied that particular types of methods are more appropriate than others for evaluating health promotion, in part because they are more likely to facilitate participation and empowerment. Traditional evaluation approaches (e.g., experimental designs, quantitative surveys using standardized measures) are often characterized as not conducive to the goals of health promotion, perhaps because they may reinforce the marginalization already experienced by particular population groups (Springett, 2001).

Although we agree that, in general, this may be true, in our experience, no one method or approach is appropriate in all circumstances and methods that some health promotion advocates suggest are inappropriate, may in fact be quite effective. Our findings suggest that a survey, for example, used well, can be both empowering and participatory, depending on the context, circumstances, and population. Similarly, Greene (1994) argues that it is not the methods used that are critically important but rather how they are used. Conversely, some methods, on the face of it, may appear participatory but are not. This was the situation in Case 1, in which a tool to measure assets can be assumed to be more empowering than focusing on deficits, but could potentially have the opposite effect.

Vulnerability

The importance of participation and empowerment and the ways in which these are facilitated is considerably more important with vulnerable or marginalized populations than with mainstream groups. Participating in an evaluation can have negative consequences for vulnerable groups, particularly if they are not always participating in a completely voluntary way. It is important to be aware that participation in health promotion programs and their evaluations may actually have negative consequences for some participants. This was particularly true in the programs for the mothers in Case 1. Participation could have been perceived as quite risky by these women when there is a danger that their responses to evaluation activities have the potential to result in children being removed from the home. To achieve authentic participation with vulnerable groups requires painstaking care to develop trusting relationships and this may take a very long time.

Also important to consider is that the reliability and validity of particular methods may be compromised when applied to vulnerable populations because of the potential for negative consequences. A complete understanding is necessary of the ways in which the evaluation may appear to be testing or judging or otherwise imposing a set of standards on families or youth who have a history of low self esteem, economic disadvantage or who feel they have little self determination. For vulnerable populations there are many more reasons to distrust anything that appears to be, at best a research project that will benefit someone else, and at worst an authoritative critique of their life.

Evaluation as Intervention

In traditional approaches to research, researchers have long recognized that the process of measurement can affect the outcome, thus potentially introducing a bias. They develop sophisticated designs to try to control for measurement effects. In health promotion evaluation, we do not consider this effect a bias. Rather, we try to develop evaluation frameworks that allow us to take advantage of the evaluation as intervention, while also accounting for it in our findings.

As Springett points out, "the boundary between the 'intervention' and the social process or context in which it occurs is often blurred" (Springett, 2001, p. 140). So too is the boundary between evaluation and intervention. In both of our cases, aspects of the evaluation influenced some outcomes, and thus were deliberately or incidentally a part of the intervention. In the School Based Project, the student participation in data analysis and interpretation resulted in feelings of empowerment. This in turn, led to new actions that contributed to changes in the school environment that were later conducive to the empowerment of other students. Thus, the original students' participation became a part of the intervention although not initially planned that way. In Case 1, evaluation strategies were deliberately designed to reinforce particular effects thus becoming an ongoing part of the intervention.

Health promotion involves multiple strategies at multiple levels, none of which occur in a linear way. In fact, from an ecological perspective, there is an ongoing iterative and reciprocal relationship between the individual (or group), their own and others' actions, and the environment. Because there is no clear linear or unidirectional relationship between input and outcome, it makes little sense to worry about contaminating or biasing the intervention with evaluation measures or processes.

All evaluations have the potential to affect those involved. In health promotion practice it behooves the practitioner or evaluator to ensure that the evaluation has a positive effect. Indeed, as illustrated above, there are many opportunities for the evaluation to contribute to and enhance the intervention and to further the empowering intentions of the projects. On the other hand, the simplest and most innocuous of methods may have very negative and unanticipated consequences. Thus, evaluation is not a neutral process. It has an impact on participants that goes beyond the impact of the health promotion intervention. The elements of the evaluation that may constitute an important intervention may not be recognized. At times, this intervention may be desirable, and at other times not, so it is important for evaluators to think about it and take this into account in the analysis. There is no one way to do this, and no particular principle that can be named, but critical reflexivity on the part of the evaluator is essential.

Way of Being of the Practitioner/Evaluator

In most instances, aligning health promotion principles and evaluation starts and ends with the practitioner's way of being in the community. It is not about the choice of methods or tools, but rather it depends on the ability of the practitioner to develop a way of being that participants experience as authentic. Reason points out that we "need the support of the community in order to follow a discipline" (Reason, 1994, p. 40). In other words, without the community we are not able to engage in our practice of health promotion. Relationships and our way of being in the world are health promoting.

Conclusion

Through the discussion of the above evaluation issues it should be clear that health promotion work invariably involves field work. As most practitioners would attest, field work is exciting and engaging partly because of the many challenges it presents. One of the greatest challenges is managing the power dynamics. As described earlier, part of the role of the researcher is to develop the ability of others to take charge of decisions that affect their lives including the evaluation processes. Yet the researcher has to serve the double purpose of being responsible for empowering practices while serving the larger goal of producing relevant knowledge for many stakeholders (e.g., funders, community members, staff, the scientific community).

We have tried to illustrate that there are appropriate and non-appropriate approaches to evaluating health promotion but we would also argue that this is not a simple dichotomy. For us the most important issue is the vulnerability of the population with whom one is conducting the evaluation and that appropriateness refers more to the process of how it is conducted rather than a specific method. A researcher with the ability to be creative and flexible is able to adapt what might appear to be non-participatory methods into collaborative tools and to use the process as a means of empowerment. We make the exception for methods such as randomized control trials but these are not usually part of the tool kit of health promotion evaluators. Conversely, a researcher can inadvertently introduce disempowering practices into participatory approaches.

We do, however, want to emphasize the importance of a participatory and empowering approach. For researchers/evaluators the consequences of a flawed research design are far less than for those with whom we are collaborating. The evaluation takes place in the lived space (Bollnow, 1961) of community members. This lived space encompasses social, historical, past and future relationships. For the evaluator, the evaluation is a point in time whereas for the community members there may be grim consequences for being involved that profoundly affect their future. In Case 1, the process or the results of the evaluation could have resulted in mothers losing the custody of their children; in Case 2 the coordinators could have lost their jobs. It is not a distant activity for them but rather a living through something that teaches them something about themselves and their world in such a way as to alter their understanding about themselves (Kugelman, 2004).

What we have described as the evaluator's or the coordinator's way of being in the community encompasses a consciousness of all the contingencies in the context of the participants' lives as well as an awareness of the cultural locatedness of our theories and methods (Murray, 2004). In the same way that health promotion principles guide us to consider the social and economic conditions of health, our evaluation theories and practices should lead us to engage with community members to understand how these conditions manifest themselves in their everyday lives and how we can develop preventative practices together. Stam has written that communities in need of preventative practices are "real consumers of knowledge and care but also crucibles of wisdom and knowledge" (Stam, 2004, p. 28), but if that knowledge is to be harnessed it will not be along the lines of some universal functional model far removed from the community members' experience.

A lack of congruence between health promotion principles and evaluation practices not only is methodologically unsound, but also approaches unethical conduct given the potential for residual negative effects left in the researcher's wake. In addition, it is clear from the examples in the two cases described above that in those situations where there was greater congruence between principles and practice there was better data. Thus, not only are ethical principles at stake but also better science.

References

Arnstein, S. (1969). A ladder of citizen participation. *Journal of the American Institute of Planners, 35*(4), 216–224.

Becker, A. B., Israel, B. A., Schultz, A. J., Parker, E. A., & Klem, L. (2002). Predictors of perceived control among African American women in Detroit: Exploring empowerment as a multilevel construct. *Health Education and Behavior, 29*(6), 699–715.

Bollnow, O. F. (1961). Lived space. *Philosophy Today, 5*, 31–39.

Butterfoss, F. (2006). Process evaluation of community participation. *Annual Review of Public Health, 27*, 323–340.

Clark, D. L. (1981). *Rational planning in curriculum and instruction*. Washington, DC: National Education Association.

Flick, U. (2006). *An introduction to qualitative research* (3rd ed.). London: Sage Publications.

Foucault, M. (1980). *Power/knowledge*. Brighton: Harvester.

Freire, P. (1970). *Pedagogy of the oppressed*. New York: Continuum Press.

Glaser, B., & Strauss, A. (1967). *The discovery of grounded theory*. Strategies for qualitative research. Chicago: Aldine.

Green, L. W., & Kreuter, M. W. (1991). *Health promotion planning: An educational and environmental approach*. Mountain View, CA: Mayfield Publishing Company.

Greene, J. (1994). Qualitative program evaluation: Practice and promise. In N. K. Denzin & Y. S. Lincoln (Eds.), *Handbook of qualitative research*. Thousand Oaks: Sage Publications.

Gregory, A. (2000). Problematizing participation: A critical review of approaches to participation in evaluation theory. *Evaluation, 6*(2), 179–199.

Hall, S. (2001). Foucault: Power, knowledge and discourse. In M. Weatherall, S. Taylor, & S. J. Yates (Eds.), *Discourse theory and practice: A reader* (pp. 72–81). London: Sage Publications.

Hargreaves, A. (1994). *Changing teachers, changing times*. Toronto: Ontario Institute for Studies in Education.

Jayaratna, N. (1994). *Understanding and evaluating methodologies: NIMSAD A systematic framework*. London: McGraw-Hill.

Kotilla, W. (2005). *Youth and ecological restoration project final report*. Victoria, Queen Alexandra Hospital Foundation. Retrieved on January 31, 2006 www.queenalexandra.org/

Kugelman, R. (2004). Health and illness: A hermeneutical phenomenological approach. In M. Murray (Ed.), *Critical health psychology* (pp. 44–57). Basingstoke, England: Palgrave Macmillan.

Labonte, R. (1993). *Health promotion and empowerment: Practice frameworks*. Toronto: Centre for Health Promotion, University of Toronto and Participaction.

Labonte, R., & Laverack, G. (2001). Capacity building in health promotion, Part 2: whose use? And with what measurement? *Critical Public Health, 11*(2), 129–138.

Laverack, G. & Wallerstein, N. (2001). Measuring community empowerment: A fresh look at organizational domains. *Health Promotion International, 16*(2), 179–185.

Lewin, K. (1952). *Group decision and social change*. In G. E. Swanson, T. M. Newcomb, & E. L. Hartley (Eds.), *Readings in social psychology*. New York: Henry Holt.

Louis, K. S., & Miles, M. B. (1990). *Improving the urban high school: What works and why*. New York: Teachers College |Press.

MacDonald, M., & Green, L. W. (2001). Reconciling concept and context: The dilemma of implementation in school-based health promotion. *Health Education and Behavior, 28*(6), 749–768.

Miles, M., & Huberman, M. (1994). *Qualitative data analysis: An expanded sourcebook*. Thousand Oaks: Sage Publications.

Miller, G., Mullett, J., & VanSant, D. (2006). *Community youth development: An evaluation of four communities, province of British Colombia*. British Colombia: Community Youth Development Coalition-BC.

Murray, M. (2004). Conclusion: Towards a critical health psychology. In M. Murray (Ed.), *Critical health psychology* (pp. 222–229). Basingstoke, England: Palgrave Macmillan.

Nyswander, D. (1955). Education for health: Some principles and their applications. *Health Education Monographs, 14*, 65–70.

Pavis, S., Constable, H., & Masters, H. (2003). Multi-agency, multi-professional work: Experiences from a drug prevention project. *Health Education Research, 18*(6), 717–728.

Paul, A., & Lefkovitz, B. (2006). Engaging youth: A how-to guide for creating opportunities for young people to participate, lead and succeed. *Sierra Health Foundation*. Accessed July 10, 2006. http://www.sierrahealth.org/programs/reach/docs/Engaging_Youth_Report.pdf

Potvin, L., Cargo, M., McComber, A. M., Delormier, T., & Macaulay, A. C. (2003). Implementing participatory intervention and research in communities: Lessons from Kahnawake Schools Diabetes Prevention Project in Canada. *Social Science and Medicine, 56*(6), 1295–1305.

Queen Alexandra Foundation. (2004). Strategic Investment Initiatives Fund (SIIF) Grants. www.queenalexandra.org

Rahman, M. A. (1993). *People's self development*. London: Zed Books.

Reason, P. (1994). *Participation in human inquiry*. London: Sage Publications.

Rebein, C. C. (1996). Participatory evaluation of development assistance: Dealing with power and facilitative learning. *Evaluation, 2*, 151–172.

Schwandt, T. (2001). *Dictionary of qualitative inquiry* (2nd ed.). Thousand Oaks: Sage Publications.

Simovska, V. (2004). Student participation: a democratic education perspective – experience from the health promoting schools in Macedonia. *Health Education Research, 19*, 198–207.

Speer, P. W., Jackson, C. B., & Peterson, N. A. (2001). The relationship between social cohesion and empowerment: Support and new implications for theory. *Health Education and Behavior, 28*, 716–732.

Springett, J. (2001). Appropriate approaches to the evaluation of health promotion. *Critical Public Health, 11*, 139–151.

Stake, R. (1995). *The art of case study research.* Thousand Oaks: Sage Publications.

Stam, H. J. (2004). A sound mind in a sound body: A critical historical analysis of health psychology. In M. Murray (Ed.), *Critical health psychology* (pp. 15–30). Basingstoke, England: Palgrave Macmillan.

Themessl-Huber, M. T., & Grutsch, M. A. (2003). The shifting locus of control in participatory evaluations. *Evaluation, 9*, 92–111.

Tjora, A. H. (2006). Writing small discoveries: An exploration of fresh observers' observations. *Qualitative Research, 6*, 429–451.

Strauss, A., & Corbin, J. (1997). *Basics of qualitative research.* Thousand Oaks: Sage Publications.

Wallerstein, N. (2006). *What is the evidence on the effectiveness of empowerment to improve health?* Copenhagen, WHO Regional Office for Europe. (Health Evidence Network Report; Accessed February 18, 2006 http://www.euro.who.int/Document/E88086.pdf.)

Wang, C., & Burris, M. A. (1997). Photovoice: Concept, methodology, and use for participatory needs assessment. *Health Education and Behavior, 24*(3), 369–387.

World Health Organization. (1986). *Ottawa charter for health promotion.* Ottawa: World Health Organization, Health and Welfare Canada, Canadian Public Health Association.

Chapter 10
Formative Evaluation and Community Empowerment Among American Indian/Alaska Natives

C. June Strickland, Felicia Hodge, and Lillian Tom-Orme

While reports on progress in achieving Healthy People 2010 objectives show minor decreases in some areas for American Indian and Alaska Native (AI/AN) populations, significant disparities still remain in chronic disease prevention/management such as mental health concerns (youth suicide and domestic violence), cancer, and diabetes (Casper et al., 2005; CDC, 2003; Edwards, 2001; Robin, Chester, Rasmussen, Jaranson, & Goldman, 1997; Strickland, 1997; Swan and Edwards, 2003). The burden of health disparities is especially heavy for AI/AN populations according to the Centers for Disease Control and Prevention (CDC, 2003). In this discussion, we will focus on our research in priority areas among AI/AN populations such as suicide prevention, cancer prevention and diabetes. Our aim is to highlight the importance of formative evaluation and qualitative approaches such as feasibility studies and focus groups combined with community based participatory research (CBPR) in laying the foundation for successful outcome and impact research that builds community capacity. Such approaches in health promotion evaluation are deemed crucial in balancing power, assuring culturally appropriate work to address community needs, and in addressing health inequalities in work with vulnerable populations.

Formative Evaluation, Cultural Appropriateness and Empowerment

In the behavioral sciences it is well recognized that evaluation may be both formative/process oriented and summative that includes both outcome and impact (Anderson & McFarlane, 2004; Butterfoss, Francisco, & Capwell, 2001; Williams, Belle, Houston, Haire-Joshu, Auslander, 2001; Lafferty & Mahoney, 2003). Green and Lewis (1986) note that the term, formative evaluation, "refers to the provision of short-loop diagnostic feedback about the quality and implementation of and immediate response to – methods, activities, or programs" (p. 27). Windsor,

C.J. Strickland
University of Washington, Seattle, WA, USA

L. Potvin, D. McQueen (eds.), *Health Promotion Evaluation Practices in the Americas*,
DOI: 10.1007/978-0-387-79733-5_10, © Springer Science+Business Media, LLC 2008   179

Baranowski, Clark, and Cutter (1984) distinguish between formative and process evaluation and suggest that formative evaluation produces information during the developmental stages of a health education program and that process evaluation provides information during the implementation. Both Green and Lewis (1986) and Windsor, (1984) note that focus groups, and pilot studies, pre-testing and seeking feedback through observations, participant observation and interviews with those involved in program implementation are all research methods that are a part of formative and process evaluation strategies. Formative and process evaluation focus on the work in progress and seek to answer questions about how appropriate the materials are for the intended population in the intervention, management issues in terms of the utilization and training of key personnel, the process of implementation, details such as the size and shape of the room, time allotted for activities, to name a few (Anderson & McFarlane, 2004; Butterfoss et al., 2001; Williams et al., 2001; Lafferty & Mahoney, 2003).

Huff and Kline (1999) note that the selection of an appropriate evaluation approach in Native Communities is dependent on a number of factors such as the stakeholders' concerns, the potential use of the information, the epistemological framework, the values that guide the work, and most importantly, the Native community perspectives on all these issues. In this discussion, we will highlight our work in formative and process evaluation and provide illustrations of evaluation that has provided the foundation for more culturally appropriate intervention design and that has also contributed to community empowerment.

Cultural appropriateness is crucial in successful health promotion programs in Native communities and formative evaluation is key to the design of culturally appropriate interventions. Stanhope and Lancaster (2002) suggest that cultural appropriateness in community health means that care is designed for the specific client, family, or community based on an understanding of cultural norms and values and supports empowerment. Likewise Clark (2006) speaks of the importance of cultural appropriateness in community health work and cautions against cultural stereotyping that may occur with individuals, families, and groups. Strickland, Squeoch and Chrisman (1999) provide an example of what it means to be culturally appropriate in one Native community in their publication on the Wa' Shat Longhouse practices and the relation to cancer prevention intervention among Yakama Indian women. Formative evaluation, including the use of focus groups provided needed information about social interactions and normative behaviors that were crucial in intervention design.

Evaluation Practices to Enhance Culturally Appropriate Interventions and Community Empowerment

In this discussion, we will consider research that falls into the category of formative and process evaluation that enhances cultural appropriateness, lays the foundation for more successful intervention design and outcome evaluation with Indian people, and supports community empowerment. Included in this discussion are feasibility efforts and focus group work in which community-based participatory research methods and/or philosophy were also employed to enhance community voice. In some study examples, multiple approaches were employed. In all we emphasize the importance of involving the community and the importance of community-based participatory research. We will also show how the formative evaluation approaches have led to successful outcome evaluation research.

Feasibility Pilot Research

Feasibility research aims to address practical issues in program implementation and thus is considered a formative evaluation method (Creswell, 1994; Mitchell & Jolly, 1992). In feasibility efforts, the researcher aims to answer crucial questions about the potential for implementing an intervention and formulated in terms of recruitment, personnel needed and preparation of personnel, appropriateness of materials, and outcome instruments and measurements (Creswell, 1994). The following example of research in suicide prevention provides greater understanding of the importance of feasibility pilot efforts.

In a five year National Institute of Nursing Research (NINR) funded research effort (Strickland, 2002), the goal was to determine the feasibility of implementing two intervention approaches to reduce AI/AN youth suicide risk and to gain insights into the cultural context in which suicide risk occurs. The study involved both qualitative and quantitative methods; both interventions examined had been found to be efficacious in reducing suicide risk among non-Indian populations.

In the first phase of the study, efforts were directed toward gaining understanding of the implementation issues in a six-week education program to provide coping and skills training through the Coping and Skills Training Program (CAST). The study was conducted in a rural reservation community in the Pacific Northwest; the tribe wanted the program to be conducted in tribal facilities in the community rather than the schools and aimed to provide transportation for students to attend. In this pilot evaluation effort, that took place over a three-month period, extensive observation field notes were taken (Burgess, 1999; Sajik, 1990). Research efforts were focused on formative evaluation in the examination of feasibility implementation issues such as recruitment, the cost in time, travel, and potential adjustments in the curriculum that might be needed to make it culturally appropriate.

The first obstacle encountered was recruitment. The screening risk survey instrument did not seem to work well. In one month, only 20 students were identified as being eligible to begin the program. It was recognized that we could reach all our potential pool and not be able to pilot another phase of the program, the individual counseling program. It was decided that we would proceed with only six students to implement the group education program. The next obstacle encountered was transportation. The tribe had thought that it would be able to transport students from over a 40-mile distance to the program each week. In reality, we had to drive about one and one-half hours to the reservation and then devote another one to two hours driving to locate and get students to the program. The cost in time and travel was extensive. The program was to be implemented each week for a six-week period; on several occasions, it was not possible to offer the program as planned due to a community event that superceded the program. For example, a death in the community resulted in all programs being closed. It was possible to complete the six-week program but not in six weeks. Another problem encountered was program participants. In one case, one of the students who had screened in as eligible for the intervention attended about half of the sessions; his mother sent another brother, who was younger and who had never been screened into the program, for about half of the sessions. It would have been culturally inappropriate to turn this young man away and thus we were only able to track data on five of the six young people in the program. Yet another obstacle was the curriculum. While most sessions worked well, one in particular that was designed to address coping with anger and communications in personal interactions did not. In this session, when students were asked to discuss situations that made them angry, they focused on racism and intergenerational pain. For example, one student stated: "I'm pissed as hell with the rape of our land." The coping training was not designed to address intergenerational pain and anger.

From this formative evaluation, it was determined that the travel costs, difficulties in staying on schedule, and obtaining adequate numbers to conduct outcome evaluation were major obstacles to implementation of this intervention in this community and revisions would be needed in the CAST program to make it more culturally appropriate. We decided to focus on the individual intervention counseling instead.

The intervention counseling took place in schools near the reservation in a Pacific Northwest Indian community during the regular school year. In this work, we achieved over a 95% recruitment and retention rate (Strickland, 2002) and were indeed able to collect sufficient data to measure outcomes. A few minor adjustments were made where there was flexibility in the protocol to make it more culturally appropriate. In this respect, rather than making telephone calls to families of youth found to be at high suicide risk, home visits were made; the message about the risk was reframed in a positive way to prevent bringing the spirit of suicide into the community and the word "suicide" was never used in the program title. This intervention built on previous formative evaluation and emphasized community values in that youth became committed to helping other youth and their community. Culturally appropriate community recognition and ceremonies were provided for these youth who participated in the program.

Focus Groups and Community-Based Participatory Research

As an introduction to the discussion of focus groups and CBPR work, let us first consider the cultural issues in implementing focus groups with Indian people and the key concepts in CBPR. This will be followed by examples of evaluation research in which multiple methods were used including focus groups and CBPR. It is important to recognize that conducting focus groups in an Indian community is very different from work in non-Native communities. From many years of conducting focus groups among Indian people in the Pacific Northwest, Strickland (1999) suggests that the researcher should be mindful of the level of acculturation and communication patterns of the group to be involved in a focus group, and that the guidelines for conducting focus groups may have to be modified. She found among the Indian people of the Pacific Northwest that it was important to allocate three to four hours for the focus group work and to have ample food and gifts. Time needed to be allocated to allow the community to respond in a Talking Circle fashion in which each individual speaks. It was possible to tape record the work but the tape recorder needed to be kept going throughout the work. After a Talking Circle pattern of communication, refreshments were provided, and after eating the groups engaged in an interactive discussion of the questions. Strickland (1999) also noted that participants may not respond directly to the questions asked but rather respond to what is triggered by the questions. Demanding that everyone speak can be culturally inappropriate. More traditional elders may need to be invited to participate in several focus groups before they will speak. In her work, Strickland (1999) also found that time also needed to be allocated at the end of the work for elders to speak if he or she felt inclined. Since almost everyone in the tribal communities was related, it was not reasonable or possible to hold to the recommendation that participants not be related. While these findings may apply to only the populations of Indian people in the Pacific Northwest, these findings serve to raise the awareness of the importance of designing focus group work to be culturally appropriate.

Community-based participatory research (CBPR) has become recognized as crucial to the assurance of the involvement of the community in research, addressing primary community issues, and balancing inequities in power in addressing the concerns of vulnerable populations (Strickland et al., 1997; Strickland, 2005, 2006). Key elements include the following: (a) involvement of the people in the identification of the research question; (b) creation of a stable decision-making team based in the community; (c) shared funding with the community; (d) involvement of the community in all phases of the study from identification of the need to implementation, data analysis and disseminations; and (e) community capacity building (Reason, 1994; Strickland, 2006; Stringer, 1996). CBPR may be a research method or a philosophical underpinning (Reason, 1994; Stringer, 1996). In either case, involvement of the community, community capacity building and empowerment is enhanced with CBPR. The following examples, drawn from cancer prevention evaluation efforts with Native people, in which CBPR has been combined with focus groups and feasibility efforts, illustrates the strengths of combining CBPR with formative evaluation to enhance community empowerment and also contribute to the design of culturally appropriate approaches that have an impact.

In work in cancer prevention screening, Strickland (2003, 2005) and Hodge & Stubbs (1999) provide insights into the use of formative evaluation to lay the foundation for translating theory into the design of culturally appropriate interventions.

Involving the community in the intervention design through the use of CBPR, the use of focus groups, and pilot formative evaluation feasibility work was found to be crucial.

Strickland (2003, 2005) invested a number of years in adapting a clinical trial that had been found to be efficacious in influencing women to conduct breast self-exam (Strickland, 1997) and expanded it to include cervical cancer screening from other research in which it was found important to offer women's health programs rather than just breast or cervical cancer screening education (Strickland, 1997). Funding was obtained initially from the University of Washington School of Nursing to support the CBPR planning team, to conduct focus groups over a one-year period, and to develop the protocol and identify culturally appropriate approaches and materials. Additional funding was obtained from IESUS (Institute for Ethnic Studies in the United States) to conduct a pilot study (Strickland, 2005). This was a community-based participatory study that focused on feasibility issues and employed focus groups as well.

In this work, a community-based planning group was established. This group included health providers in the tribal clinic, the health administration, community health nurses and community health representatives (CHRs), a member of the records department, a research assistant member of the community, representatives of the population to be involved in the study, and the American Indian Outreach Coordinator for the Pacific Northwest Cancer Information Service. Some meetings were also held with community elders to gather their perspectives on the population to be involved in the study and procedures for implementation. The research assistant, a Native member of the community, was oriented to the study and trained to obtain consent forms, conduct interviews, and recruit study participants. She also supported the facilitation of the focus group work. Meetings were held with the CBPR planning team almost monthly during the study. The tribal council had approved the study through a tribal resolution as well as the Institutional Review Board. Procedures for dissemination of results were developed with the health administration.

Community based participatory research often leads to work in identifying and obtaining funding from a number of resources to address tribal needs and thus the relationship may span a number of studies. One example of a cultural adaptation drawn from this study (Strickland, 2003, 2005) provides greater understanding of how formative evaluation can contribute to the design of more culturally appropriate interventions. In previous research (Strickland, 1997), it was recognized that commitment to do breast self-examination had a positive and significant impact on engaging in the practice among non-Native people. This was achieved by having study participants sign a written contract. When this was discussed in the planning team and in focus group work with the tribal community (Strickland, 2003, 2005), the community suggested that it would be more appropriate to have the study participants stand and pledge to the community and the grandmothers that they would engage in the practice. In this community, written contracts held little value; the spoken word and commitment to the people and the elders held more value.

Much like the suicide prevention work, in this cancer prevention work, through the use of focus groups, we were able to identify the population to be included in the intervention, the appropriate materials to use in the education effort, and issues in implementation. In work with the CBPR planning team, we were able to identify recruitment issues, additional training needs of tribal research assistants in collecting data, and costs that had not been anticipated.

Hodge & Stubbs (1999) conducted intervention research to address healthy lifestyle behaviors related to cancer prevention and illustrate the complexities and commitment needed to adapt behavioral science theories in Indian communities. Their work illustrates well the importance of formative evaluation and feasibility efforts to design culturally appropriate interventions. Hodge, Pasqua, Marquez and Geishirt-Cantrell (2002) demonstrates the use of traditional approaches of communication and learning, such as story telling and other oral traditions that can be of significance for use in intervention projects. Using the Talking Circle as a method of communication and support in a cervical cancer screening project, Hodge & Stubbs (1999) found that American Indian women do not necessarily adopt positive health behaviors for themselves unless the behaviors are linked with concerns for the family and modeling the positive behaviors in the community.

Hodge's work in California (Wellness Circle, NINR 1997–2003) illustrates the investment needed to assure culturally appropriate outcome evaluation instrumentation and further illustrates the value of the Talking Circle as formative evaluation in intervention design. In this effort, she reports on the cultural constructs of wellness in an environment of high risk behaviors. Employing Talking Circles among Native groups at 13 rural reservation sites (N = 403) allowed for an increased dialogue in a non-threatening environment (Wellness Circles, NINR 1997–2003). This approach further facilitated communications among group members and encouraged the adoption of healthy lifestyle recommendations. The intervention curriculum merged knowledge of health risk, healthy lifestyles, and traditional illness beliefs in a manner that encouraged thoughtful consideration of illness and wellness in American Indian culture. In addition, it served to empower members by facilitating self-help approaches to wellness.

In yet another study, Hodge & Stubbs (1999) evaluated the efficacy of culturally appropriate psychosocial counseling and support intervention on adherence to cervical cancer screening and follow-up recommendations for American Indian women. This study validated self-reported screening behaviors through data abstraction. Staff were trained to conduct data abstraction. An easy to use abstraction form was developed for this difficult task. The intervention, which involved a series of group support meetings coupled with story telling, reinforced the preventive measures of cancer screening and proved to be successful. This resulted in a significant pre-test to post-test improvement (p = .0001) in the areas of knowledge, attitudes, and practices (Pap smears) compared to control groups.

From her research and extensive familiarity with the research literature in cancer prevention, Hodge suggests that it is important to test and implement specific evidence based practices (modified for cultural appropriateness) and that such protocols need to be integrated into the routine clinical care at large American Indian hospitals, health centers and related reservation based satellites. She notes that as a "new" illness, cancer has only recently begun to receive recognition as a health problem requiring intervention among American Indians.

Tom-Orme (1988, 1994) has devoted much of her career to diabetes research in AI/AN communities. Her perspectives and research work further illustrate the importance of involving the community, designing programs that are useful for the community, and complexities in undertaking research in Indian communities that is aimed at addressing outcome and impact evaluation. Her work also illustrates the importance of formative evaluation in the design of appropriate interventions.

Tom-Orme notes that any research conducted in an AI/AN community must be approved by a locally sanctioned tribal group or committee. Some of these review bodies may be formal institutional review boards, while others are composed of the tribal health boards or a designated committee. Because health related research in AI/AN communities is ubiquitous and tribal or local community concerns are not always represented, American Indian and Alaska Native communities have begun to request that intervention research be planned jointly with the local people. An AI/AN Tribal Health Research Advisory Council is currently being formed through the Department of Health and Human Services in accordance with the government-to-government relationship (personal communications, C. Grim, 4/24/06). This Council aims to achieve the following: (a.) obtain input from tribal leaders on health research priorities; (b.) provide a forum where agencies can coordinate their research activities; and (c.) provide a forum to disseminate information about AI/AN research. Culturally competent health promotion research and interventions are considered to be of utmost importance to AI/AN populations if disparities in chronic disease and mental health are to be addressed and decreased.

From her work, Tom-Orme recognizes that funding agencies may be most often interested in data-driven outcome evaluation research but tribal communities prefer a combination of both qualitative and quantitative research methods that provide direct service to the community as it is being implemented. In addition, from her experience, Tom-Orme recognizes that tribes want intervention research instead of more studies that describe the increasing rates of disease. Of particular interest are those studies that emphasize health protectors and traditional methods that promote health.

Hodge's work in diabetes research also illustrates the importance of involving the community and utilizing culturally appropriate approaches in research (Hodge & Geishirt-Cantrell, 2005). Involving the community assures a flow of information and feedback evaluation that contributes to more culturally appropriate interventions and meaningful outcome evaluation. In a study of diabetes among the Sioux and Winnebago of South Dakota and Nebraska, she evaluated the impact of peer educators in the provision of health education sessions with adults who had diabetes (Hodge, Welty, DeCora, & Geishirt-Cantrell, 2003). Peer facilitators were found to be instrumental in providing education information in rural, isolated communities. Culturally appropriate education materials were designed to provide accurate information on diabetes, nutrition, and the importance of exercise in a group support model. These materials also promoted healthy lifestyles at the individual, family, and community levels. The intervention resulted in significant reductions in fatalistic attitudes about diabetes prevention, onset, treatment, and control (Hodge & Geishirt-Cantrell, 2005).

In discussing some of the research in which she is involved, Tom-Orme provides information about the Education and Research Towards Health (EARTH) study and provides an example of outcome evaluation that was based on previous formative work that formed the foundation for the intervention. She suggests that the national prospective cohort study called EARTH is an excellent example of research that involved the community from the ground up. In this study, a touch screen computerized questionnaire is used to collect self-reported evaluation data on diet, physical activity, health and lifestyle, history of disease, and medications. At the end of the study visit, participants receive immediate feedback about how they reported their health-related activities in the questionnaire and from lab tests. The participants receive either a congratulatory note or suggestions on needed lifestyle changes. This approach provides immediate feedback information to participants and is being well received. As an etiology study, it will also provide information on impact and outcomes as well as describe the process of implementation and participant satisfaction. As a cohort and prospective study, this work will also supply current data to provide to the participating tribes for immediate use in health planning.

In the EARTH study (Slattery et al., 2006), it was found that about 11% of the study participants from this Southwest tribe spoke only the Native language and 60% spoke both English and the Native language in the home. Thus language was recognized as an important issue in intervention design. In this work, it became necessary to translate the study questionnaire to the local language so that questions could be better understood and thus higher quality data obtained.

Conclusion

In these formative evaluation research efforts in suicide prevention, cancer prevention and diabetes, one may see that formative evaluation is crucial in successful intervention design in work with Native communities. Formative evaluation in which the community is involved, Community-based Participatory Research, focus groups to make cultural adaptations, and pilot feasibility efforts are all important parts of the formative evaluation process and provide much needed information before embarking on full-scale intervention outcome evaluation. These efforts allow the researcher to address issues such as recruitment, the translation of the theory to culturally appropriate interventions, and the design of culturally appropriate instruments for the collection of baseline and follow-up data. While such efforts require considerable researcher time, travel, and expense to develop and implement, one may see that investing in laying this foundation is crucial to the design of interventions that will result in adequate recruitment of participants in interventions, the design of culturally appropriate assessment instruments and interventions, and ultimately success in outcome/impact evaluations. Such approaches also enhance community capacity and empower communities to address their own health concerns. Community members are involved in the decision-making in CBPR planning groups and focus groups, and are hired to conduct interviews and facilitate focus group work. The costs to conduct extensive formative evaluation can be a major barrier if researchers do not have adequate institutional support, funding, and structures that reward such efforts.

From these efforts we have learned the following lessons: (a) do conduct pilot feasibility studies (formative evaluation) in trying to adapt intervention protocols in AI/AN communities that have been found to be efficacious in other populations; (b) do follow the tribal rules and regulations about all approvals for evaluations; (c) do work with key informants from the community and learn about cultural values, issues, systems, structures, and daily life in conducting research in tribal communities; (d) do work with CBPR planning teams and hire and train personnel from the community to support implementation; (e) do expect to make changes in instruments, language, procedures, etc.; (f) do recognize that there are different patterns of communications in groups in AI/AN communities and that has an effect on research methods and data collection. In this work we have learned the importance of involving the community through CBPR planning teams, building on cultural patterns of communication in the design of culturally appropriate instruments and intervention approaches, and the importance of formative evaluation in addressing key implementation issues. We also recognize that investment in extensive formative evaluation research is costly in time, resources, and sometimes requires extensive travel to remote tribal communities. Funding to sustain community planning groups between grants and academic institutional support is crucial to this effort.

In this discussion, we have focused primarily on formative/process evaluation and provided examples of feasibility studies, focus group work, and community-based participatory research in American Indian communities. In so doing we have shown the importance of formative research to the design of more culturally appropriate outcome evaluation work. We have also shown the importance of formative evaluation approaches in building community capacity, balancing power, and including the community in the decision-making process.

By providing examples from our research in major areas of concern such as suicide prevention, cancer prevention, and diabetes, we have highlighted the lessons learned and recognized challenges and barriers to this work such as time, travel, funding, and institutional support, but have also shown that investment in formative evaluation and qualitative methods provides the important foundation for successful interventions. Greatly needed is support for continued formative evaluation and qualitative approaches to design culturally appropriate interventions that involve and empower the people and address the major areas of health concern such as mental health, cancer prevention, and diabetes.

References

Anderson, E., & McFarlane, J. (2004). *Community as partner: Theory and practice in nursing* (Chapters 12 & : 273–310). New York: Lippincott Williams & Wilkins.

Burgess, R. G. (Ed.). (1999). *Field research source book and field manual*. New York: Routledge, Chapman & Hall, Inc.

Butterfoss, F., Francisco, V., & Capwell, E. (2001). Evaluation in practice: Stakeholders participation in evaluation. *Health Education and Practice, 2*, 114–119.

Casper, M. L., Denny, C. H., Coolidge, J. N., Williams, G. I Jr., Crowell, A., Galloway, J. M., et al. (2005). *Atlas of heart disease and stroke among American Indian and Alaska Natives*. Atlanta, GA.: U.S. Department of Health and Human Services, Centers for Disease and Prevention and Indian Health Service.

Centers for Disease Control (2003). Findings from the Behavioral Risk Factor Surveillance System, 1997–2000. *Morbidity and Mortality Weekly Report Surveillance Summaries, 8*(52), SS-7.

Clark, M. J. (2006). *Community health nursing: Caring for populations* (5th ed.). Upper Saddle River, NJ: Prentice Hall.

Creswell, J. W. (1994). *Research design: Qualitative and quantitative approaches*. Thousand Oaks, CA: Sage.

Duran, E., & Duran, B. (1995). *Native American pos-tcolonial psychology*. State University of Albany, N.Y.: New York Press.

Edwards, B. (2001). A national perspective on cancer surveillance & measuring health disparities. American Indian/Alaska Native Leadership Initiative Biennial Conference: Changing Patterns of Cancer Care in Native communities. Scottsdale, Arizona.

Green, L., & Lewis, F. (1986). *Measurement and evaluation in health education and health promotion*. Palo Alto, CA: Mayfield.

Grim, C. (2006). Presentation at the 18th Annual Indian Health Service Research Conference. April 24, 2006. Phoenix, Az.

Hodge, F., & Stubbs, H. (1999). Talking circles: Increasing cancer knowledge among American Indian women. *Cancer Research and Therapy., 8,*:103—111.

Hodge, F. S. & Geishirt-Cantrell, B. (Submitted 2005). *The burden of illness: Deferred cancer screening among rural California Indians*. University of California, Los Angeles (Unpublished manuscript).

Hodge, F. S., Pasqua, A., Marquez, C. A., Geishirt-Cantrell, C. (2002). Utilizing traditional Storytelling to promote wellness in American Indian communities. *Journal of Transcultural Nursing, 13*(1), 6–11.

Hodge, F. S., Welty, T., DeCora, L., & Geishirt, B. (2003). *Changing diabetes fatalism among Plains American Indians*. University of California, Los Angeles (Unpublished manuscript).

Huff, R. & Kline, M. (1999). *Promoting health in multicultural populations: A handbook for practitioners*. Thousand Oaks, CA: Sage.

Lafferty, C., & Mahoney, C. (2003). A framework for evaluating comprehensive community initiatives. *Health Promotion and Practice, 4,*(1), 31–50.

Mitchell, M., & Jolly, J. (1992). *Research design explained*. Philadelphia, PA: Harcourt, Brace, Jovanovich College Publishers.

Reason, P. (1994). Three approaches to participative inquiry. In N. K. Denzin & Y. S. Lincoln (Eds.), *Handbook of qualitative research*. Newbury Park, CA: Sage.

Robin, R W, Chester, B., Rasmussen, J K, Jaranson, J M, & Goldman, D. (1997). Factors influencing utilization of mental health and substance abuse services by American Indian men and women. *Psychiatric Services, 48*(6), 826–834.

Sajik, R. (1990). Field notes: *The making of anthropology*. NY: Cornell University Press.

Stanhope, M. & Lancaster, J. (2002). *Foundations of community health nursing*. St. Louis, Missouri: Mosby.

Strickland, C. June (2006). Challenges in community based participatory action research implementation: Experiences in cancer prevention with Pacific Northwest Indian tribes. *Cancer Control, 13*(3), 230–236.

Strickland, C. J. (1997). Suicide among American Indian, Alaska Native, and Canadian Aboriginal Youth. *International Journal of Mental Health, 25*(4), 11–32.

Strickland, C. J. (1999). Conducting focus groups cross-culturally: Experiences with Pacific Northwest Indian people. *Public Health Nursing, 16*(3), 190–197.

Strickland, C. J. (2002). *Suicide Prevention among Pacific Northwest Indian Youth*. National Institute of Nursing Research (NINR) Final Report. Seattle, WA: University of Washington School of Nursing.

Strickland, C. J. (2003). *Pacific Northwest American Women's Health Screening Program: Program Development Phase using a CBPR approach*. Seattle, WA. (Proposal funded through the University of Washington School of Nursing Research and Intramural Program).

Strickland, C.J. (2005–2006). *Pacific Northwest American Indian Women's Health Screening: Feasibility Implementation Phase*. Seattle, WA (Proposal funded through the University of Washington Institute of Ethnic Studies of the United States (IESUS).

Strickland, C. J., Feigl, P., Upchurch, C., King, D., Pierce, H., Grevstad, P., et al. (1997). Improving breast self-examination compliance: A Southwest Oncology Group randomized trial of three interventions. *International Journal of Preventive Medicine, 26*, 320–332.

Strickland, C. J., Squeoch M., & Chrisman, N. (1999). Health promotion and cervical cancer prevention among Yakama women of the Wa'Shat Longhouse. *Journal of Transcultural Nursing, 10*(3), 190–196.

Strickland, C. J., Walsh, E., & Cooper, M. (2006). Healing the impact of colonialization: Pacific Northwest Indian elder's perspectives on suicide prevention. *Journal of Transcultural Nursing, 17*(1), 5–12.

Stringer, E. T. (1996). *Action research: A handbook for practitioners*. Thousand Oaks, CA: Sage.

Slattery, M. L., Schumacher, M. C., Lanier, A. P., Edwards, S., Edwards, R., Murtaugh, M. A., et al. (2006). A prospective cohort of American Indians and Alaska Natives: Study design, methods, and implementation. *American Journal of Epidemiology*, Advance access, June 22.

Swan, J. and Edwards, B. (2003). Cancer rates among American Indians and Alaska Natives. *Cancer, 98*(6), 1262–1272.

Tom-Orme, L. (1988). Chronic disease and social matrix: A Native American diabetes intervention. *Recent Advances in Nursing, 22*, 89–109.

Tom-Orme, L. (1994). Traditional beliefs and attitudes about diabetes among Navajo and Utes. In J. R. Joe & R. S. Young (Eds.), *Diabetes and disease of civilizations: Impact of culture in indigenous people*. New York: Mouton de Gruyter.

Windsor, R., Baranowski, T., Clark, N., & Cutter, G (1984). *Evaluation of Health Promotion and Education Programs*. Palo Alto, CA.: Mayfield Publishing Co.

Williams, J., Belle, G., Houston, C., Haire-Joshu, D., Auslander, W. (2001). Process evaluation methods of a peer delivered health promotion program for African American women. *Health Promotion and Practice, 2*, 135–154.

Chapter 11
Intersectoral Approaches to Health Promotion in Cities

Nicholas Freudenberg

The health problems facing the world today increasingly require complex solutions in which public health interventions must work across sectors and levels of organization. Cities – where two-thirds of the global population is expected to live by 2030 – especially face challenging health conditions like cardiovascular disease, diabetes, obesity, avian flu, infant mortality, and depression and social conditions like concentrated poverty, rising inequality, and declining public infrastructures. These problems demand that effective health promotion measures must integrate efforts within the health care, education, environmental protection, housing, nutrition and economic development sectors.

In this chapter, I will examine intersectoral approaches to health promotion, describe the rationale and characteristics of this strategy, and then examine the strategies used to evaluate intersectoral work and the methodological and organizational challenges to evaluation that this approach poses. I define intersectoral health promotion interventions as organized activities that seek to improve well-being by influencing multiple determinants of complex health problems that operate across sectors and levels of organization (WHO, 1986a, 1997). Sectors are functional areas such as education, employment and health care; levels describe hierarchical arenas of social interaction such as individuals, families, communities and jurisdictions. Intersectoral interventions seek to make changes in different systems in order to achieve defined public health goals. These goals can address one or multiple health problems. In some cases the *health* outcomes of intersectoral interventions are unintended or secondary benefits of initiatives designed to achieve economic, educational or other goals.

Planners and implementers of intersectoral interventions need to appreciate the unique challenges their approach poses to evaluation while evaluators need to grasp the contextual influences on implementation if they are to design valid, implementable and policy-relevant evaluation studies. Since successful evaluation requires practitioners and evaluators to find a common language so they can collaborate, this chapter is addressed to both.

N. Freudenberg
City University of New York, New York, NY, USA

L. Potvin, D. McQueen (eds.), *Health Promotion Evaluation Practices in the Americas*,
DOI: 10.1007/978-0-387-79733-5_11, © Springer Science+Business Media, LLC 2008   191

Even though intersectoral work is used in both urban and non-urban settings, this chapter focuses on examples from cities because so many people already live in cities, rapid urbanization is further concentrating the world's population in urban areas, and because urban complexity creates unique opportunities and challenges for both implementation and evaluation of this approach.

Complexity is evaluators' greatest challenge – if interventions had only a few dimensions, influenced only a single outcome, and operated in uniform and easily described environments, the job of evaluators would be easy. Intersectoral health promotion in cities presents complexity on every front. Thus, understanding the contextual variables that influence cities and intersectoral interventions becomes an evaluator's first task, a prerequisite for solving the more familiar tasks of choosing outcomes, designing evaluation studies, collecting data and interpreting findings.

History of Intersectoral Health Promotion

Just as evaluators need to understand the dynamic spatial characteristics of the settings in which they work, so too must they appreciate the temporal changes in the types of interventions they evaluate. After World War II, the dominant approach to international public health became large-scale categorical campaigns that targeted specific diseases (Commission on Social Determinants of Health, 2007). The successful campaign to eliminate small pox and the failed efforts to eradicate malaria illustrate this model (Litsios, 1997). In the 1960s and 1970s, in part in response to these top-down single sector approaches, other more grass-roots, community-based and intersectoral models emerged in the developed and developing worlds. These new approaches emphasized health education and disease prevention and targeted changes in social conditions as well as medical care (Commission on Social Determinants of Health, 2007). In 1976, Halfdan Mahler, then Director-General of WHO, proposed the goal of "Health for All by the year 2000". "Health for all," he said, "implies the removal of obstacles to health – the elimination of malnutrition, ignorance, contaminated drinking water and unhygienic housing – quite as much as it does the solution of purely medial problems" (Mahler, 1981).

Two international health conferences crystallized the themes in this new approach that played out in the 1980s. The 1978 International Conference on Primary Health Care in Alma Alta declared that primary health care should be the foundation of health systems and that health work had to be fully integrated with other efforts to improve living conditions (Cueto, 2004; WHO/UNICEF, 1978). In 1986, the First International Conference on Health Promotion formulated the Ottawa Charter for Health Promotion, which identified key perquisites for health: peace, shelter, education, food, income, a stable eco-system, sustainable resources, social justice and equity (WHO, 1986b). The charter defined health promotion as "the process of enabling people to increase control over, and to improve their health." The key activities for health promotion were to build healthy public policy, create supportive environments, strengthen community action, develop personal skills, and reorient health services (WHO, 1986b). Implicit in the Ottawa Charter's broad scope was an understanding that successful action required collaboration across sectors and among various constituencies including government, the private sectors, nonprofits and grassroots organizations (Commission on Social Determinants of Health, 2007).

In the 1990s, the ambitious vision and mission embodied in the goal of Health for All and the statements from the Alma Alta and the Ottawa meetings confronted what came to be known as the Washington Consensus or neoliberalism (Coburn, 2000). In this view, liberalization of restrictions on the free market was the best strategy for economic development and social improvement. Its chief proponents were the United States government, the World Bank and the International Monetary Fund. By promoting free trade, removing restrictions on the flow of capital, privatizing health and social services and reducing government regulation, neoliberals believed that any short-term pain these strategies imposed would contribute to long-term gains. While neoliberalism also advocated an intersectoral approach, it was business rather than government that took the lead and the goal of coordinated planning was to reduce rather than enhance public sector participation in key policy decisions. This difference between the bottom-up approach to intersectoral health promotion implied in "health for all" and the top-down, business-directed approach of neoliberalism continues to divide advocates of intersectoralism.

In the current decade, critics of neoliberalism charge that it undermined rather than supported improved well-being, enhanced inequality and hurt the most disadvantaged groups such as women and children most (de la Barra, 2006). In response to these criticisms, several international organizations proposed a new focus on poverty reduction as a key goal. In this view, concerted but narrowly focused global action was needed to overcome the limitations of the market in solving social and problems. The Millennium Development Goals (MDG) are an example of this approach (United Nations, 2007). They propose eight cross-cutting goals aimed at poverty and hunger, universal primary education, gender equality, child mortality, maternal health, HIV/AIDS and other diseases, environmental sustainability, and global partnership for development (United Nations, 2007). By choosing targeted goals, emphasizing global and national action, and focusing on reducing poverty rather than inequality, the MDGs represent a new focal point for intersectoral health promotion. How frontline and national public health professionals locate health promotion initiatives within the context of MDGs and how they respond to the progressive critics of the top-down MDG approach will play an important role in shaping the future of intersectoral health promotion in the current period.

What is the implication of this history for evaluators? In health promotion, as in other fields, defining outcomes of interest is always a political as well as a scientific task. The changing views on the goals and scope of health promotion in the last several decades demonstrate that broader global forces shape the context in which interventions are constructed, implemented and evaluated. An evaluator who is unaware of the meaning of a specific project's goals, activities and outcomes to the various stakeholders (e.g., international funders, national public health officials, municipal leaders, local residents) is ill equipped to carry out a valid and policy-relevant evaluation.

Significance of Intersectoral Health Promotion

Intersectoral health promotion has the potential to contribute to solving a wide range of health problems. This approach is particularly useful for addressing problems whose causes or consequences manifest themselves in different sectors (e.g., the impact of air pollution on respiratory health). It is useful for addressing what have been called "wicked problems" (Rittel & Webber, 1973) that are resistant to solution with categorical interventions. However, even relatively straightforward (at least conceptually) medical problems like getting antiretroviral or tuberculosis medications to those who need them may require interventions that address health care, water, housing, transportation, international commerce, and employment sectors.

The case for intersectoral approaches to health promotion can be found within several theoretical and conceptual frameworks. Systems theories hold that a system as a whole is an appropriate object of study and that change at one level or in one sector requires understanding of the system itself in order to achieve desired results and avoid unintended consequences (von Bertalanffy, 1968). Ecological models of health promotion emphasize the importance of considering different levels of influence and their interactive effects on health (Green, Richard, & Potvin, 1996; Richard, Potvin, Kishchuk, Prlic, & Green, 1996; Stokols, 1996). Scholarship on social determinants of health posits that social conditions influence multiple health and social outcomes and that underlying social structures often serve as the fundamental cause of prevalent inequities in population health (Link & Phelan, 1995; Marmot & Wilkinson, 1999; Tarlov, 1996). Advocates for intersectoral approaches emphasize their desire to address these deeper causes. For example, the Milan Declaration on Healthy Cities (1990), adopted by the European Healthy Cities projects, stated: "We pledge our political support for the strengthening of intersectoral action on the broader determinants of health and for exploring with our city councils or other city authorities ways to make health and environmental impact assessment part of all urban planning decisions, policies and programmes." Recent interest in reducing or eliminating disparities in health provides additional support for intersectoral approaches since achieving this goal will require actions at multiple levels of organization and across diverse sectors (Satcher & Rust, 2006).

Solving complex problems often require the participation of those constituencies who are affected by the problem. Intersectoral approaches bring these parties together and engage them in a process of forging solutions that address the diverse perspectives. As the Athens Declaration for Healthy Cities (1998) put it: "Health is promoted most effectively when agencies from many sectors work together and learn from each other. Health is everyone's business. We pledge our political support for unlocking the health potential of all stakeholders in our cities' future, including the specific needs of men, women, children, and minority populations" (Athens Agenda for Healthy Cities, 1998).

Public health interventionists recognize participation as a characteristic of effective programs (Israel, Eng, Schultz, & Parker, 2005) and good governance as a prerequisite for such participation (Jeffrey, 2006). Reviews on coalitions and partnerships suggest strategies for building intersectoral alliances for action and the renewed interest in community-based participatory research offers methods of engaging a variety of relevant stakeholders in the planning, implementation and evaluation of intersectoral interventions (Butterfoss, 2006; Fear & Barnett, 2003; Israel et al., 2005; Minkler & Wallerstein, 2003).

Sustainable development is another field that can contribute insights into considering the long-term consequences of intersectoral work and into the task of scaling up interventions (von Schirnding, 2005). For evaluators, the theoretical foundations of a specific intersectoral interventions can inform the development of logic models (Lafferty & Mahoney, 2003), theories of change (Connell, Kubisch, Schorr & Weiss, 1995), or "grounded theories" (Glaser & Strauss, 1967) that can serve as a framework for the design of evaluations.

Characteristics of Intersectoral Interventions

Intersectoral health promotion initiatives (IHPIs) differ on a variety of key characteristics including their objectives, level of intervention, intensity and duration of their activities, and their goals around replicability and sustainability. Specifying these differences can help planners to consider the decisions they must make in designing these interventions and evaluators to choose appropriate assessment methods.

Scope of Objectives

IHPIs differ in the scope of their objectives. Some identify a single health objective (e.g., increasing physical activity) and work across sectors (e.g., health, transportation, parks and recreation, etc.) to achieve that goal. Others, like the European Healthy Cities Projects, choose multiple health outcomes and work across sectors to achieve these goals (WHO Healthy Cities Network, 2003). Another option is to choose objectives that cut across sectors, e.g., health, employment, community development, and criminal justice, requiring activities in different sectors to achieve different outcomes, as in *Oportunidades* in Mexico (Box 11.1).

Box 11.1 *Oportunidades*, **a program to reduce poverty in Mexico.** In 1997, Mexico initiated a national program to reduce poverty and improve health by providing "conditional cash transfers" to families to send their children to school, use preventive health services, and improve diet. Based on the belief that coordinated services across sectors would enhance the impact of single-sector activities, *Oportunidades* was soon expanded from rural areas, where it began, to Mexico's cities. (Skoufias, Davis & de la Vega, 2001; Levine 2004) Designed to reach the extremely poor, the program provides cash incentives that can increase a family's income by 25%. Evaluation studies have shown measurable improvements in school attendance, use of health services and nutrition. *Oportunidades* illustrates an intersectoral approach to improving health that begins at the national level, involves services from several sectors, and regards health as only one outcome among many.

Generally, interventions with more objectives and operating in more sectors are more complex and require additional planning, coordination and resources for both implementation and evaluation. One of the challenges in these kinds of interventions is uniting sectors with different interests and end goals. Interventions like the Detroit Partnership (Box 11.2), whose objectives cut across several sectors, involve representatives of each relevant sector in the planning and evaluation process.

Box 11.2 The Detroit Community-Academic Partnership Established in 1995 as an urban research center (URC), its partnership involves the University of Michigan Schools of Public Health, Nursing, and Social Work, the Detroit Department of Health and Wellness Promotion, nine community-based organizations, and a hospital system. It aims to improve the health and quality of life of low-income families and communities in urban Detroit through interdisciplinary, collaborative, community-based participatory research (Schulz et al., 2002; Israel et al., 2001; Lantz, Viruell-Fuentes, Isfael, Softley, & Guzman, 2001). The URC has interacted with municipal agencies addressing health, the environment, housing, police and others. The center has trained community health workers to serve as resources within several Detroit neighborhoods. The URC is a model of intersectoral health work that was initiated by university researchers but is now directed by community representatives from several urban neighborhoods.

Level of Intervention

Interventions take place and seek to bring about changes at different levels of social organization, from individuals and families to communities, cities, nations and the world. Some IHPIs may operate solely at the individual or family level, seeking to change individual behavior that cuts across sectors, e.g., health care utilization and school attendance, while others like the Millennium Development Goals (United Nations, 2007) require action at the village, national and global levels. Multi-level interventions are more complex than those confined to a single level and require additional planning, coordination and resources. Evaluators may find ecological theories and models useful for designing their evaluation (Elder et al., 2007; Long John, 2004).

Interventions operating across sectors at only one level, e.g., the municipal, will require horizontal integration – engagement with representatives of others sectors working at that level. Multi-level interventions will also require vertical integration with representatives of one or more sectors working at other levels. Programs such as *Oportunidades* in Mexico (Box 11.1) require both types of integration. To some extent, the demands of each type of integration pull planners in different directions (Stern & Green, 2005). Horizontal integration may require grassroots, bottom-up approaches since the participants themselves have to find the motivation to join together across sectors. Vertical integration may be more likely to originate in national governments, which have the authority to convene participants in a top-down approach. In either case, participants themselves must be convinced of the value of collaboration to sustain projects. IHPIs that require high levels of both horizontal and vertical integration especially face difficult challenges. Evaluators of multi-site intersectoral interventions may benefit from developing methods of measuring horizontal and vertical integration systematically in order to assess its contribution to success.

Intensity and Duration of Interventions

IHPIs vary in the intensity and duration of their activities. Some carry out a few activities and have limited contact with any constituency while others have intense engagement with one or more populations. Similarly, some initiatives are time-limited campaigns that carry out activities that seek to achieve their goals in a specific time frame while others intend to be ongoing activities. In general, IHPIs that are more intense and of longer duration have greater potential to reach goals of public health significance but planners are always concerned about identifying a point of diminishing returns when additional increments of intensity and duration no longer produce cost-effective benefits. Developing standardized metrics for describing the intensity and duration of interventions could contribute to a more systematic body of evidence on the value of additional increments of intervention.

Sustainability and Replicability

Related to the previous point, IHPIs differ in whether they seek to achieve sustainability and replicability or whether they are time and place specific, ending once they have achieved a goal. While public health researchers and policy makers value sustainability and replicability, practitioners often must respond to an emerging need and move on either when that need has been met or their attention is diverted by a new need. These differences in sustainability and replicability have important implications for the type of evaluation appropriate to a particular intervention. It is worth noting that sustainability and replicability may not need to be considered for a time and place-specific intervention that succeeds in solving a problem. But when the characteristics of a problem are such that it is likely to recur at other times or in other places, intervention planners must consider sustainability and replication. Whatever the longer term goals, however, evaluators can always provide program implementers with systematic feedback that can improve performance at a specific place and time.

Models for Intersectoral Work

Recent scholarship provides one foundation for new approaches to intersectoral health promotion; current practice, always a vital starting point for new initiatives, provides another. In this section, I review models for intersectoral health promotion and offer a few examples of each. These models are not mutually exclusive but vary in key ways. As shown in Table 11.1, these models differ in the level at which they seek change and their key participants. To date, empirical evidence is lacking as to whether these models pose unique evaluation challenges. However, evaluators may find it helpful to consider whether interventions within a model offer insights that can avoid repetition of mistakes. For example, by choosing outcomes that can be measured using existing municipal data sources, evaluators working at this level may be able to save the expense of collecting their own data to assess intervention effects.

Global Models

Global programs work in several countries and regions around the world, combining local and national efforts. For example, the World Health Organization's Healthy Cities project operates at the global, regional, national and local levels (Awofeso, 2003; Goldstein, 2000; Harpham, Burton, & Blue, 2001). At the higher levels, the organization provides technical assistance, guidance and information exchanges to participants. It may also initiate vertical integration across levels. At the local level, Healthy Cities projects bring together key players from city government, neighborhood and civic groups and professional organizations.

Table 11.1 Models of intersectoral health promotion interventions

Model	Level of change	Key goals	Participants	Examples
International alliances	Global policy; distribution of resources	Mobilizing international action; reallocating global resources; creating global networks	International organizations, national NGOs*, national governments	Millennium Development Goals; World Social Forum; WHO Healthy Cities
National programs	National policy or programs in one or more sectors	Integrating actions to solve national problems across sectors	National governments NGOs*	Cities for Life(Peru) CDC PATCH
Municipal (or regional)	Municipal policy and services	Integrating actions and policies to solve municipal problems across sectors	Municipal governments, NGOs*, business, labor	Healthy Cities projects, Local Agenda 21 projects
Grassroots	Community or neighborhood policy or services, norms or behavior	Integrating action across sectors at community level	Local NGOs, local government, informal neighborhood associations	Neighborhood-based health promotion programs

*NGO = non governmental organization

From a different political perspective, the World Social Forum and Global Health Watch bring together activists and some government leaders to consider alternatives to the development and health policies advocated by Western-dominated international organizations (Global Health Watch, 2006). Evaluators of global interventions need to select measures and devise measurement strategies that are feasible in the different settings where the program is offered or else account for differences in context and methods.

National Models

Either national governments or national NGOs lead and support efforts to promote health across regions. The Cities for Life Forum in Peru (Box 11.3) is an example. National models usually seek both vertical integration with local efforts and horizontal integration across sectors. Support from the central government can give these programs the needed credibility and resources. On the other hand, governments that are unpopular or seek to use a health promotion initiative to impose an ideological agenda may make it more difficult for an intervention to reach or engage its target populations. National initiatives may be able to use existing national data to evaluate outcomes and when the program is sponsored by the national government it might be willing to provide the resources and personnel for evaluation.

Box 11.3   Cities for Life Forum, Peru Cities for Life Forum is a national network of 83 institutions including municipalities, civil society organizations and universities in 29 cities in Peru. The organization defines its vision as "an expression of sustained development... to offer the inhabitants adequate life standards, through equal opportunities for a healthy, secure, productive and liveable life" (Miranda, 2004). Its participants engage in activities at the local, municipal and national levels to develop capacity for environmental health promotion and management, to support sustainable urban development and to improve environmental quality. A National Assembly of representatives from municipalities makes overall policy decisions and local chapters plan their own activities to improve health and environmental conditions and also to promote democracy and good government (Miranda, 2004). Programs include a national campaign to ban use of asbestos in Peru, municipal and national "participatory budgeting" exercises, building sustainable houses in a low-income Lima neighborhood, and university-based training programs for environmental management (Hordij, 2005; Miranda, 2004).

Municipal Models

Several characteristics of cities make them particularly suited for intersectoral approaches to health promotion but also require adaptation of this strategy to the urban setting (Freudenberg, 2006). Table 11.2 describes some of the ways cities differ from non-cities and lists the implications for program implementation and evaluation.

City government or citywide NGOs bring people together across cities and sectors to address identified problems. In some cases the group itself chooses the problems to address and sets priorities for actions; in others the convening body (e.g., the Mayor's Office) brings people together around an already defined problem. Recently some city health departments have begun to develop health objectives that require action across sectors (e.g., NYC Take Care New York, San Francisco Five Year Prevention Plan) (Freudenberg, 2006). In these situations, municipal staff may also be involved in monitoring the success of these multisectoral efforts, analyzing their policy implications, and advocating for policy change based on the findings.

Grass Roots Mobilization

In grass roots mobilization, community or neighborhood organizations come together to address problems they have defined that require action across sectors. As Hasan, Patel, and Satterthwaite (2005) have noted, "there is a huge physical, conceptual and institutional distance between the individuals, households, and

Table 11.2 How cities different from non-cities

Characteristic	Health consequences	Implications for intersectoral intervention	Implications for evaluation	Selected references
Population density	Overcrowding, availability of social support, biological and social contagion, environmental stress	Public health programs can reach large sectors of the population efficiently	Increases opportunities for participants in an intervention to have a variety of interactions with others, potential confounders with intervention impact; impact of interventions may vary by population density	Galea, Freudenberg, & Vlahov, 2005; Liu, Wilson, Qi, & Ying, 2007
Population diversity	Creates opportunities for multiple social networks; increases potential for intergroup conflict	Necessitates tailoring interventions to meet the needs of different subpopulations	Single intervention can affect different sub-populations in different ways, complicating evaluation	Des Jarlais, Padian, & Winkelstein, 1994; Noar, Benac, & Harris, 2007; Ryan, Skinner, Farrell, & Champion, 2001
Rich array of social and human resources	Dense social networks, many community organizations, numerous formal and informal service providers available to support individuals and communities	Key assets for intersectoral urban health promotion; may make it easier to operate in multiple sectors, even with limited resources.	In one view, resources seen as "noise" that must be excluded from an analysis of intervention impact; another view sees them as potential intervention enhancers, creating the necessity of describing and measuring them systematically	James, Schultz, & van Olphen, 2001; Kretzmann & McKnight, 1993; Schulz, Parker, Israel, Allen, Decarlo, & Lockett, 2002

Table 11.2 (continued)

Characteristic	Health consequences	Implications for intersectoral intervention	Implications for evaluation	Selected references
Complexity	Multiple systems interact; pluralistic political structures create competing stakeholders; cities linked to other sociopolitical levels, such as neighborhoods, metropolitan regions, and nation-states	Simple interventions are rarely sufficient to solve problems, many programs have unintended as well as intended outcomes, generalization from one setting to another can be problematic; contextual complexity requires intervention complexity	Makes traditional methods of evaluation imported from the natural and biomedical sciences less relevant since many confounding influences cannot be controlled; suggests more flexible approaches to evaluation, including the development of problem-oriented theories of change	Connell et al., 1995; Bodstein, 2007
High levels of inequality	Inequality associated with poor health	Interventions may reinforce or widen disparities in health. Since they often further advantages the better off; intersectoral interventions can make disparity reduction an explicit goal.	Assess changes in health disparities as possible unintended consequences of interventions that end up benefiting those already better off.	Link & Phelan, 1995; Minkler, 1994
Health interventions need to attract and retain support of policy makers and residents to influence population health	Politics rather than need may drive resource allocation; few public health problems can be solved within the time span of the election or budget cycles in which policy makers operate, making support unstable	Health interventions compete for support with other interventions; public health planners need to operate effectively in scientific, economic, and political arenas to win the means to implement the policies and programs they advocate	Assessing process as well as outcomes of intersectoral interventions may help to identify biological, environmental, economic and political pathways by which activities lead or fail to lead to intended outcomes.	Freudenberg, 2006

communities facing serious deprivation, and the decision-making processes and management of the official development assistance agencies" (p. 17). Grass roots organizations can close this gap by putting community residents in the driver's seat, giving them the power to define the problem and devise solutions (Burra, 2005). For example, the West Harlem Environmental Action Coalition is an environmental justice group that seeks to protect residents of one New York City neighborhood against environmental threats to health and to reduce disparities in environmental exposure in New York City (Vasquez, Minkler, & Shepard, 2006). It has worked in housing, transportation, environmental protection and other sectors. For evaluators, grassroots coalitions may offer easier access to participants who have personally experienced the problems the intervention seeks to address and enjoyed the benefits of the intervention. However, the capacity of smaller NGOs to collect data, adhere to standard intervention protocols or sustain interventions through unstable funding may be limited, complicating the work of evaluators.

Intervention and Analytic Strategies for Intersectoral Work

For the most part, intersectoral health promotion uses the same intervention strategies as unisectoral work, e.g., community mobilization, public education, community development, staff training, small groups, etc. However, a few intervention and analytic methods may prove particularly suitable for implementing and evaluating health promotion programs that work across sectors. These include health and environmental impact assessment, portfolio planning, and various participatory strategies.

Health Impact Assessment of Public Policy

Health impact assessment of public policy, a tool being developed in Europe, may help to bring these questions into the policy arena. (Cole & Fielding, 2007; Kemm, 2001; Morrison, Petticrew & Thomson, 2001). To avoid repeating costly mistakes, municipal health officials and public health researchers can monitor the health impact of public policy more systematically and develop new and more effective ways to advocate for the health of the public (Parry & Stevens, 2001). Since intersectoral work is based on the premise that action in one sector may have health consequences, health impact assessment may help both to plan and evaluate intersectoral initiatives (Dannenberg et al., 2006). Recent efforts to use health impact assessment to consider the health consequences of various transportation policy options in London, England illustrate this potential (Mindell, Sheridan, Joffe, Samson-Barry, & Atkinson, 2004). In another example, urban planners and city officials in Bologna, Italy assessed the health and environmental effects of a market that collected and distributed to homeless and poor people, almost expired food from supermarkets. By distributing food from nearby markets, the project reduced transportation costs, improved nutrition and served as an economic development project. Documentation of these intersectoral impacts provided support for the proposal (Healthy Cities 21st Century, 2005).

Portfolio Evaluation

Recently, some health economists have developed methods for analyzing the optimal "portfolio" of health interventions that best use available resources for maximal impact on health. (Bridges & Terris, 2004; Sendi, Al, Gafni, & Birch, 2003, 2004). This approach allows officials to consider different levels of risk in investing in one program as opposed to another (e.g., high risk and high payoff interventions compared with lower risk and lower payoff ones). This method uses a single numeric, whether dollars, mortality, years of productive life lost, or others to compare the value of different intervention strategies. Just as financial investors seek a portfolio of investments balanced in risk, payoff, sector of the economy and region of the world, so public health officials may want to review their portfolio of interventions to assess whether they are investing public resources wisely.

This technique has particular relevance to intersectoral initiatives since rarely will a single intervention strategy be sufficient to address the multiple determinants of a complex health problem that operate within different sectors. Use of a single evaluative metric (e.g., cost or mortality) also facilitates considering the value of interventions across sectors. While further work is needed before portfolio evaluation can be applied to an assessment of the interventions in a particular municipality, such an exercise might help municipal or national health departments to clarify assumptions, highlight choices, and diversify the range of public health interventions now offered in most cities.

Participatory Approaches

Since intersectoral interventions often operate across levels and sectors, including the variety of constituencies that have a stake in the problem and its solution can enhance intervention effectiveness and support. Methodologies that have been proposed to achieve this goal include community-based participatory research, participatory action research, and participatory planning (Kapiriri et al., 2003; Minkler & Wallerstein, 2003; Naylor, Wharf-Higgins, Blair, Green, & O'Connor, 2002). Of particular importance is engaging representatives of each sector and level in the planning process in order to ensure that their points of view are addressed in the planning process. Several recent works provide detailed guidance on the operational and methodological challenges of implementing participatory strategies (Israel et al., 2005; Minkler & Wallerstein, 2003).

On the implementation side, participatory budgeting, a process by which various constituencies across sectors participate in setting priorities and allocating municipal budgets can assist intersectoral initiatives to gain the wisdom of diverse stakeholders and also promote more democratic approaches to problem-solving (Hordij, 2005). For example, the Cities for Life Forum in Peru (Box 11.3) used participatory budgeting as a method of promoting democratic governance.

Participatory approaches also have the potential to address unequal power dynamics within intersectoral interventions. While intersectoral and participatory theories emphasize the importance of including relevant constituencies in the planning, implementation and evaluation process, they do not in themselves address the power imbalances among these groups. In fact, most health and development initiatives do not include the most affected individuals or communities in meaningful decision-making roles (Hasan et al., 2005) and being "at the table" has meaning only if one has the power to influence decisions. While no single action can correct these inequities, participatory approaches that support the creation of, invite to the table and concede meaningful power to strong organizations of poor people can create an environment for more democratic health promotion policies and programs.

On the evaluation side, participatory approaches also have value, although they are often time consuming and labor intensive. By including the perspectives of diverse stakeholders in defining research questions, planning evaluation design, collecting data and analyzing findings, evaluators can gain a deeper understanding of the pathways by which interventions make a difference, the meaning of findings and their implications for policy and practice. If evaluators regard community participation as a façade – a necessary but painful public relations exercise – they miss opportunities to do richer and deeper scientific inquiry.

Challenges to Intersectoral Heatlh Promotion

Intersectoral health promotion initiatives face a variety of implementation challenges that warrant systematic consideration. These problems are inherent in the organizational and conceptual complexity of such interventions and have implications for both practitioners and evaluators.

Starting Point of Collaboration

Planners of IHPIs must determine the extent to which health problems versus other problems are the starting point of collaboration. If health is the starting point, then health organizations are logical and credible conveners. In the *Agita Sao Paulo* program (Box 11.4), for example, the health benefits of increased physical activity were the intervention's primary rationale. Other sectors such as schools and employers were involved in order to implement the range of project activities rather than because of their inherent interest in physical activity. In contrast, the Millennium Development Goals project (United Nations, 2007) has economic, justice and educational objectives as well as health aims. Thus, health organizations were one more player at the table and not the central force driving the process.

Box 11.4 *Agita São Paulo Agita São Paulo* is a multi-level, community intervention designed to increase physical activity among the 37 millions residents of the 645 municipalities in the state of São Paulo in Brazil (Matsudo et al., 2002, 2003). Founded in 1996 by the regional health department and university-based researchers, *Agita São Paulo* works with local governments, employers, schools and other organizations. Programs target students, workers and senior citizens using a transtheoretical model of stages of behavior change (Prochaska et al., 1994). In its first decade, *Agita São Paulo* has sponsored three main types of activities: (1) "mega-events", designed to reach at least one million people, through events organized on holidays (e.g. Carnival, International Labor Day, etc.), media coverage, and educational materials; (2) actions conducted with partner organizations such as schools, employers or senior citizens centers; and (3) ongoing partnerships with more than 300 institutions in which the *Agita Sao Paulo* provides information, materials and technical assistance designed to help partners enhance their physical activity programs. More than 50 municipal governments in Sao Paulo have established *Agita* committees to plan, and carry out local programs.

When health professionals initiate IHPIs, they need to weigh the advantages and disadvantages of making health the starting point. On the one hand, health is often a compelling issue of interest to a variety of constituencies and action to improve health has a social legitimacy that few openly oppose. On the other hand, some constituencies may be more motivated to join efforts to, for example, promote economic development or to reduce social inequities. Deciding how to "frame" the problem has critical implications for who will join and who can provide leadership.

In some cases, reframing the problem is the starting point of intersectoral collaboration. To illustrate, a public health organization in New York City wanted to portray high school dropout as a public health issue in order to broaden support for policy action to reduce dropout. Through dialogue with education groups, the campaign decided to focus on school-based health interventions that could contribute to reducing school dropout – a frame that gave equal weight to health and educational outcomes (Public Health Association of NYC, 2005). Reframing the issue helped to create common ground across sectors.

Evaluators need to understand the priorities of an initiative's sponsors and design an evaluation that maximizes the opportunity of documenting success or failure in the most important sectors. Given limited evaluation resources, it may be necessary to select a few outcomes for evaluation, at the risk of missing other significant outcomes. On the other hand, a distinctive feature of intersectoral initiatives is their potential to bring about unanticipated changes or changes across sectors. For example, in the Detroit Academic Community Partnership (Box 11.2) each intervention contributed to strengthening community cohesion, itself an important determinant of health. Had evaluators not considered this outcome across different interventions, they may have missed documenting an important benefit. Where possible, evaluators of intersectoral interventions may want to dedicate at least some resources to what has been called "goal free" or "illuminative" evaluation (Scriven, 1993), a method that allows researchers to discover unintended or unexpected consequences.

Bureaucratic and Organizational Issues

Intersectoral initiatives face bureaucratic and organizational challenges. Most government agencies and even many non-governmental organizations operate categorically – addressing one problem or type of problem or having responsibilities in one sector. Thus, their decision-making processes and organizational infrastructures support categorical approaches. When intersectoral intervention teams propose new decision-making or institutional structures that better meet their needs, they may encounter passive or active resistance from those more familiar or comfortable with the status quo. For example, in the United States, many municipalities have begun to develop intersectoral approaches to improving health and social outcomes for those returning home from jail or prison. To achieve success requires coordination of criminal justice, health, vocational, economic development and housing officials. (Freudenberg, Rogers, Ritas, & Nerney, 2005; Re-entry Policy Council, 2005). Yet in few city governments do these officials report to a single boss, thus there may be no mandate to take action across sectors. In addition, the savings in one sector, e.g., in the jail system due to lower reincarceration, may not accrue to that agency, discouraging even supportive officials from taking action for fear of losing resources. Several critiques of the Healthy Cities model note the difficulty of convincing municipal governments to take ongoing responsibility for coordinating intersectoral interventions (Awofeso, 2003; Milewa & de Leeuw, 1996).

A further complication of these bureaucratic problems is the challenge of ensuring both vertical and horizontal integration of IHPIs. In some cases, an existing entity such as the municipal or national government has clear authority for horizontal integration, at least across public agency sectors. But an initiative that requires integration among public and private partners or among participants without prior experience working together may lack any entity that has the authority or credibility to convene stakeholders. In such cases, it may be difficult to maintain accountability for defined goals. One solution is to create a process that builds intervention-specific accountability – a time consuming task.

Every public health endeavor requires resources and the resources available determine the scope of the project. In categorical interventions, usually one participant is responsible and accountable for providing or assembling needed resources such as money and staff. In intersectoral interventions, however, frequently many agencies and sectors are expected to contribute resources, again complicating questions of accountability and oversight. On the one hand, having multiple partners may increase the potential pool of resources. On the other hand, however, as public priorities or leadership of private agencies changes, support for an intersectoral initiative may diminish, making it more difficult to win the resources needed to accomplish objectives across sectors.

For evaluators, the challenges of working across levels and sectors may require researchers to enter domains outside their field of expertise. For example, a health researcher studying the health impact of a jail reentry program may be unfamiliar with the meaning and measurement of common criminal justice outcomes measures, e.g., recidivism. In such cases, evaluation teams may need to include investigators from several disciplines in order to avoid mistakes or a time-consuming learning curve.

Balance Between Process and Content

Finally, every IHPI must find the right balance between investing time, effort and resources in the *process* of creating a collaborative, defining governance, and engaging and sustaining the participation of old and new partners and the *content* of achieving desired health outcomes. If insufficient attention is devoted to process, participants may drop out or narrow their scope of activities. However, if the initiative does not deliver on outcomes, funders and government may drop their support. Unfortunately, there is no generic formula to determine the proper balance between these two. At best, intersectoral planning teams that are aware of this dilemma can review this balance periodically and make corrections as needed. Evaluators can play a useful role by documenting the process of addressing the changing balance between these two and providing the feedback needed for corrective action.

Evaluating Intersectoral Health Promotion

Evaluators of intersectoral health promotion programs face all the traditional scientific and logistical problems that evaluators of other types of interventions face. Several recent reviews provide an overview of these issues (Butterfoss, 2006; Evans, Adam, et al., 2005; Evans, Lim, Adam, & Edejer, 2005; Jackson & Waters, 2005; Ogilvie, Egan, Hamilton, & Petticrew, 2005). Here I focus on some of the unique issues that evaluators of IHPIs face.

Appropriate Outcome Measures

Evaluators know that clear objectives are the foundation for good evaluation. In IHPIs, however, defining measurable objectives may be especially difficult. In some cases, an intervention's sponsors may agree on broad goals such as improving well-being for a city's residents, but differ on what dimensions of well-being are most important. For example, in a recent Mayoral intersectoral initiative to reduce poverty in New York City (New York City Commission on Economic Opportunity,

2006), public health officials were asked to identify interventions that could reduce poverty by improving health. For city officials, the primary outcome of interest was a reduction in the city's poverty rate and in dependence on public benefits. For health officials, the objectives were reducing teen pregnancy, improving management of chronic diseases, and so on. While in theory it would be possible to measure all possible outcomes, in practice agreeing on evaluation priorities for this initiative proved to be difficult. While all parties acknowledged the linkages among these outcomes, they differed on their relative priority and therefore on how best to judge success.

In other cases, intersectoral interventions may choose to focus on less quantifiable goals such as improving social justice, reducing disparities in health, or increasing political participation in setting health policy. At least in the short term, it may be difficult to define measures that fully reflect the breadth of these goals. This may force project sponsors either to narrow their goals – at the risk of trivializing their broader objectives – or to adopt a more process-oriented evaluation, perhaps less likely to convince policy makers to provide additional support. Some critics of the Healthy Cities projects have asserted that the emphasis on process evaluation has failed to provide evidence that this approach in fact improves health or reduces disparities while supporters respond that the mobilization around health is itself a success (Goldstein, 2000; Harpham, et al, 2001; Milewa & de Leeuw, 1996).

Value and Limits of Theory

Public health researchers emphasize the importance of developing interventions based on social science theories, arguing that this approach leads to clearer conceptualization of the mechanism by which interventions succeed and defining the relevant evaluation questions (Glanz, Rimer, & Lewis, 2002). In practice, however, most social science theories focus on one level of organization (e.g. individuals or communities) or are grounded in work in a single sector (e.g., the health belief model in the health care system). As a result, few theories provide the breadth to inform interventions that cross levels or sectors. Thus, interventions often choose a theory more narrow than its scope. For example, *Agita Sao Paulo* (Box 11.4) is based on the transtheoretical model, which seeks to explain only individual behavior, although the intervention itself works in multiple systems to bring about institutional change. Some investigators have addressed this problem by blending theories from different levels or sectors into a more complex whole. While this approach has its merits, it limits the potential for assessing theoretical constructs across interventions. If every intervention requires a unique theory, the development of a theoretical framework for intersectoral interventions becomes problematic.

Appropriate Comparisons Groups

Many intervention researchers have argued that randomized clinical trials, the gold standard for individual-level interventions, are not appropriate for community or policy level interventions (MacDonald, Veen, & Tones, 1996; Ziglio, 1997). In some cases, health promotion evaluators have randomized communities or jurisdictions into different arms of a trial but this is expensive and contextual differences among different sites may skew results. Moreover, given the complexity of many intersectoral interventions and the importance of tailoring interventions to specific settings, finding appropriate comparisons can be difficult. One solution may be to make multiple comparisons, e.g., a city to itself before and after intervention, the intervention city to one or more comparable cities, and communities within a city which have been exposed to varying levels of intervention intensity. In those fortuitous cases where each comparison leads to the same conclusion, the weight of the evidence can provide stronger support for intervention effectiveness.

Collecting Data Across Sectors and Levels

By definition, intersectoral interventions work across sectors and levels, making the collection of standardized data difficult. For individual level measures, it may not be possible to match data from two or more systems (e.g., health, public assistance and criminal justice) if common identifiers are lacking. Simply gaining access to such datasets can prove to be time consuming or pose significant confidentiality issues. For community-level measures, different sectors may use different boundaries for municipal districts, again making it difficult to match summary statistics (e.g., poverty rate and rates of HIV infection) from different agencies. At regional or global levels, differences in definitions of variables of interest, or accuracy or completeness of data can make comparisons difficult. For example, nations differ even in their definitions of urban and rural, making comparisons of effectiveness in these two settings problematic.

Integrating Findings from Different Levels and Sectors

Even when useable data can be extracted from different sources, integrating findings across levels and sectors can pose additional challenges. The development of multilevel analytic methods allows evaluators to assess the independent effects of individual, community and contextual factors on outcomes of interest (Diez Roux, 2000; Galea & Schulz, 2006), making various techniques for multilevel or hierarchical modeling of potential value to intersectoral evaluators. Where valid data from these different levels are not available, evaluators are concerned both about ecological fallacies, where changes in population characteristics are inappropriately applied to individuals, and atomistic fallacies, where changes in environments are inappropriately attributed to individuals.

In some cases, evaluation of intersectoral interventions requires assembling data from a variety of sources and levels to make a "weight of the evidence" argument. For example, a variety of evaluation activities suggest that *Agita Sao Paulo*

(Box 11.4) has been successful in increasing levels of physical activity. Regular surveys show increases in levels of population physical activity; public opinion polls showed increasing awareness of the program and an increase in levels of physical activity associated with awareness and several smaller studies show increases in physical activity among program participants (Matsudo et al., 2003). Together, these data provide persuasive evidence of program effectiveness.

Interdisciplinary Intersectoral Evaluation Teams

Intersectoral interventions require interdisciplinary teams for evaluation as well as for planning and implementation. Evaluation expertise is needed within each sector involved in the intervention, at each level of intervention, in the various methodologies selected for use, and for the health outcomes of interest. Including community residents and policy makers in planning and carrying out the evaluation ensures that their questions of interest are addressed and their experiences with the problem inform the evaluation design and methods, as illustrated by the work of the Detroit Urban Research Center (Box 11.2). To date, evaluation of health promotion interventions has often focused on biological and behavioral outcomes rather than social or population health changes (Rush, Shiell, & Hawe, 2004), suggesting the need for additional expertise at higher levels of organizations.

Disseminating Findings to Influence Policy and Practice

Evaluation studies have multiple audiences: intervention participants and beneficiaries, funders, government, advocates and global institutions. Planning an evaluation so as to reach these key constituencies requires an understanding of their questions and concerns. For intersectoral interventions, policy makers and practitioners in different sectors may bring different questions to an evaluation, forcing evaluators to conduct sector-specific assessments. Developing processes of participation for each stage of an intervention, from planning to interpreting findings to communicating with policy makers, can help to ensure that evaluation results will have an impact (WHO European Working Group, 1998).

Cost-Benefit and Cost-Effectiveness Analyses

Increasingly, policy makers expect evaluators to consider the economic as well as the health consequences of health promotion interventions (Evans, Lim, et al., 2005; Rush et al., 2004). For intersectoral programs, this requires consideration of costs and benefits in a variety of sectors. Often, the benefits of IHPI are realized in a longer time frame than policy makers usually consider, and, as mentioned, the benefits do not always accrue to the sector or agency that bears the costs. Thus, evaluators need to find ways to present relevant information to decision-makers at the appropriate level and to make a strong case as to why investment now can save lives and money in the future.

Evaluators are also expected to consider the impact of their intervention on other sectors and the common monetary metric that cost benefit analyses use facilitates comparison across sectors (Niessen, Grijseels, & Rutten, 2000). This approach to health impact assessment can supplement previously described methods that use measures of mortality or morbidity as their outcomes.

In summary, evaluators of intersectoral interventions face a variety of unique methodological, operational and political challenges. By including representatives of all concerned constituencies in the evaluation process; by creating interdisciplinary, intersectoral evaluation research teams; by learning from the growing literature on health impact assessment and multilevel research methods; and by incorporating cost-benefit analyses, evaluators can contribute to more informed decisions about intersectoral health promotion initiatives.

Recommendations

This review of the planning, implementation and evaluation of intersectoral approaches to health promotion with a focus on urban settings has described the potential benefits of this approach and also some of its limitations and obstacles. I conclude with a few suggestions for future research and practice.

Develop Theories and Models that Link the Literature on Social Determinants of Health to Intersectoral Health Promotion

In the last decade, researchers have again focused attention on the social determinants of health and the necessity of addressing these fundamental causes in order to improve health in both the developed and the developing world (Irwin & Scali, 2005). To date, however, the research on determinants and the evaluation studies of interventions have been mostly separate; the former focused more on social science theories, the latter on empirical atheoretical studies or individual-level psychological theories. As a result, intersectoral interventions have lacked a conceptual framework that explained the pathways and mechanisms by which activities led to changes at various levels and within different sectors.

While an empirical approach to intersectoral health promotion encourages close attention to the all-important context, it also is difficult to translate into guidance to planners of new interventions. Moreover, it encourages interveners to fall back on the more familiar and acceptable individual-level approach to health promotion. For these reasons, developing theories and models that can link the understanding of social determinants of health to action to modify these determinants across sectors is a high priority.

Standardize Outcome Measures for Health Promotion Through Consensus Process

One concrete step towards a more systematic literature would be to reach agreement on the definitions and measurement of common outcomes measures. For example, differences in defining what it means to have access to clean water or appropriate sanitation in various developing nation urban and rural areas has led researchers to reach different conclusions about the impact of interventions from the same data (McGranahan & Satterthwaite, 2006). While no body has the authority to impose such definitions, bringing researchers and practitioners together to propose standards can help to create more useful guides to practice and evaluation.

Evaluate More Systematically

Despite the plethora of evaluation studies of health promotion interventions, the body of literature on the impact of intersectoral initiatives is scant. Much of the literature that does exist focuses on process evaluation – useful but not very persuasive to policy makers. The challenge is to develop systematic methodologies less structured than the Cochrane Reviews or the Guide to Community Preventive Services (Zaza, Briss & Harris, 2005) but more organized than the anarchy of the peer-reviewed and grey literatures. The problem with the former is that the restrictions on study inclusion and the formal analytic methods exclude many relevant studies (Truswell, 2005) and may particularly exclude those that cross sectors. More loosely structured reviews, on the other hand, may not produce findings that can apply across settings or yield insights that can actually guide practice.

What is lacking is any systematic approach to choosing which interventions to evaluate at what level of rigor in order to provide the knowledge needed for guiding policy and practice. While intersectoral health promotion interventions are not unique in this respect, their potential value in addressing the major health problems facing urban populations and the complexity of evaluating across sectors and levels make this a fruitful arena for developing more systematic approaches. International organizations such as the World Health Organization, the International Union for Health Promotion and Education or the Millennium Development Fund can play a role in initiating such a process.

Look for Ways to Use Existing Social, Human and Cultural Capital to Support Intersectoral Health Promotion

In the foreseeable future, health promotion is unlikely to attract the financial support it needs to achieve its potential. Military, economic development, medical care and educational sectors, to name a few, will almost always be more successful in winning resources from those in power. Thus, to achieve success, health promotion will need to find other ways to gain the resources it needs. Fortunately, a variety of other sources are available. In fact, intersectoral approaches to health promotion may be uniquely qualified to attract the social, human and cultural capital that can contribute to success (Hancock, 2001; Hawe & Shiell, 2000; Khawaja & Mowafi, 2006; Wakefield & Poland, 2005). While these forms of capital are not a substitute for direct financial support for health promotion from government and business, they can stretch the reach of under-funded programs and contribute other positive outcomes in their own right. By framing problems broadly, by linking efforts to promote health to those to increase social justice and reduce inequity, and by rooting interventions within the communities that will benefit, intervention planners can attract more of the resources needed to achieve their objectives. On another level, by creating interventions that build social, human and cultural capital, health promoters can create the virtuous circles that support sustainable health promotion. Evaluators can contribute to this process by including measurement of such changes in their evaluation plan.

Redefine Sustainability and Replicability

A persistent critique of health promotion is that successful programs are rarely brought to scale and many are not even sustained in their original setting. In recent years, researchers have begun to study the process of bringing successful interventions to scale (Chopra & Ford, 2005; Johns & Torres, 2005; Vassall & Compernolle, 2005), making recommendations such as distinguishing between scaling up in rural and urban areas, assessing the adequacy of human resources needed for scaling up, and considering the administrative costs of bringing programs to scale.

Another approach to the problem has been to re-think the meaning of sustainability and replicability for complex interventions in dynamic settings where contextual factors may limit traditional methods. For example, in assessing the question of scale in achieving the Millennium Development Goals, Hasan et al. (2005) suggest that "going to scale is not achieved through expanding one standard initiative but through supporting a large number of local initiatives, and through supporting city or municipal authorities that want to support community-driven approaches on a city-wide scale" (p. 16). This may be an especially useful way to address sustainability and replicability for intersectoral initiatives where local conditions are best addressed through local planning. By rethinking the meaning of these terms, evaluators can design studies that may contribute to wider dissemination of successful interventions.

In summary, intersectoral health promotion initiatives promise deeper solutions to the complex health problems facing the world today and especially its cities. This approach has the potential to develop health promotion interventions that can match the complexity, multifaceted and dynamic nature, and political dimensions of the health and social problems that face the growing proportion of the world's urban population. However, what makes intersectoral health promotion initiatives promising – their multiple partners, multilevel activities, flexibility and comprehensiveness – also makes them difficult to define, implement, evaluate and sustain. By learning how to negotiate these complexities, health promotion planners and evaluators can contribute to the realization of the vision of health for all.

References

Agenda 21. (2003). Indicadors 21. Indicadors locals de sostenibilitat a Barcelona. Documents 8. Ajuntament de Barcelona. Retrieved August 15, 2007 from http://64.233.161.104/search?q=cache:8jFnt3oDatgJ:www.bcn.es/agenda21/A21_text/indicadors/Int_indicators.doc+Healthy+cities+Barcelona&hl=en&gl=us&ct=clnk&cd=5

Athens Agenda for Healthy Cities. (1998). Retrieved August 15, 2007 from www.euro.who.int/AboutWHO/Policy/20010917_1

Awofeso, N. (2003). The Healthy Cities approach– reflections on a framework for improving global health. *Bulletin of the World Health Organization*, 81(3), 222–223.

Bodstein, R. (2007). The complexity of the discussion on effectiveness and evidence in health promotion practices. *Promotion & Education*, 1(Suppl), 16–20.

Bridges, J.F., & Terris, D.D. (2004). Portfolio evaluation of health programs: A reply to Sendi et al. *Social Science & Medicine*, 58, 1849–1851.

Burra S. (2005). Towards a pro-poor framework for slum upgrading in Mumbia, India. *Environment and Urbanization*, 17(1), 67–88.

Butterfoss, F.D. (2006). Process evaluation for community participation. *Annual Review of Public Health*, 27, 323–340.

Chopra, M., & Ford, N. (2005). Scaling up health promotion interventions in the era of HIV/AIDS: Challenges for a rights based approach. *Health Promotion International*, 20(4), 383–390.

Coburn, D. (2000). Income inequality, social cohesion and the health status of populations: the role of neoliberalism. *Social Science & Medicine*, 51, 135–46.

Cole, B.L., & Fielding, J.E. (2007). Health impact assessment: a tool to help policy makers understand health beyond health care. *Annual Review of Public Health*, 28, 393–412.

Commission on Social Determinants of Health. (2007). *A conceptual framework for action on the social determinants of health* (2nd ed.). Geneva: WHO.

Connell, J.P., Kubisch, A.C., Schorr, L.B., & Weiss, C.H. (Eds.). (1995). *New approaches to evaluating community initiatives: Concepts, methods, and contexts*. Washington, DC: Aspen Institute.

Cueto, M. (2004). *The origins of primary health care and selective primary health care*. Joint Learning Initiative: JLI Working Papers Series.

Dannenberg, A.L., Bhatia, R., Cole, B.L., Dora, C., Fielding, J.E., Kraft, K., et al. (2006). Growing the field of health impact assessment in the United States: An agenda for research and practice. *American Journal of Public Health*, 96(2), 262–270.

de la Barra, X. (2006). Who owes and who pays? The accumulated debt of neoliberalism. *Critical Sociology*, 32(1), 125–161.

Des Jarlais, D.C., Padian, N., & Winkelstein, W. (1994). Targeted and universal strategies for preventing HIV transmission. *New England Journal of Medicine*, 331,1452–1453.

Diez Roux, A.V. (2000). Multilevel-analysis in public health research. *Annual Review of Public Health*, 21, 171–192.

Elder, J.P., Lytle, L., Sallis, J.F., Young, D.R., Steckler, A., Simons-Morton, D., et al. (2007). A description of the social-ecological framework used in the trial of activity for adolescent girls (TAAG). *Health Education Research*, 22(2), 155–165.

Evans, D.B, Adam, T., Edejer, T.T., Lim, S.S., Cassels, A. & Evans, T.G. (2005). WHO Choosing Interventions that are Cost Effective (CHOICE) Millennium Development Goals team. Time to reassess strategies for improving health in developing countries. *British Medical Journal*, 331(7525), 1133–1136.

Evans, D.B., Lim, S.S., Adam, T. & Edejer, T.T. (2005). Choosing Interventions that are cost effective (CHOICE) Millennium Development Goals Team. Evaluation of current strategies and future priorities for improving health in developing countries. *British Medical Journal*, 331(7530), 1457–1461.

Fear, H., & Barnett, P. (2003). Holding fast: the experience of collaboration in a competitive environment. *Health Promotion International*, 18(1), 5–14.

Freudenberg, N. (2006). Interventions to improve urban health. In Freudenberg, N. Galea, S., & Vlahoveds, D. (Eds). *Cities and Population Health* (pp. 294–326). Nashville: Vanderbilt University Press.

Freudenberg. N., Rogers, M., Ritas, C., & Nerney, M. (2005). Policy Analysis and Advocacy: An Approach to Community-Based Participatory Research. In Israel, B., Eng, E., Schultz, A., & E. Parker (Eds.). *Methods in community-based participatory research for health* (pp. 349–370). San Francisco: Jossey-Bass.

Galea, S., Freudenberg, N., Vlahov, D. (2005). Cities and population health. *Social Science & Medicine*, 60(5), 1017–33.

Galea, S. & Schulz, A. (2006). Methodological considerations in the study of urban health: How do we best assess how cities affect health? In Galea, S., Freudenberg, N., & D. Vlahov (Eds). *Cities and Population Health* (pp. 277–293). Nashville: Vanderbilt University Press.

Glanz, K., Rimer, B. K., & Lewis, M. L. (2002). *Health behavior and health education: Theory, research, and practice* (3rd ed.). New York: Jossey-Bass.

Glaser, B.G. & Strauss, A. (1967). *The Discovery of grounded theory: Strategies for qualitative research.* Edison, NJ: Aldine.

Global Health Watch. (2006). *Global Health Watch 2005–2006.* Retrieved August 15, 2007, from http://www.ghwatch.org/2005report/ghw.pdf

Goldstein G. (2000). Healthy cities: overview of a WHO international program. *Reviews on Environmental Health*, 15(1–2), 207–214.

Green L.W., Richard, L., & Potvin, L. (1996). Ecological foundations of health promotion. *American Journal of Health Promotion*, 10(4), 270–281.

Hancock, T. (2001). People, partnerships and human progress: Building community capital. *Health Promotion International*, 16(3), 275–280.

Harpham, T., Burton, S., & Blue, I. (2001). Healthy city projects in developing countries: The first evaluation. *Health Promotion International*, 16(2), 111–125.

Hasan, A., Patel, S., & Satterthwaite, D. (2005). How to meet the Millennium Development Goals (MDGs) in urban areas. *Environment and Urbanization*, 17(1), 3–15.

Hawe, P. & Shiell, A. (2000). Social capital and health promotion: A review. *Social Science & Medicine*, 51(6), 871–885.

Healthy Cities 21st Century. (2005). Introducing health impact assessment in Bologna, Italy: A case study. Geneva: World Health Organization. Retrieved August 15, 2007, from http://www.euro.who.int/Document/Hcp/HIA_toolkit_5.pdf

Hordijk, M. (2005). Participatory governance in Peru: Exercising citizenship. *Environment and Urbanization*, 17(1), 219–239.

Irwin, A., & Scali, E. for the WHO Commission on Social Determinants of Health. (2005). Action on the social Determinants of health: Learning from previous experiences. Geneva: WHO. Retrieved August 15, 2007, from http://www.who.int/social_determinants/resources/action_sd.pdf

Israel, B., Eng, E., Schultz, A., & Parker, E. (2005). *Methods in community-based participatory research for health.* San Francisco: Jossey-Bass.

Israel, B.A., Lichtenstein, R., Lantz, P., McGranaghan, R., Allen, A., Guzman, J.R., et al. (2001). The Detroit community-academic urban research center: Development, implementation, and evaluation. *Journal of Public Health Management and Practice*, 7(5), 1–19.

Jackson, N., & Waters, E. (2005). Guidelines for systematic reviews in health promotion and public health taskforce. Criteria for the systematic review of health promotion and public health interventions. *Health Promotion International*, 20(4), 367–374.

James, S.A., Schultz, A.J., & van Olphen, J. (2001). Social capital, poverty, and community health. In Saegert, S., Thompson, P. & Warren, M. (Eds.). *Building social capital in urban communities*, (pp. 165–188). Thousand Oaks, CA: Sage; 2001.

Jeffery, J. (2006). Governance for a sustainable future. *Public Health*, 120(7), 604–608.

Johns, B., & Torres, T.T. on behalf of WHO-CHOICE. (2005). Costs of scaling up health interventions: A systematic review. *Health Policy & Planning*, 20(1), 1–13.

Kapiriri, L., Norheim, O.F., & Heggenhougen, K. (2003). Public participation in health planning and priority setting at the district level in Uganda. *Health Policy & Planning*, 18(2), 205–213.

Kemm, J. (2001). Health impact assessment: A tool for healthy public policy. *Health Promotion International*, 16, 79–85.

Khawaja, M., & Mowafi, M. (2006). Cultural capital and self-rated health in low income women: Evidence from the Urban Health Study, Beirut, Lebanon. *Journal of Urban Health*, 83(3), 444–458.

Kretzmann, J.P.,& McKnight, J.L. (1993). *Building communities from the inside out: A path towards finding and mobilizing community's assets*. Chicago: ACTA.

Lafferty, C.K., & Mahoney, C.A. (2003). A framework for evaluating comprehensive community initiatives. *Health Promotion Practice*, 4(1), 31–44.

Lantz, P.M., Viruell-Fuentes, E., Israel, B.A., Softley, D., & Guzman, R. (2001). Can communities and academia work together on public health research?: Evaluation results from a community-based participatory research partnership in Detroit. *Journal of Urban Health*, 78(3), 495–507.

Levine, R. (2004). *Millions saved: Proven successes in global health*. Washington, DC: Center for Global Development.

Link, B.G., & Phelan, J. (1995). Social conditions as fundamental causes of disease. *Journal of Health and Social Behavior*, 35(special issue), 80–94.

Litsios, S. (1997). Malaria control, the cold war, and the postwar reorganization of international assistance. *Medical Anthropology*, 17(3), 255–278.

Liu, G.C., Wilson, J.S., Qi, R., & Ying, J. (2007). Green neighborhoods, food retail and childhood overweight: Differences by population density. *American Journal of Health Promotion*, 21(4), Suppl, 317–325.

Longjohn, M.M. (2004). Chicago project uses ecological approach to obesity prevention. *Pediatric Annals*, 33(1), 55–7, 62–63.

Macdonald, G., Veen, C., & Tones, K. (1996). Evidence for success in health promotion: suggestions for improvement. *Health Education Research*, 11(3), 367–376

Mahler, H. (1981). The meaning of "health for all by the year 2000." *World Health Forum*, 2(1), 5–22.

Marmot, M., & Wilkinson, R. (1999). *Social determinants of health*. New York: Oxford University Press.

Matsudo, V., Matsudo, S., Andrade, D., Araujo, T., Andrade, E., de Oliveira, L.C., et al. (2002) Promotion of physical activity in a developing country: The Agita Sao Paulo experience. *Public Health Nutrition*, 5(1A), 253–261.

Matsudo, S.M., Matsudo, V.R., Araujo, T.L., Andrade, D.R., Andrade, E.L., de Oliveira, L.C., et al. (2003). The Agita Sao Paulo Program as a model for using physical activity to promote health. *Revista Panamericana de Salud Pública*, 14(4), 265–272.

McGranahan, G., & Satterthwaite, D. (2006). A developing world perspective: Health and deficiencies for provision for water and sanitation in urban areas of Africa, Asia, and Latin America and the Caribbean. In Galea, S., Freudenberg, N. & Vlahoveds, D. (Eds) *Cities and Population Health* (pp. 194–205). Nashville: Vanderbilt University Press.

Milan Declaration on Health Cities. (1990). Retrieved August 15, 2007, from http://www.euro.who.int/AboutWHO/Policy/20010927_8

Milewa, T., & de Leeuw, E. (1996). Reason and protest in the new urban public health movement: An observation on the sociological analysis of political discourse in the 'healthy city.' *British Journal of Sociology,* 47(4), 657–670.

Mindell, J., Sheridan, L., Joffe, M., Samson-Barry, H., & Atkinson, S. (2004). Health impact assessment as an agent of policy change: Improving the health impacts of the mayor of London's draft transport strategy. *Journal of Epidemiology and Community Health,* 58(3), 169–174.

Minkler, M. (1994). Challenges for health promotion in the 1990s: Social inequities, empowerment, negative consequences, and the common good. *American Journal of Health Promotion,* 8(6), 403–413.

Minkler, M., & Wallerstein, N. (Eds.). (2003). *Community-based participatory research for health.* San Francisco: Jossey-Bass.

Miranda, L. (2004). Cities for life revisited: Capacity-building for urban management in Peru. *Environment and Urbanization,* 16(2), 249–261.

Morrison, D., Petticrew, M., & Thomson, H. (2001). Health Impact Assessment and beyond. *Journal of Epidemiology and Community Health,* 55(4), 219–220.

Naylor, P.J., Wharf-Higgins, J., Blair, L., Green, L., & O'Connor, B. (2002). Evaluating the participatory process in a community-based heart health project. *Social Science & Medicine,* 55(7), 1173–1187.

New York City Commission on Economic Opportunity. (2006). Increasing Opportunity and reducing Poverty in New York City. Retrieved August 15, 2007, from http://www.nyc.gov/html/om/pdf/ceo_report2006.pdf

Niessen, L.W., Grijseels, E.W., & Rutten, F.F. (2000). The evidence-based approach in health policy and health care delivery. *Social Science & Medicine,* 51(6), 859–869.

Noar, S.M., Benac, C.N., & Harris, M.S. (2007). Does tailoring matter? Meta-analytic review of tailored print health behavior change interventions. *Psychological Bulletin,* 133(4), 673–693.

Ogilvie, D., Egan, M., Hamilton, V., & Petticrew, M. (2005). Systematic reviews of health effects of social interventions: 2. Best available evidence: How low should you go? *Journal of Epidemiology and Community Health,* 59(10), 886–892.

Parry, J., & Stevens, A. (2001). Prospective health impact assessment: Pitfalls, problems, and possible ways forward. *British Medical Journal,* 323, 1177–1182.

Prochaska, J.O., Velicer, W.F., Rossi, J.S., Goldstein, M.G., Marcus, B.H., Rakowski, W., et al. (1994). Stages of change and decisional balance for 12 problem behaviors. *Health Psychology,* 13(1), 39–46.

Public Health Association of NYC. (2005). *Defining a Common Education and Health Policy Agenda for the 2005 NYC Election.* Retrieved August 15, 2007, from http://www.phanyc.org/files/Education%20Report7.24.05.pdf

Re-entry Policy Council. (2005). Charting the safe and successful return of prisoners to the community. Retrieved August 15, 2007, from www.reentrypolicy.org

Richard, L., Potvin, L., Kishchuk, N., Prlic, H., & Green, L.W. (1996). Assessment of the integration of the ecological approach in health promotion programs. *American Journal of Health Promotion,* 10(4), 318–328.

Rittel, H., & M. Webber. (1973). Dilemmas in a General Theory of Planning. *Policy Sciences,* 4(2), 155–169.

Rush, B., Shiell, A., & Hawe, P. (2004). A census of economic evaluations in health promotion. *Health Education Research,* 19(6), 707–719.

Ryan, G.L., Skinner, C.S., Farrell. D., & Champion, V.L. (2001). Examining the boundaries of tailoring: The utility of tailoring versus targeting mammography interventions for two distinct populations. *Health Educucation & Research,* 16, 555–566.

Satcher, D.,& Rust, G. (2006). Achieving health equity in America. *Ethnicity & Disease,* 16(2), Suppl 3, 8–13.

Schulz, A.J., Parker, E.A., Israel, B.A., Allen, A., Decarlo, M., & Lockett, M. (2002). Addressing social determinants of health through community-based participatory research: The East Side Village Health Worker Partnership. *Health Education & Behavior,* 29(3), 326–341.

Scriven, M. (1993). *Hard-won lessons in program evaluation: New directions for program evaluation*. Nashville: Jossey-Bass.

Sendi, P., Al, M.J., Gafni, A., & Birch, S. (2003). Optimizing a portfolio of healthcare programs in the presence of uncertainty and constrained resources. *Social Science & Medicine*, 57, 2207–2215.

Sendi, P., Al, M.J., Gafni, A., & Birch, S. (2004). Portfolio Theory and the alternative decision rule of cost effectiveness analysis: Theoretical and practical considerations. *Social Science & Medicine*, 58, 1853–1855.

Skoufias. E., Davis, B., & de la Vega, S. (2001). Targeting the poor in Mexico: An evaluation of the selection of households into PROGRESA. *World Development*, 29(10), 1769–1784.

Stern, R., & Green, J. (2005). Boundary workers and the management of frustration: A case study of two Healthy City partnerships. *Health Promotion International*, 20(3), 269–276.

Stokols, D. (1996). Translating social ecological theory into guidelines for community health promotion. *American Journal of Health Promotion*, 10(4), 282–298. Review.

Tarlov, A. (1996). Social determinants of health: The sociobiological translation. In Blane, D., Brunner, E., & R. Wilkinson (Eds.), *Health and social organization* (pp. 71–93). London: Routledge.

Truswell, A.S. (2005). Some problems with Cochrane reviews of diet and chronic disease. *European Journal of Clinical Nutrition*, 59(Suppl 1), S150–154.

United Nations. (2007). *Millennium Development Goals report 2007*. New York: UN. Retrieved August 15, 2007 from http://unstats.un.org/unsd/mi/mi_goals.asp

Vasquez, V.B., Minkler, M., & Shepard, P. (2006). Promoting environmental health policy through community based participatory research: A case study from Harlem, New York. *Journal of Urban Health*, 83(1), 101–110.

Vassall, A., & Compernolle, P. (2005). Estimating the resource needs of scaling-up HIV/AIDS and tuberculosis interventions in sub-Saharan Africa: A systematic review for national policy makers and planners. *Health Policy*, 79(1), 1–15.

von Bertalanffy, L. (1968). *General system theory: Foundations, development, applications*. New York: George Braziller.

von Schirnding, Y. (2005). The World Summit on Sustainable Development: Reaffirming the centrality of health. *Global Health*, 1. Retrieved August 15, 2007, from http://www.globalizationandhealth.com/content/1/1/8

Wakefield, S.E., & Poland, B. (2005). Family, friend or foe? Critical reflections on the relevance and role of social capital in health promotion and community development. *Social Science & Medicine*, 60(12), 2819–2832.

WHO Healthy Cities Network. (2003). Phase IV(2003–2008) of the WHO Healthy Cities Network in Europe: Goals and Requirements. Copenhagen: World Health Organization Europe. (2003).

World Health Organization European Working Group on Health Promotion Evaluation. (1998). Health promotion evaluation: recommendations to policy makers: Report of the WHO European Working Group on Health Promotion Evaluation. Copenhagen: WHO Regional Office for Europe (Document EUR/ICP/IVST 05 01 03).

World Health Organization. (1986a). *Intersectoral Action for Health*. Geneva: WHO.

World Health Organization. (1986b). *Ottawa charter for health promotion*. Geneva: WHO. Retrieved August 15, 2007, from http://www.euro.who.int/AboutWHO/Policy/20010827_2

World Health Organziation. (1997). *Intersectoral action for health: A cornerstone for health for al in the 21st century*. Geneva: WHO.

Zaza, S., Briss, P.A., & Harris, K.W. (Eds.). (2005). *The Guide to Community Preventive Services: What works to promote health?* New York: Oxford University Press.

Ziglio, E. (1997). How to move towards evidence-based health promotion interventions. *Promotion & Education*, 4(2), 29–33.

Chapter 12
The Participatory Evaluation of Healthy Municipalities, Cities and Communities Initiatives in the Americas

Marilyn Rice and Maria Cristina Franceschini

Activities addressing the basic determinants of health have increased significantly, yet social and economic inequities continue to erode health conditions for many population groups. This is the reason why health promotion must continue to focus on bridging gaps among and within countries. Creating a healthy and supportive setting, also known as the settings approach, continues to be the most used health promotion strategy. Proven, cost-effective health promotion strategies can protect and improve the health of all persons. Determinants of poverty and equity, and their influence on health can be addressed through creating sustainable public policies and laws, developing supportive environments, building public-private partnerships, strengthening networks, mobilizing the media and other means of communication, and promoting an active role of municipal and local governments in health promotion and development. This article describes experiences and summarizes the main lessons learned from the application of a participatory evaluation methodology to three Healthy Municipalities, Cities and Communities initiatives in Brazil and Peru.

The Healthy Municipalities and Communities (HMC) Movement in the Americas

The Pan American Health Organization (PAHO) defines health promotion based on the Ottawa Charter (1986), which states that health is "the process of enabling and empowering people to take control over and improve the determinants of health." Health is promoted in the social context of people's daily lives, and is supported by public policies that affect social conditions and life styles, and these in turn give shape to healthy behaviors. PAHO developed and introduced the Healthy Municipalities, Cities and Communities (HMC) strategy in the 1990s to improve and promote local health and development. This strategy is being actively implemented in 18 of the 35 countries and three territories of the Americas.

M. Rice
Pan American Health Organization, Washington D.C

L. Potvin, D. McQueen (eds.), *Health Promotion Evaluation Practices in the Americas*,
DOI: 10.1007/978-0-387-79733-5_12, © Springer Science+Business Media, LLC 2008
221

The orientation of the Healthy Municipality, City or Community strategy is to ensure continuous improvements in the underlying conditions that affect the health and well-being of its members. This is achieved by facilitating joint action among local authorities, community members and key stakeholders aimed at improving their living conditions and quality of life. Based on the notion of health as having a good quality of life, the actions of the HMC strategy focus more on the underlying determinants of health than on their consequences in terms of disease and illnesses (PAHO, 2002).

HMC is based on the premises that (1) various systems and structures governing social, economic, civil and political conditions, as well as the physical environment, can impact individuals' and communities' health; and that (2) health is inherently linked to an individual's capacity to act in the community and society to which he/she belongs. HMC strives to create a synergy between these two premises: promoting individual actions and society's response. The ultimate goal is to enable processes that allow people to take control over their own health while improving equity, social participation, accountability and responsive local governance.

The evaluation of health promotion strategies, such as HMC, has been recognized by the international community as critical to strengthening the capacity of institutions and communities to promote measures that are effective and coherent with the needs and priorities of the population. Due to the complexities of evaluating social and developmental interventions, there is a scarcity of information regarding evaluation and effectiveness in developing countries. In addition, existing evaluation tools and methodologies have not appropriately captured changes in central health promotion elements (social participation, community empowerment, intersectorial collaboration, equity, etc.), nor have they provided insights into the multiplying effect of working with various determinants of health in a coordinated manner.

PAHO's Evaluation Initiative

In 1999, PAHO established a Healthy Municipalities Evaluation Working Group formed by evaluation experts from leading institutions in the Region working on issues related to health promotion and local development. The Working Group was comprised of governmental, non-governmental and academic sectors from countries throughout the Region, including Argentina, Brazil, Canada, Chile, Colombia, Ecuador, and the United States. The Group met periodically for several years to develop tools and resources to support investment in health promotion. Drawing upon resources developed mainly by, English-speaking countries, the Working Group selected elements most relevant for the settings in the Region, as well as those reflecting the most relevant principles. The Working Group agreed that specific evaluation tools, frameworks and evidence of effectiveness were needed to support health promotion and similar initiatives. Building upon these recommendations, the Evaluation Working Group developed a series of evaluation tools, among them, a *Participatory Evaluation Guide for Healthy Municipalities, Cities and Communities*.

A participatory evaluation is considered to be an appropriate methodology because it reflects the principles of the HMC strategy, recognizes the complexities of HMC as a local development initiative, and facilitates the development of capacities, learning and empowerment. The process of conducting a participatory evaluation stimulates autonomy and community self-determination as it allows communities to improve their ability to resolve their own problems (PAHO, 2006).

In a participatory evaluation, the key stakeholders are involved in all phases of the process, including the design, implementation, management, interpretation, and decision-making about the evaluation and its results. The methodology implies more than the application of participatory techniques to conventional approaches for monitoring and evaluation. It requires:

- Participation of key stakeholders in all phases of the process.
- Negotiation and consensus about what to evaluate and how results will be interpreted and utilized.
- Continuous learning that results in capacity building and incorporation of lessons learned in the decision-making process.
- Flexibility to adapt to a continuously changing environment (PAHO, 2006).

The *Participatory Evaluation Guide for Healthy Municipalities, Cities and Communities* provides guidance and tools to HMCs to evaluate their own efforts, and contribute to the evidence base of the strategy's effectiveness. The Guide provides recommendations on evaluation processes and tools, as well as a mechanism to showcase and document the rich, extensive, and varied experiences and results related to the HMC strategy.

The Guide offers an evaluation framework that incorporates essential elements of HMC, and other health promotion initiatives, such as intersectoral collaboration, social participation, capacity building, individual physical and material conditions, health determinants, and community capacity, among others. The Guide orients users through a step-by-step process to design and implement continuous cycles of monitoring and evaluation throughout the life of an HMC initiative. The methodology supports the documentation and analysis of changes and accomplishments in terms of processes, outcomes and results, and guides users on how to communicate and act on the results to improve their HMC initiative. A Facilitator's Guide and training modules have been developed to support training activities in the application of the Guide.

When conducted in a truly participatory manner, the methodology proposed in the Guide promotes accountability and motivates continuous and active participation from all stakeholders. Since the participatory evaluation process is based on the commitment and dedication of all stakeholders, it is expected that the process will create a sense of common interest among those involved and produce positive changes in their community.

Nevertheless, as with most collaborative and participatory efforts, the participatory evaluation methodology has some inherent challenges. Bringing together and building consensus among people from various backgrounds, sectors, institutions and groups that often have different, if not conflicting, needs, agendas and interests, can be complex and time-consuming. The flexibility and openness required in the participatory evaluation process can also be perceived as less effective and objective compared to traditional approaches by those who are used to working with such approaches.

The Guide is a unique resource for the Region, providing an alternative orientation for evaluation that reflects the underlying health promotion principles of many long-term initiatives. Built upon philosophies of health promotion operating throughout the Region for decades, and incorporating additional elements from traditional evaluation models, the Guide affords an opportunity for HMCs to provide the information necessary to improve their initiatives while continually building capacity through participation. This dual approach has not previously been available to HMCs in the Region of the Americas.

Selected Countries' Experiences with the Participatory Evaluation Methodology

During 2004–2006, the *Participatory Evaluation Guide for Healthy Municipalities, cities and Communities* was introduced into several countries in the Americas through formal trainings conducted by PAHO in collaboration with country partners. Following the trainings, several communities in various countries of the Americas applied the participatory evaluation methodology to their HMC initiatives. This section describes three experiences that took place in Brazil and Peru.

The Application of the Participatory Evaluation Guide in the Campinas Region, State of São Paulo, Brazil[1]

Since 2003, the Network of Potentially Healthy Municipalities (NPHM) has been working with municipalities of the Campinas region, in the state of São Paulo, in the southeast region of Brazil, to support their efforts to implement the HMC strategy. The Network, spearheaded by the University of Campinas (UNICAMP), comprises over 30 municipalities, accounting for about two million inhabitants of the Campinas Region. The NPHM's objectives are to (1) support, promote and monitor HMC strategies through the construction of public policies, participation from all sectors, and the development of sustainable initiatives; (2) support local governments in the implementation of integrated initiatives; and (3) improve capacity among managers, technical staff, academia, organizations and society that have as a common goal to promote improvements in quality of life through health promotion.

During 2004, a series of workshops were conducted to introduce the *Participatory Evaluation Guide for Healthy Municipalities, Cities and Communities* to mayors of the Campinas region. The main goal of these workshops was to introduce

---

[1] The information about this experience was compiled from Sperandio et al. (2006).

participants to the core concepts and methodology, and to discuss the applicability of participatory evaluation to some of the initiatives taking place in the region. Ten municipalities participated in this effort. Participants also included municipal managers and experts of various technical areas.

During these workshops the different sections of the Guide were presented followed by an in-depth discussion on how the concepts and steps proposed could be applied to the context of their HMC experiences. As a result, the workshops provided participants with a very rich opportunity to discuss, exchange and reflect on their experiences with the HMC strategy. Participants reported that the Guide concretely helped them to consider the consequences of their actions more consistently, stimulating interest in the issue of evaluation and an in-depth reflection about health promotion activities being implemented in their communities.

An interesting characteristic of these initial discussions was the myriad of interpretations given by participants of health promotion-related concepts presented in the Guide, such as intersectoral collaboration, participation, empowerment, etc. Acknowledging that the diversity of opinions could have direct implications for the planning and implementation of the evaluation process, participants engaged in a productive and positive dialogue to reach consensus on the interpretations given to the material. At the conclusion of the workshops, participants assumed the commitment to introduce the Guide to their communities, and, in collaboration with other community stakeholders, to develop and apply a participatory evaluation plan adapted to their local realities. In the following months, these participants reported back on their experiences and lessons learned from the application of the Guide.

One of the first observations made by participants when applying the Guide to their HMC initiatives was that the methodology proposed emphasized various aspects of health promotion that had been overlooked in previous evaluation efforts. This brought up a "difficulty" for the evaluation as participants realized that their HMC initiatives had not appropriately taken into account those health promotion elements during their planning stages (for example, programs were not intersectoral), and, therefore, presented a real challenge for evaluation. As a result, communities reported the need to first engage in a process of discussion and reflection on how to revise the planning and implementation processes of health promotion initiatives in order to more appropriately incorporate some of the missing health promotion principles and, in a subsequent phase, conduct an appropriate evaluation.

The political timing of the application of the Guide was described as sensitive, since it occurred right before the local elections. This generated uncertainty about who would still be present to follow up on the initiatives, or even if initiatives would continue. The municipalities' experiences demonstrated how the transitory nature of local political decisions can weaken programs and public policies, particularly when there is a change of political parties. Such situations emphasize the need to form strong coalitions among all sectors of society to strengthen and sustain the HMC initiative and its evaluation.

The Campinas experience demonstrated that moments of political and administrative transition can have considerable impact on work conducted at the community level. It can cause delays and losses (including financial) since the time necessary to explain and get agreement on the continuation of programs can be very long. This has consequences for the evaluation of programs being implemented, and especially for programs conducted by a previous administration that are not continuing under the new one.

Another challenge faced by those applying the *Participatory Evaluation Guide to Healthy Municipalities, Cities and Communities* in the Campinas Region was the establishment of an intersectoral Evaluation Subcommittee, whose role was to take charge of the planning and implementation of the evaluation process. Particularly challenging were the cases in which municipal managers were not totally on board with the program and/or its plan of action. Lack of support from those in charge of the budget and general management of health promotion initiatives can seriously impair the ability of the remaining stakeholders to undertake the evaluation initiative. It also decreases the probability that the results of the evaluation will be taken seriously and utilized in the planning and implementation of future initiatives. This underscores the need to guarantee buy-in from all relevant stakeholders in order to launch and sustain the initiative, as well as the need to continuously promote awareness among all stakeholders of the objectives and benefits of the participatory evaluation.

Those participating in the Campinas experience also highlighted that the methodology presented in the Guide was new to most of the health secretariats of the municipalities. As a result there was a need to generate an internal orientation throughout public institutions to discuss the new concepts and assess the degree of agreement among staff in order to incorporate the new methodology into existing programs. This was particularly true when it came to generating intersectoral collaboration and guaranteeing social participation in actions and decision-making processes. This was a slow process, as it needed to take place through meetings, forums and discussion groups, and required linking various levels of administration, questioning existing paradigms, and dealing with resistance at both individual and collective levels.

Respect for the time needed to achieve acceptance by those working in public institutions was crucial in the Campinas experience in order to put in place programs that were consistent with the communities' expectations. However, participating municipalities reported that patience is paying off and resulting in more optimal use of resources, adoption of more consistent health promotion practices, and improvements in personal motivation among public staff in the administration.

Application of the Guide in the Community of Vila Paciencia, State of Rio de Janeiro, Brazil[2]

The HMC initiative in Vila Paciencia was launched in 1999 in a poor urban community located in the state of Rio de Janeiro, Brazil. The community context is one

---

[2] Information about this experience was compiled from Becker et al. (2006).

of great poverty and social vulnerability. Created in the 1960s to shelter victims of a large flooding, the Vila Paciencia community remained as a relocation site for populations displaced from nearby shantytowns. Today, the community comprises 8000 people living under very precarious conditions with high unemployment rates, and within a context of marked repression of basic human and citizenship rights. Community life is permeated by drug trafficking, which often represents the main lifestyle alternative for unskilled and unemployed youth. Organized crime strictly controls access in and out of the community and leaves great stigma on its residents. Community organizations and the neighborhood association are weak and have not been able to become established in a sustainable manner. There has been little public investment in the area and a marked disinterest from the public sector to get involved with the community. Actions toward improving the community have been limited to those implemented by religious groups and NGOs.

The Vila Paciencia HMC initiative focused on developing community empowerment based on the principles of health promotion. The strategic approach was to incorporate the community's inhabitants in the process of developing and improving health and quality of life through (1) mobilizing and strengthening local actors and leadership, and (2) creating a network of social intervention projects aimed at solving the most pressing community problems. This was implemented through participatory workshops to identify priority issues and develop action plans based on available resources; the application of a community survey used to create a database of basic community data; concerted efforts to involve various sectors (public and private) and other stakeholders working in the community; and the organization of community participation and strengthening of community associations. Five thematic areas were defined as the focus of actions to be taken: health and education; community organization; housing and sanitation; cultural and recreational activities; and generation of employment and income. Based on these themes, 41 intervention projects were implemented from 2002 to 2004.

The next phase for the HMC initiative was to monitor and evaluate the activities undertaken during those years. During 2005–2006, the Participatory Evaluation methodology was introduced and applied to the Vila Paciencia experience. The initiative's intersectoral committee was not functioning due to the abandonment of its members resulting from their loss of interest in continuing to work in a community that did not receive sufficient resources from the local government. There were also difficulties in establishing linkages with the public sector, due to the community's "historical social isolation and lack of citizenship rights", which is marked by "structural oppression and violence." (Becker et al., 2006)

The fragile community organization did not guarantee voice to its inhabitants and there was constant tension between community desires and the interests of those regulating the community life. As a result, formal participation from the community association became impossible, since the association's president was "ousted" due to his "involvement in drug trafficking activities", which generated mistrust within the population about the participation of the local association. (Becker et al., 2006)

Due to the complexity of the situation, a decision was made to evaluate the experience by reviewing and reflecting on actions already taken since 1999 and analyzing points of convergence with the five HMC pillars proposed in the *Participatory Evaluation Guide to Healthy Municipalities, Cities and Communities* as evaluation domains (participation, intersectoral collaboration, healthy public policies, sustainability, healthy structures and good governance). The work was conducted by a team composed of three psychologists, a social worker and a medical doctor who had been working in the community and participated in the planning and implementation of the HMC initiative. Later, participants from a local community committee joined the group. It was not possible to include a representative from the public sector, given the lack of interest it demonstrated towards the community.

The group formed an Evaluation Subcommittee to lead the evaluation process. However, it was not possible to form one that was representative of the various segments of the community due to the complications of the community context described above. For the same reason, the group decided that it would not be feasible to implement all the steps proposed in the Guide. The Evaluation Subcommittee decided to focus its work on evaluating three phases of the initiative that were planned and implemented with input from the community: Community Development, Local Action, and Community Mobilization. Community participation in these phases included the development of a community assessment, defining indicators and collecting the data. The efforts of the Evaluation Subcommittee focused on determining and analyzing points of convergence between the methodology, concepts and pillars of the guide with the actions implemented by the initiative. This was done through meetings and discussions among those participating in the Evaluation Subcommittee in which they analyzed the products of each of the determined initiative phases and the process that took place.

In terms of community participation, the group concluded that the community assessment demonstrated two forms of community participation: one based on personal gains and another based on leadership and voluntarism to achieve collective goals. In relation to the healthy public policies pillar, since the initiative was spearheaded by a civil society organization, working within the context of extensive social exclusion, the conclusion was that the initiative did not result in any contribution to public policies. As for the sustainability pillar, the group concluded that community actions taken in the context of the HMC initiative had favored the incorporation of various projects in the community as well as the allocation of more financial resources. Projects that resulted from the community assessment included various trainings and community development activities, particularly activities focused on children; a community kitchen with the creation of a women's group to generate revenues; the organization of recreational activities for children, youth; development of a community committee that met on a monthly basis to discuss community issues. When analyzing the intersectorial collaboration pillar, the group concluded that through the Community Committee it was possible to incorporate representatives from the community and the university. Partners included: the local school and day care center, the neighborhood association, the Municipal Social Action Secretariat, a STD/AIDS organization, among others. As for the healthy structures and good governance pillar, the group found that as a result of the initiative, community residents had started to increase their participation (for example, creating a community kitchen, participating in health fairs, etc.).

The Vila Paciencia experience points out some of the many challenges that a participatory evaluation initiative faces due to contexts of social exclusion, poverty and violence in which the initiative might be immersed. However, as the Evaluation Subcommittee reported, the *Participatory Evaluation Guide to Healthy Municipalities, Cities and Communities* was useful in highlighting aspects of the initiative that were lacking or weak, such as participation from the public sector, and bringing about discussions on how to address the issue. The transitory nature of local political decisions and an agenda based on electoral priorities were some of the main factors inhibiting participation by the public sector. The public sector was present at the beginning of the initiative, but its participation faded through the years. Absence of this public sector's contribution led to emphasis being placed on the process of getting the community organized.

Similar to the implementation of a health promotion initiative such as HMC, the application of a participatory evaluation methodology requires joint effort from all relevant stakeholders. This was one of the main challenges in Vila Paciencia. However, the process of applying the methodology proposed in the Guide demonstrated the difficulties in gaining representation of key stakeholders, which, in turn, stimulated the group to bring about change in this arena. In this case, use of the Guide in the evaluation process actually stimulated participation in the HMC initiative.

The Guide's emphasis on intersectoral collaboration contributed greatly to the understanding of local politics and the role of different actors (public, private, community, etc.), constituting a reference for discussions and decision-making. In this initiative, intersectoral collaboration was difficult, particularly in relation to developing and maintaining the intersectoral committee and evaluation subcommittee. Upon realizing the challenge, the group decided to create a new intersectoral group centered on the construction of a new community kitchen. The new group includes representatives from the local public sector (municipal education and social development, state social assistance), and community members.

In this new phase the group decided to discuss the Guide's proposed pillars indirectly, relating them to community issues. This was aimed at facilitating comprehension of the concepts by putting them into the context of a local practical experience, using the various implementation phases of the community kitchen project. New actors have demonstrated interest in being involved with the evaluation process and have participated in the monthly meetings. It is expected that working on the evaluation will help to strengthen the work of the new intersectoral group and support the sustainability of the Vila Paciencia initiative.

The Application of the Participatory Evaluation Methodology in Peru[3]

The HMC strategy in Peru dates back to 1996 with the launching of the "Healthy Municipalities and Communities Declaration", which was coordinated by the

---

[3] Information about this experience was compiled from Red de Municipios y Comunidades Saludables del Peru (2004).

Peruvian Ministry of Health and the Pan American Health Organization (PAHO), and signed by various institutions, community-based organizations, civil society organizations, universities and local authorities. In 2003 the Peruvian Network of Healthy Municipalities was established with 29 municipalities, catalyzing the HMC process throughout the entire country. Today (2007) the network comprises over 130 municipalities and seven regional networks.

In 2004, a workshop was conducted in Peru to introduce the Participatory Evaluation methodology. Participants included technical staff from the Ministry of Health, municipal authorities and staff, health professionals, students, and representatives from NGOs and universities involved with the HMC strategy in the country.

As a result of this workshop, a series of activities and actions took place, such as the inclusion of a participatory evaluation module into the curriculum of the Health Promotion Certificate Program offered by the San Marcos University and the launching of a series of participatory evaluation processes by Proyecto Amares (a program supported by the European Community) in rural communities in Peru. In addition, participatory evaluation was incorporated into the Ministry of Health's Healthy Municipalities Program, which defines the technical norms for the HMC strategy at the national level. The municipality of Miraflores also applied the participatory evaluation methodology to their "Tai Chi in the Parks" Program. The remainder of this section describes the process and the results of the Miraflores experience.

The Miraflores' Experience: Participatory Evaluation of the "Tai Chi in the Parks" Program

The "Tai Chi in the Parks" initiative was implemented in the 1990s as a public health strategy in the municipality of Miraflores, in Lima, Peru. Today, the "Tai Chi in the Parks" Association is responsible for the maintenance, improvement and advancement of the initiative along with Tai Chi Clubs and more than 20,000 elderly people who practice Tai Chi in the municipality.

The mission of the "Tai Chi in the Parks" Program is to transform Miraflores into the municipality with the healthiest and most active elderly population in Peru, thereby, promoting healthy aging of the population. The initiative's main objectives are to incorporate the practice of Tai Chi and its philosophy as a daily, voluntary and accessible habit in the life of Miraflores' elderly population; and to achieve physical, psychological, social and spiritual development of Miraflores' elderly population through the practice of Tai Chi.

To this end, the initiative offered free Tai Chi classes during weekdays in various parks in Miraflores; supported the formation of Tai Chi clubs, which are informal Tai Chi groups, and developed a "Tai Chi in the Parks" network; promoted various community activities such as festivals, Tai Chi championships, conferences, etc.; and trained community elderly to become Tai Chi instructors, thereby increasing human resources necessary to expand the program.

During 2004–2005, the participatory evaluation methodology was applied to evaluate this experience. An Evaluation Subcommittee was formed to plan and implement the evaluation process. This group was comprised of technical staff from the municipality, the program coordinator, program participants and elderly members of the community who did not participate in the program. Initially, one of the main concerns of the group was to engage in an independent, empowering process that would not be dominated by the municipality and program managers. To address this issue, the group changed its name to "Evaluation Group" and determined by consensus who would be part of the group.

A series of meetings took place to introduce the evaluation methodology to all participants and to reach consensus on all its core concepts. These meetings were guided by a trained facilitator. Through weekly workshops, all of the Evaluation Group members were trained in the participatory evaluation methodology. Working with the elderly population was described as a facilitating factor since most of the participants were retired and had flexibility to participate in these initial meetings. The fact that most participants of the Evaluation Group were not involved with the health sector or were not health professionals was also a facilitating factor in these initial discussions. This allowed the group to be more open to explore issues related to social and psychological benefits of the program, and not to be focused on evaluating the health benefits of the program in terms of disease prevention.

Based on the process and the steps proposed in the Participatory Evaluation Guide, the group developed an evaluation plan. This included developing evaluation questions, reaching consensus on key concepts, and defining indicators, data collection methods and a work plan. The group requested that a representative from the Universidad Mayor de San Marco join the process in order to provide support and guidance related to the data collection and analysis processes.

When planning for the evaluation, the group came across a major issue, which was that the "Tai Chi in the Parks" Program had not been planned and implemented in a participatory manner. It had also not fully taken into account core health promotion principles (such as intersectorial participation), which posed a challenge in applying the evaluation framework proposed by the Participatory Evaluation Guide. However, engaging in the participatory evaluation process had the positive impact of highlighting these deficiencies and mobilizing the group to search for solutions. In order to address these issues, the group approached its problems from different perspectives and took into account the factors that might facilitate or hinder the participation of other stakeholders.

The Evaluation Group reported facing many challenges in its work. Some of the group's participants demonstrated great resistance to the idea of implementing a participatory methodology due to ingrained concerns and negative ideas related to actions taken with the input of the community. There were fears of excessive criticism and an increase in "demands" by the community if offered the opportunity to participate. The data collection and analysis phase of the process suffered delays due to difficulties in coordinating the work with the technical staff from the Ministry of Health and the university, who were providing technical guidance in these matters. The Evaluation Group also reported initial discrepancies related to the various interpretations given by the group to the concept of health promotion and other core concepts related to the evaluation. In addition, turnover of key personnel in the municipality caused major delays in the implementation process.

Other challenges faced by the group included difficulties with data analysis (due to low technical capacity among participants) and lack of flexibility and openness on the part of some group members in listening and engaging in a true dialogue. Having a good facilitator was reported as a key aspect of the process to guide the discussion and help the group reach conclusions.

During site visits for data collection the group identified various issues such as difficulties with sound systems, and the need to limit the access of dogs to the parks during the Tai Chi classes. The group quickly passed this information on to those responsible for the program coordination, and they in turn were able to work with the parks management to solve these problems. Seeing the results of their efforts highly motivated the participants of the Evaluation Group to be more involved in the process. Many manifested an interest in evaluating other aspects of the "Tai Chi in the Parks" Program and learning more about the participatory evaluation methodology. As a result, a series of workshops were conducted to identify other key aspects of the program and to define priorities for the next round of evaluation. These workshops were organized by the Evaluation Group itself, which included a skilled facilitator to help participants identify the main strategic lines to be addressed. This turned out to be an important opportunity to bring together program managers and program beneficiaries to participate in the process. Dialogue and participation was also strengthened and provided a broader vision for the program.

The Evaluation Group devised two strategies to broaden the evaluation process: (1) to incorporate the San Marcos National University, to provide technical support in the processes related to the evaluation, and (2) to engage the current Evaluation Group in the evaluation of other programs aimed at the elderly population in the municipality. The participatory evaluation brought about significant changes in the way programs are planned in the municipality, particularly with respect to involving various stakeholders and sectors, and requiring participatory planning and evaluation as part of how programs are devised and implemented.

Discussion

Health promotion has advanced significantly in the past few decades, accompanied by an increasing interest in evaluating its effectiveness. Participatory evaluation holds great promise for helping to generate this evidence and promote understanding of the factors that affect, positively and negatively, the advances of health promotion in the Region.

The experiences described above highlight some of the challenges posed by the complex and multidimensional local and national contexts into which participatory evaluation is introduced. Factors affecting the success of evaluation initiatives were identified at various levels (individual, institutional, political, community, etc.). These factors intertwine and impact each other in very complex ways, a fact that was reflected in the municipalities' experiences in implementing participatory evaluation.

Political context and timing were two of the main factors affecting the evaluation process. Given the strong emphasis of initiatives like HMC on the active involvement of local authorities and the public sector, election periods and political transitions can cause major delays (if not termination) of initiatives, shortage and/or change of personnel and funds, and great uncertainty about the future of the initiatives. This highlights the importance of establishing strong coalitions among all sectors of society to strengthen and sustain the HMC initiatives and their evaluation. A stronger and broader base of support can provide continuity and sustainability to such initiatives during these transitional periods.

Being able to work in a truly intersectorial manner poses another challenge for most health promotion initiatives and their evaluation, yet it is an important factor affecting sustainability of these efforts. Lack of support from critical stakeholders, such as municipal program managers or key personnel at public institutions, can seriously deter or isolate the advancement of the initiative. It can also jeopardize the possibility that the evaluation results will be taken into consideration by all relevant stakeholders, hence threatening the likelihood that results will be used to improve the initiative.

All experiences reported that the participatory evaluation process was lengthy and time consuming. This is due to various factors, such as bringing together a variety of stakeholders from various backgrounds, sectors and interests; reaching consensus on core concepts and paradigms; and working through institutions and organizations with rigid and bureaucratic structures and work cultures. The various levels of knowledge and literacy among those involved also affected the time it took to complete the process.

Recognizing the time needed for institutions, organizations and individuals to adapt and accept a new methodology is crucial. The implementation of a participatory evaluation often requires great changes in how organizations and institutions function and work. However, given the appropriate consideration and time, people become motivated and apply dedicated efforts to implementing these new programs and methodologies. Achieving this acceptance, particularly from public institutions and their staff is critical in order to put in place programs that are consistent with the communities' expectations, make optimal use of resources, more effectively incorporate health promotion practices, and improve personal motivation among public staff and other stakeholders.

The experiences described in this chapter also reflected a general lack of understanding about the concept of health promotion (often considered an approach to disease prevention) and the participatory evaluation methodology. This can have a direct impact on the planning of the evaluation since how people understand key concepts will shape the design, data collection, analysis and presentation of results of the evaluation. The introduction of the *Participatory Evaluation Guide to Healthy Municipalities, Cities and Communities* can play an important role in addressing these issues by serving as a catalyst to engage people in a joint reflection and learning process.

Also reported were concerns related to the benefits of conducting a participatory evaluation, particularly related to the time it takes to conduct the process and the usefulness of the data it will produce. Resistance by key institutions to applying a participatory evaluation methodology was also common. It is important to address these concerns and take into account the challenges faced by stakeholders coming from institutions with rigid and bureaucratic structures, that often do not have a policy that enables or facilitates coordination with other institutions or working in an intersectorial manner. It is also important to take into account that these stakeholders are often under great pressure to produce results in a short period of time.

Concerns arose about working with the community, often expressed as fear of receiving negative comments, prejudice against actions taken with "too much" input from community members, and the possibility that the process would generate "unrealistic demands" made by community members. This can be particularly true of communities in which, traditionally, programs and approaches were implemented from the top-down and truly representative and participatory mechanisms for community participation were scarce or non-existent. However, the experiences described above suggest that the process itself of engaging in a participatory evaluation and having the opportunity to engage with other community stakeholders resulted in positive changes in attitudes and perspectives related to the potential of community participation.

Working with institutions with rigid and bureaucratic structures can also pose a challenge for participatory evaluation. Barriers include lack of institutional support or excessive bureaucracy, lack of coordination among public sector institutions, strict guidelines regarding the use of funds, and conflicts among the different actors involved (federal, state, municipal). High turnover of personnel at all levels and institutions can be particularly disruptive. Public sector personnel are frequently transferred to another state or unit/program within their institutions and it is often the case that in their new posts they are no longer in a position to follow through with the initiatives for which they were previously responsible. On the positive side of working with institutions, the process of engaging in participatory evaluation can open communication channels with other levels and sectors providing valuable inputs for the evaluation process, and clearing a path for exploring new modes of intersectoral collaboration.

Working with institutions also offers the opportunity to routinize processes and methodologies within work plans, programs, curriculums, etc. For example, the inclusion of the participatory evaluation methodology into the curriculum of the San Marcos National University's Health Promotion Certificate Program, in Peru, provides an ongoing opportunity to build capacities and increase technical knowledge among professionals working in the field. Institutions can often have a far-reaching impact with the potential to promote and support the implementation of health promotion activities, their evaluation and the allocation of resources for these priorities.

Having strong, sustained and dynamic leadership is central to the sustainability of an evaluation initiative. Active commitment and engagement from institutions both at the local and national levels is key to the success of such initiatives, as is collaborative work among them. National and regional HMC networks can be central in these efforts, given their potential far-reaching connections to municipalities throughout a country or region, as well as their connection with key stakeholders that can support the evaluation process.

Conducting a participatory evaluation can be an empowering process by itself, as the experiences described demonstrate. Merely by engaging in the planning and implementation of the participatory methodology, communities and stakeholders were more willing and interested in participating and maintaining this participation. The process itself also provided a very rich opportunity to discuss, exchange and reflect on countries' experiences with the HMC strategy. These discussions brought to light the various interpretations that participants gave to health promotion concepts and principles. This often resulted in a productive and positive dialogue among participants in order to reach consensus on the various concepts and principles utilized in their evaluation processes.

The *Participatory Evaluation Guide to Healthy Municipalities, Cities and Communities* was developed to respond to a direct need expressed by those implementing the HMC Strategy and other health promotion programs. However, once the methodology was made available and applied, most stakeholders reported not being ready to implement such an innovative approach to evaluation. Primarily, stakeholders came to a realization that their HMC and health promotion programs and initiatives had not appropriately taken into account key health promotion principles (such as intersectorial collaboration or community participation).

The application of the participatory evaluation approach made an important contribution to these initiatives, as it shed light on the gaps in their efforts and mobilized those involved to confront the problems and reflect on how to address them. This is stimulating many municipalities to review their planning and implementation processes in order to more appropriately incorporate health promotion principles. As a result, the community groups and institutions involved in this initiative are engaged in re-examining and reorienting their planning and implementation processes in order to more effectively apply the participatory evaluation methodology in the future. Thus, engaging in the participatory evaluation process has served as a catalyst to generate intersectoral and participatory processes essential to the development of HMC initiatives.

Participants in the three experiences described above reported that engaging in a participatory evaluation was highly motivating and revitalizing, concretely stimulating those involved to look at their actions more consistently, and promoting interest in the issue of evaluation. The participatory evaluation experience strengthened capacities among those involved, generated commitment to follow health promotion principles, strengthened alliances among key stakeholders, and emphasized the potential of participatory evaluation as a decision-making tool. As such, participatory evaluation holds great promise for contributing to the advancement of health promotion in the countries of the Region.

References

Becker, D., Edmundo, K., Nunes, N., Mattos, A., Marques, R., & Bonato, D. (2006). "CEDAPS/Rio de Janeiro: a iniciativa de Vila Paciência" In M. Akerman & R. Mendes (Eds.),

Avaliação Participativa de Municipios, Comunidades e Ambientes Saudáveis: a trajetória brasileira – memória, reflexões e experiencia. São Paulo, Brazil: Midia Alternativa.

Pan American Health Organization/World Health Organization (2002) *Healthy Municipalities and Communities: Mayor's Guide for Promoting Quality of Life.* Washington, DC: Pan American Health Organization/World Health Organization.

Pan American Health Organization/World Health Organization (2006) *Guía de Evaluación Participativa para Municipios y Comunidades Saludables.* Lima, Peru: Pan American Health Organization/World Health Organization.

Red de Municipios y Comunidades Saludables del Peru (2004) *Experiencia de Aplicación de la Guía de Evaluación Participativa en el Peru.* Washington, DC: Report submitted to the PAHO Healthy Municipalities Evaluation Working Group.

Sperandio, A. M., Correa, C., Rodriguez, E., & Bueno, R. M. (2006) A experiência de aplicação do Guia de Avaliação Participativa em uma Rede de Municipios: um processo em desenvolvimento. In M. Akerman & R. Mendes (Eds.), *Avaliação Participativa de Municipios, Comunidades e Ambientes Saudáveis: a trajetória brasileira – memória, reflexões e experiencia.* São Paulo, Brazil: Midia Alternativa.

Chapter 13
Evaluating Health Promotion in Rio de Janeiro, Brazil: An Integrated Local Development Project

Regina Bodstein

This chapter discusses the strategies used to evaluate implementation of a health-promotion project in the Manguinhos neighborhood of Rio de Janeiro, Brazil. The principles of health promotion and the concept of sustainable and intersectoral local development provided the underlying guidelines for the program. Aimed at addressing local determinants of health, and the social, environmental, cultural and economic dimensions of quality of life, the Integrated Local Development Project was supported by, and led to, community mobilization and participation (Ferreira & Buss, 2002; Buss & Ramos, 2000). In this chapter we discuss the challenges of evaluating a program that brought about change in various settings and at various levels. Specifically, it affected teaching and research at the National School of Public Health; it led to reorienting the healthcare model of the National School of Public Health's Academic Health Center; it triggered intense community mobilization; and it resulted in a new intersectoral dialogue focusing on improved quality of local life in Manguinhos (Bodstein, Zancan, & Estrada, 2001; Bodstein & Zancan, 2003; Hartz, Ramos, & Marcondes, 2002; Zancan et al., 2002).

In 1999 the Brazilian National School of Public Health of the Foundation Oswaldo Cruz, the Brazilian Association of Collective Health, and the Canadian Association of Public Health developed a technical cooperative agreement to support the integration of health promotion into Brazilian public health policy and programs, which led to the creation of the Integrated Local Development Project. The project sought to develop a new public health paradigm on primary health care and on health promotion by linking health promotion theory, research, and training with public health practice (Canada-Brazil/HPIA, 2003).

The National School of Public Health, a leading institution for public health teaching and research in Brazil, had experience with many community health projects that were based on understanding the local determinants of health. These included an Open University project to improve environmental and health conditions, Health-Promoting Schools, Physical Activity for Residents, Acupuncture and Homeopathy, "Alimentação Viva" Project, Program for Healthcare in the Elderly,

R. Bodstein
Department of Social Science at the National School of Public Health (ENSP), Fundação Oswaldo Cruz, Rio de Janeiro, Brazil

L. Potvin, D. McQueen (eds.), *Health Promotion Evaluation Practices in the Americas*,
DOI: 10.1007/978-0-387-79733-5_13, © Springer Science+Business Media, LLC 2008   237

and STD/AIDS (Buss & Ramos, 2000; Ferreira & Buss, 2002; Zancan, Bodstein, & Marcondes, 2002).

The School's history of working in the neighborhood of Manguinhos, a favela (shanty town) bordering campus, contributed to the evolution of a comprehensive conception of improved quality of life and local development in Manguinhos, and for reflecting on health-promotion principles in public policies, services, teaching, and research in the health sector (Carvalho, Bodstein, Hartz, & Matida, 2004; Ferreira & Buss, 2002). The Integrated Local Development Project sought to share exemplar health promotion practices and to disseminate these in Brazil by way of three strategies : (1) enhancing the capacity of the School of Public Health's Academic Health Center and the community to develop, implement, and evaluate health promotion strategies; (2) strengthening health promotion within the School's programs in public health; and (3) disseminating health promotion and population health concepts and project results throughout Brazilian, Canadian, and international public health networks. The first activity in this Canadian-Brazilian collaboration was the implementation of a project to address root determinants of health and intersectoral collaboration called the Integrated Local Development Project in Manguinhos. At the same time, the project received timely support from the Brazilian

Table 13.1 Evaluation of the Integrated Local Development Project

Dimensions and Issues	Evaluation Strategies
Degree of health-promotion principles incorporated by the practitioners and researchers;	Semi-structured and self-applied questionnaire
Importance of family health team to reinforce social orientation practices at Academic Health Center	Interviews with professionals in family health-program team
Process of partnership and intersectoral agenda formation addressing social determinants of quality of life in Manguinhos	Direct and systematic observation of interactions and discussions in coordination meetings Activities notes
Identification of strategic actors, communities associations, and cleavages	Community participatory diagnosis
Impasses in the creation of Local Development Forum	Direct and systematic observation of meetings and workshops; notes from Forum discussions
Mapping social initiatives and equipments in the communities	Field survey and interviews with key actors and social organizations in the communities
Identification of an existing set of solidarity and collaboration at the community level (leaderships involved in cultural, educational, and sports activities)	Mapping of activities and social organizations Content analysis
Conflicting interests and impasses in the implementation process	Content analysis of decision-making process

Source: Bodstein & Zancan, 2002; Bodstein & Zancan, 2003; Canada-Brazil/HPIA, 2003; FCDDH, 2000; Hartz et al., 2002.

Association of Collective Health to develop a leadership position in the debate about public health in the country, and support from the Brazilian Research and Projects Financing Agency (ABRASCO, 2002).

In this chapter we describe the key dimensions and evaluation strategies of the project in Manguinhos (see Table 13.1). We center this discussion on negotiation in intersectoral actions vis-à-vis community participation in an integrated local development agenda.

Local Development and Health Promotion in Manguinhos

In Brazil, a framework for Sustainable and Integrated Local Development originated in the mid-1990s and was based on the Economic Commission for Latin America and the Caribbean model that postulated that development presupposes a participatory, equitable, and sustainable process (CEPAL, 1991). The process involves a concept of "local development as a social process combining economic growth with redistribution and improvement of the community's quality of life" (Buss & Ramos, 2000, p. 15), and intersectoral policies in relation to social support network organizations in a given social and territorial space. The proposal included employment and income generation (e.g., micro-credit and cooperatives), housing, sanitation, health, and education, among other components, and was based on participatory diagnosis of the problems and needs in a given local territory or community (Agenda 21, 1992; CEPAL, 1991; Oficina Social, 1998). Local development projects occurred in small communities and municipalities (counties) in Brazil and they prioritized mechanisms for employment and income generation through public-private partnerships (Buss & Ramos, 2000; Krutman, 2004). Up until the late 1990s, local development projects in large metropolitan areas and slum communities were uncommon and posed a major challenge for the proposed model.

The initial approach of the Integrated Local Development Project in Manguinhos in 1999 called for establishing a group, led by the Brazilian National School of Public Health, that consisted of representatives from academic institutions, state and municipal secretariats, and large state-owned and private companies with the aim of integrating actions to improve quality of life in Manguinhos. As the proposal evolved, the coordinating group saw the need for a team focused specifically on monitoring and evaluating the project. School of Public Health researchers involved in health promotion and education, and who had direct links with the implementation of the Integrated Local Development Project, designed the evaluation proposal.

The willingness and availability to participate in the coordination meetings was crucial, since there was consensus concerning the need to monitor the planning of actions, their spin-offs, the decision-making process, and community participation in the implementation of the program. Thus, the evaluation team was integrated into the Integrated Local Development Project coordination team, participating as observers in the majority of the decisions.

Evaluative Perspectives

The Integrated Local Development Project evaluators wanted to determine how health promotion principles have been implemented or translated in the School of Public Health practices and to understand the particular ways in which integration of health promotion occurred at the School (Hartz et al., 2002). A semi-structured, self-applied questionnaire was used to collect information on opinions of the professionals involved in the cooperative agreement concerning teaching, research, and reorientation of the Academic Health Center. In addition, curriculum and scientific output of the School were also examined (Hartz et al., 2002). Analysis of the resulting material showed that the introduction of health promotion concepts actually reinforced various principles and practices already in place at the School of Public Health in general and at the Academic Health Center in particular. Interviewees, however, perceived major challenges in the proposal for a dialogue that linked teaching, research, and intervention through health diagnosis and action on the local determinants of the health or disease. Tensions between healthcare practices and health-promoting practices were reported. Lack of intersectoral actions and dialogue among scattered initiatives and projects at the School itself and in the Academic Health Center was perceived as a problem.

Health Promotion as Local Development

Evaluators of the Integrated Local Development Project sought to analyze the Manguinhos initiative from a perspective that viewed health promotion as local development based on the social determinants. This analysis looked at the decision-making process, which involved a wide range of stakeholders and intersectoral actions, in an innovative proposal for community participation (Bodstein et al., 2001). The group in charge of evaluation faced a complex intervention in various settings, with numerous stakeholders and partnerships, and which developed in two major dimensions, namely, intersectorality and the social space of mobilization and participation by local community members.

Intervention Complexity and Context

In a social and territorial context of extreme poverty and violence, it was important to focus on evaluation of the program implementation's dynamics (Denis & Champagne, 1997; Hartz, 1999; Potvin, Haddad, & Frohlich, 2001; Potvin & Richard, 2001; Rootman, 2001). In the face of a comprehensive and multi-focal intervention addressing determinants of health and based on active collaboration of social agents, evaluation aimed exclusively at effects and impacts was obviously not adequate (Chen, 1990; Connell & Kubish, 1998; Pawson & Tilley, 1997; Thurston & Potvin, 2003). Instead, it was understood that the evaluation should capture the complexity of the intersectoral collaboration and community participation and examine obstacles to collaborative actions that might put at risk the program's implementation and results.

A literature on the evaluation of the Health Action Zones (deprived sub-regional units) in England in the 1990s was useful to the extent that the design, principles, and objectives bore similarities to the Manguinhos experience, despite the evident differences in context and levels of social inequality between the two countries. In the British case (unlike the Manguinhos project), the initiative stemmed from action planned at the central level by the National Health Service aimed at a systemic approach to health inequalities. The Health Action Zones program had a seven year implementation timeframe and specific budget allocation; in short, its execution and subsequent evaluation occurred at the central level (Barnes, Matka, & Sullivan, 2003; Sullivan, Barnes, & Matka, 2002; Sullivan, Judge, & Sewell, 2004; Springett, 2005).

In the Integrated Local Development Project in Manguinhos, growing violence and its impact on both quality of life and patterns of sociability and collective action were key issues (Bodstein & Zancan, 2002; Jackson et al., 2003; Peres et al., 2005; Wacquant, 2001; Zaluar, 1997). The evaluative approach sought to analyze *context* and identify the principal processes and practices of *strategic actors* who could potentially hinder or even prevent intersectoral actions and community participation. In the Manguinhos case the attempt was to identify processes that historically hindered collaboration in a locality with a particularly harsh struggle for political space and resources. The issue was to evaluate a set of processes triggered by an intervention in a highly conflictive social space. Thus, the evaluation had to acknowledge that social programs are undeniably social systems and that programs work by introducing new ideas and/or resources into an existing set of social relationships (Pawson, 2003; Pawson, 2002; Pawson & Tilley, 1997; Sullivan et al., 2002). The evaluation approach concentrated on what appeared essential in the program's conceptualization: the dynamics of implementation through mechanisms and strategies for community participation and negotiation of an agenda for multi-sector and integrated development.

Evaluators as Participants

The evaluation team worked with the coordinating body and participated in meetings where the program decisions were made. This was crucial from the evaluators perspective because it allowed them to document, in locus, the formation of a decision-making space that constituted an innovative process resulting from the composition and breadth of the membership. As observers, the evaluation group could analyze the numerous difficulties and impasses in the implementation of intersectoral decisions, integration of agendas, and agreement on actions at both the government and community levels.

Lessons Learned in an Intersectoral Approach

The initial approach for the Integrated Local Development Project was the formation of partnerships and establishment of an intersectoral group that convened important sectors of the public administration together with stakeholders from institutions that were highly motivated to get involved in the project. A large share of the proposal's initial success was due to a municipal policy called the "macro-function" – a plan to integrate various municipal departments sharing related activities – and to participation of the Municipal Health Department's Family Health Program in Manguinhos. The School of Public Health and the funding agencies played key roles in defining the program's guidelines, forming a steering committee that coordinated program actions and provided credibility and some prospects for sustainability.

In addition to the steering committee, several specific thematic groups were established to address basic quality of life issues in Manguinhos (e.g., health, environment, housing, sanitation). The severity of the housing problem, with dangerous and degraded dwellings, made developing a housing project the priority on the local agenda. Negotiations around this project gained enormous political visibility and nearly dominating the entire Integrated Local Development Project agenda. Conflicting interests emerged among local political groups, leading to allegations of serious manipulation of the roster of families to benefit from the project. Meanwhile, resources needed for housing and basic sanitation issues necessitated major public investments and technical support, involving long and cumbersome negotiations with funding agencies and other administrative sectors. It became clear that the issues addressed were long-standing and relatively intractable and that such issues served to foment disagreement and demobilize large segments of the community that were lobbying for an immediate solution.

The presence of an evaluation group in the program steering committee allowed close monitoring of implementation difficulties from the project's onset. One difficulty was that the representatives from different sectors brought a pre-defined agenda to the steering committee meetings. Instead of negotiating an agenda with shared objectives, previously determined, sector-specific goals were merely juxtaposed. Negotiation on priorities and reflection on agreements for intersectoral actions adapted to local conditions did not actually occur, thus exposing both a lack of previous experience with this level of intersectoral action and a lack of effective collaboration on specific goals. This entire process confirmed what has been found in extant evaluation literature: coalitions are easy to build in principle, but difficult to maintain when it comes to making them work together and develop common goals (Weiss, 1998). While the Integrated Local Development Project was successful in planning and initiating intersectoral negotiation, it lacked sustainability and effective collaboration (Bodstein & Zancan, 2002).

Reorientation of the Academic Health Center

Present in 95% of Brazil's municipalities and counties, the Family Health Program is a strategic and priority program of the Brazilian Federal government that has focused on strengthening and restructuring primary health care since the mid-1990s. The Family Health Program emphasizes not only individual care but health promotion based on community participation and intersectoral actions. Two Family Health Program teams were set up in Manguinhos, generating a series of community activities in the program that were based on health promotion principles. Involvement of the School of Public Health's Academic Health Center in this effort was enormously important. First, it guaranteed a concrete space for articulating the action and interests of professionals, researchers, and community representatives. Second, by providing the local population with primary health care for more than 30 years, it gave the School and the Integrated Local Development Project widespread credibility and recognition in the community. Here primary health-care practitioners and researchers could integrate health promotion into health care practices.

The presence of the Family Health Program in Manguinhos was crucial to a discussion within the Integrated Local Development Project on reorientation of health-care services and it contributed decisively to mobilizing the community. Community mobilization took place mainly through a diagnosis of the local health problems, and registration of families to be served by the Family Health Program. Community representatives were involved in the selection and training of young residents who became "community health agents" as part of the Family Health Program's multidisciplinary teams. Acting as a formal link between professionals and the local population, community health agents are a fundamental component of the Family Health Program's objective to reorient healthcare services. Their role in the program is to visit registered families and support improvement in their health and living conditions.

Interviews with professionals on the Family Health Program teams during the evaluation process highlighted the difficulties faced by community health agents and program teams in the development of health education and health promotion activities. Some of these difficulties hindered actions in reorienting the care-based, curative, clinical model toward a more health promoting strategy of action (Senna, Mello, & Bodstein, 2002). Professionals reported that the population's demand for medical care, together with a pervasive conception of health in terms of disease and illness, contributed to the difficulty of reorienting healthcare model.

On the other hand, because of their proximity to the health and social problems in the Manguinhos community, community health agents and family health program teams were able to identify a variety of local problems that required intersectoral solutions. The Family Health Program strategy, according to health-promotion principles, posed the need for intersectoral actions at the level of Academic Health Center management and routine provision of care. As a result, the group responsible for management of the health unit, a partner in the entire process of negotiating the Integrated Local Development Project, was redefined to integrate members from other administrative sectors, with the intention of sharing responsibility for decisions related to local health-related issues (Reis & Vianna, 2002).

The evaluation group found that negotiation of intersectoral action is extremely challenging at the service-level because it requires a large investment in time and energy by management professionals and practitioners. As previous literature has noted, very often social service agencies are linked together weakly, with each agency giving high priority to its own goals and interests and low priority to those of other agencies (Chen, 1990). Implementation of intersectoral actions in the Academic Health Center revealed the difficulty of maintaining partnerships and collaborative work in relation to the demand for integrated solutions to both specific, short-term issues as well as long-term, structural ones.

Municipal Government Involvement

Despite managers' motivation and commitment to the project, the role of the municipal government fell far short of what was expected. Most notably the municipal government was not able to fully address the demands for basic urban infrastructure and public security in Manguinhos and huge problems and precarious conditions remained unsolved. There was low adherence by some sectors of the public administration in the implementation of the Integrated Local Development Project in Manguinhos, and several important institutional stakeholders withdrew their involvement in the program. The project coincided with an election campaign for the Rio de Janeiro Mayor's Office and City Council, which hampered the dialogue, partnerships, and collaborative work between the program and the municipal government. Thus, the proposal for macro-level intersectoral action and partnership with large private enterprises from the region failed to reach fruition and lasted for less than a year.

The Manguinhos evaluation showed that "Coalitions are easy to form under a vague and noble goal because each member can find some reason or motive to participate. Conversely, operative goals, involving the details of resource allocations or value trade-offs, only highlight differences among coalitions and enhance the conflicts between them" (Weiss, 1998). It further illustrated intersectoral dialogue can be impeded by a highly politicized setting – as might be expected in an antipoverty program (Shadish, Cook, & Leviton, 1991; Weiss, 1972; Weiss, 1998). Finally, it shows that intersectoral action can be undermined by institutional fragmentation and administrative discontinuity.

From the onset, the evaluative process showed clearly that while it was important for community mobilization that the program addresses projects and issues of great political visibility, it also demonstrated that the program was never fully implemented due to potential conflicts associated with entrenched interests. In the case of the Manguinhos project, these issues contributed to demobilization.

Participation and Socio-Cultural Mediation

The original conceptualization of the Integrated Local Development Project explicitly valued community perspective, empowerment, and genuine participation, as opposed to a token participation that would have merely legitimized the proposed intervention (Ferreira & Buss, 2002). It was clear to policymakers that success in the implementation of the project in such an adverse socioeconomic setting hinged on broad community mobilization and adherence to the proposal by organized sectors. The mobilization strategy used "rapid participatory diagnosis" to create a Local Development Forum. A participatory diagnosis was conducted by the Bento Rubião Foundation Center for Human Rights (FCDDH, 2000) and consisted of an extensive field survey with a series of interviews and contacts to identify key leaders, organizations, and stakeholders for studying the communities' history, identity, and cultural characteristics. It also mobilized and brought together the main stakeholders, interest groups, organizations, and community demands, converging in a broad mobilization and convening the Local Development Forum.

The effects and results of the community mobilization and participation translated into a significant number of meetings, assemblies, community forums, formation of committees and thematic groups, as well as in the creation of videos, booklets, and posters explaining the Integrated Local Development Project. The Forum, called "Acorda Manguinhos" or "Wakeup Manguinhos", convened for the first time more than 50 local leaders (Santos & Martins, 2002). It was a highly politicized arena and highlighted both the success of the mobilization strategy and the existence of deeply rooted conflicts and interests. The Forum revealed enormous receptiveness and high level of adherence to the project by participants, however, it also revealed the impasses and difficulties experienced by local associations. A mosaic of community associations and organizations with limited scope and little or no cooperation reflected the tensions in local associative life.

Conflicts and discord occurred in all macro-sectoral negotiation processes involving the Integrated Local Development Project agenda. The program experienced a moment of intense conflict with the weakening of the coalition and the partnerships that had originally launched the effort. The evaluation group, observing the changes brought about by the project, attempted to monitor and analyze the emerging impasses that culminated in the Forum's negotiation of a local development agenda. Together with the community leaders, women's associations, and Forum leaders, the evaluation group designed a survey of the existing social initiatives and resources in Manguinhos, with the aim to identify, publicize, and articulate sociocultural projects and resources in the community, i.e., social capital (Coleman, 1990; Putnam, 1996). The research resulted in the Guidebook of Social Resources, which detailed collaboration among the various existing initiatives in the area (Bodstein et al., 2001). This survey revealed the strong presence and importance of religious groups responsible for social interventions in the area. It also revealed fragmentation and lack of coordination among local social programs.

The Manguinhos community had a previous history of community mobilization and revitalization that involved renewed leadership and the emergence of a series of socio-cultural and health initiatives focused on youth, women, elderly, and people with HIV/AIDS, chronic non-communicable diseases, and disabilities. These initiatives promoted alternative nutritional practices, environmental education and activities, and physical activity. Analysis by the evaluation group of the rapid participatory diagnosis reports (FCDDH, 2000) identified the more pressing needs, such as housing and basic sanitation, as compared to educational and recreational activities, especially for children and youth. It also examined social capital as a mechanism for local collaboration and cultural mediation in the associative life in Manguinhos (Bodstein et al., 2001; Peres, Bodstein, Marcondes, Ramos, & Lazer, 2005; Zancan et al., 2002).

Local Associative Life in Manguinhos

A study was conducted to analyze local associative life and identify existing relationships of solidarity, cooperation, and trust. The goal was to identify explanatory factors, given the impasses for cooperation and collective action illustrated by the "Wakeup Manguinhos" Forum. This field survey interviewed main community leaders, delving into greater depth on community life, local demands and problems, and perceptions or opinions concerning the process of mobilization and participation. Analysis of the survey produced evidence of the conflict between neighborhood associations that have a monopoly over local political representation, and non-governmental associations that represent plural forms of organization and directly or indirectly challenge the political practices adopted by the Manguinhos neighborhood associations (Bodstein et al., 2001). This research also revealed the role played by local groups responsible for mediating the community's needs and demands in relation to institutions and the public sector and their support of cultural and sports activities in the community. Despite discords, these cultural mediators represented a possible source of solidarity and cooperation.

In Manguinhos, cultural mediators, together with the professionals providing social and cultural services to the local population, played a major role in linking communities and institutions and organizations, and were a source of social capital in the community. This notion of increasing community capacity in an adverse environment expands on earlier work that focuses more on the ability to work together and lobby for community improvements (e.g., Jackson et al., 2003). In the Manguinhos community, needs related to education, sports, and leisure were subsumed in the need for improvement in urban infrastructure and services. It was necessary to identify the conditions and forces that limit intervention opportunities and devise strategies to respond to these forces (Bauman, 2003; Giddens, 2002). Preoccupation with unemployment, lack of job prospects, and idleness among youth in Manguinhos was a common and strong theme in the discourse of local leaders. Recreational and cultural activities were valued by the leaders and by the population in general, because of their potential to strengthen positive sociability, affirm identity, and improve self-esteem. Through these activities, community leaders or cultural mediators gain visibility and recognition in the entire community (Alvito, 2001). Such activities are crucial for generating mechanisms that reinforce and create social capital in the community.

The survey of local associative life showed the presence of factors that constrained collective action and the capacity for horizontal collaboration. Working together collaboratively to lobby for community improvements was hindered by a marked difference in the interests of important local community organizations. Paternalistic practices and cronyism created vertical relationships of dependence and subordination in the population and its leaders in relation to political parties, institutions, and the public sector in general.

Violence Undermines Civic Life

The alarming violence that afflicts both more- and less-developed countries undermines civic life and solidarity in neighborhoods like Manguinhos (Jackson et al., 2003; Wacquant, 2001). The presence of a contingent of adults and young people who are marginalized from basic citizens' rights, discriminated against, and stigmatized turns these communities into social ghettoes (Santos & Martins, 2002). In what are viewed as dangerous areas, the stigma of violence marks the residents and particularly the young slum-dwellers, who are seen as being on the verge of criminal activity, if not already involved in it (Rinaldi, 1998). Like other prejudices, this stigma has the potential to be self-assimilated, reinforcing young people's adherence to violence and marginalization. Thus, the drug traffic and violence become a central representation of power in the slums, altering the networks of reciprocity and solidarity and the values shared by residents (Zaluar, 1997).

Initiatives that reinforce positive values and self-esteem are increasingly necessary to improve quality of life in areas with increasing violence. The evaluation of associative life made it clear that cultural mediators in Manguinhos share and are acutely aware of this problem. Mechanisms for democratization, participation, and innovation that operate in community interventions are two-way: government must be open channels for participation and expanding public space for community leaders, while community leaders must share responsibility for local action to build solidarity (Jacobi, 2002). In the case of Manguinhos, the municipal government was entirely open in the beginning as a partner in the Integrated Local Development Project, but then retreated, denying sustainability for the community's principal proposals and demands.

Reflection on Evaluation Practice

The evaluative approach described here was applied to a comprehensive health promotion and local development program in a very poor area in the city of Rio de Janeiro. The program's innovative nature and the impasses in its implementation required an evaluative approach that documented intersectoral and community dialogue over the course of the program's duration. The most striking characteristic of the Integrated Local Development Project was the community's mobilization to engage with the project's management committee that included academic institutions, sectors of State and municipal government (e.g. housing, health, and labor), private companies, and social organizations present in the community.

The fact that the evaluation team had a seat in the periodic meetings of the program's coordinating body allowed the documentation of the numerous difficulties and impasses in the implementation of intersectoral decisions, integration of agendas, and agreement on actions at both the government and community levels. The evaluative approach benefited from reflexive knowledge gained through participation in the decision-making process and debate on proposals and actions in the management committee's meetings. Knowledge of the program's design and objectives, the dilemmas in implementation within a problematic context, and the impasses that emerged in the decision-making process shaped the evaluation questions.

In essence, the evaluation centered on the principles and objectives underlying the program's construction, that is, in accordance with a comprehensive view of the social, environmental, cultural, political, and technical determinants of health. This occurred in an environment characterized by continuous negotiation. The evaluation of a program that involves multilevel processes, components, and mechanisms is by definition a complex process. Two major evaluation issues were examined: (1) the process of dialogue and negotiation of intersectoral strategies in Manguinhos, and (2) community mobilization premised on participation and consensus for an integrated local development agenda.

This evaluation revealed a conflictive organizational and participatory context that was averse to collaborative actions. A reflexive and analytical evaluation, coupled with participation in the process, was crucial to the credibility of an evaluation in which there were diverse interests and growing political conflicts. The evaluation used a contextual analysis to explain the impasse in the implementation of intersectoral and participatory actions, and to reveal the proposed program's limits. The context shaped and defined the program itself, as well as the choice of evaluation questions. These evaluation questions sought to illuminate the progressive nature of the program in relation to the difficulties in implementing action on social determinants of health. This could only be explained by understanding the associative life in Manguinhos, the complex issues (housing and basic sanitation projects), and the responsibility and role of the public sector in solving them.

The context was conceived and analyzed as a structured set of relations that define social practices and political interests and identify both supportive participants as well as those resistant to the program and the proposed changes. Use of a qualitative methodology to understand the interests shaping practices and structuring relations that were historically present in the communities was fundamental. In this sense, only by identifying and working with strategic actors in the community – cultural mediators – and using in depth interviews, could we understand conflicts in the associative life of Manguinhos.

The evaluation process demonstrated that the program's context can be defined. In the case of the Manguinhos project, there was a set of relations and interests attached to the intergovernmental sphere and also a space defined by the common and discordant interests of the community. Both displayed contradictions that were heightened by a highly politicized environment not prone to consensus. A lack of integration among governmental sectors and agencies, and the fact that each had their own interests, was an issue the evaluators observed in the program's coordination meetings. On the other hand, the Academic Health Center favored intersectoral action and social participation since it was widely used and respected by the Manguinhos community.

In addition to describing actions and obstacles, this evaluation attempted to construct an explanation for these processes based on a view of context as a space build by structured practices that shape social relations and policies, past and current. The evaluation describes structural processes that prevented full implementation of the project. Initiatives with characteristics similar to the Integrated Local Development Project depend, to a large extent, on expanding the decision-making space by mobilizing and valuing existing social relationships and social organizations acting in the local area (Barnes et al., 2003).

The evaluation process for the Manguinhos program was carried out in close proximity to the community through participation of cultural mediators. Collaboration with these strategic actors started in the participatory diagnosis phase, and eventually allowed the mapping of social spaces (or solidarity networks) and social capital in Manguinhos. This gave visibility to the socio-cultural and recreational movements existing in the area. Work with strategic actors in the community was crucial to the evaluative process. From this participatory evaluation, the contribution of the cultural mediators to community sociability and solidarity – so necessary for quality of life and decreasing local violence – became apparent, lending greater visibility to local social capital.

Conclusion

Various evaluation strategies have been discussed here in light of the diversity of dimensions and settings in the Integrated Local Development Project. We attempted to systematize the opinions of professionals at School of Public Health regarding strengthening health promotion practices. We also focused on the analysis of the program's implementation process by examining the formation of partnerships and the mobilization of various institutional and non-institutional stakeholders. This involved a systematic reflection on the project related to two central strategies for health promotion and local development: an intersectoral approach and community mobilization and participation.

This evaluation sought to focus on innovative elements in a program whose greater objective was to act on the social determinants of health in communities lacking urban infrastructure and public services and plagued by violence. The project proposed housing and basic sanitation projects, employment and income generation, reorientation of the local health center, and various initiatives to foster social inclusion and curb violence. These are complex issues, difficult to solve in the short term, and require significant public investment.

The evaluation questions tried to capture the complexity of a process involving health promotion to improve quality of life determinants in an extremely adverse social and political context. Impasses in the negotiation of a common agenda for the Manguinhos area were evident in collaboration attempts by academic institutions, various levels of government, non-governmental organizations, and the participating communities. The evaluative practice highlighted the interdependence between the program and the context, since there were frequent changes and reorientations throughout its two-year history. This was a long process of establishing a common agenda, integrating intersectoral actions in the program, and reflecting on changes and the intricate negotiations among diverse stakeholders whose political and partisan interests were always at stake. To understand the impasses arising in both intersectoral collaboration and participation by local representatives, and to explain the origin of interests and conflicts constantly at stake, we interviewed community leaders who offered insights that revealed both unity and division in local associative life.

The evaluators' participant observer role in the process of formulating and negotiating an agenda were crucial to the selection of questions and to the very choice of the evaluative approach itself. In conclusion, evaluation practice discussed here was achieved by constantly fine-tuning the Manguinhos project in response to local context, by participatory observation of the entire complex decision-making process, and by autonomy in reflecting on the impasses for cooperation and collective action.

References

ABRASCO. (2002). Oficina Pesquisa Avaliativa em Promoção da Saúde e Desenvolvimento Comunitário. In *V Congresso Brasileiro de Epidemiologia*. Curitiba, Paraná.

Alvito, M. (2001). *As cores de Acari: uma favela carioca*. Rio de Janeiro: Editora FGV.

Barnes, M., Matka, E., & Sullivan, H. (2003). Evidence, Understanding & Complexity – Evaluation in non-linear Systems. *Evaluation, 9*(3), 265-84.

Bauman, Z. (2003). *Comunidade: a busca por segurança no mundo atual*. Rio de Janeiro: Jorge Zahar Ed.

Bodstein, R., Zancan, L., & Estrada, D. (2001). *Guia de Equipamentos e Iniciativas Sociais em Manguinhos*. Rio de Janeiro: Ed. FIOCRUZ.

Bodstein, R., & Zancan, L. (2002). Avaliação das ações de promoção da saúde em contextos de pobreza e vulnerabilidade social. In L. Zancan, R. Bodstein, W. B. Marcondes (Eds.), *Promoção da saúde como caminho para o desenvolvimento local: a experiência em Manguinhos-RJ* (pp. 39–59). Rio de Janeiro: ABRASCO/FIOCRUZ.

Bodstein, R., & Zancan, L. (2003). Monitoramento e Avaliação do Programa de Desenvolvimento Local Integrado e Sustentável. *The Integrated Local Development Project*. Relatório de Pesquisa, Manguinhos.

Buss, P. M., & Ramos, C. L. (2000). Desenvolvimento Local e Agenda 21. Desafios da Cidadania. *Cadernos da Oficina Social, 3*, 13–65. Rio de Janeiro: COEP.

Canada – Brazil Technology Transfer Fundation. (2003). *The Integrated Local Development Project*. HPIA. Closing Report.

Carvalho, A. I., Bodstein, R., Hartz, Z., & Matida, A. H. (2004). Concepções e Abordagens na Avaliação em Promoção da Saúde. *Ciência e Saúde Coletiva, 9*(3).

Chen, H. T. (1990). *Theory – Driven Evaluation*. Newbury Park: Sage Publications.

Coleman, J. S. (1990). *Foundation of social theory*. Cambridge: Harvard University Press.

Connell, J. P., & Kubish, A. C. (1998). Applying a Theory of Change Approach to the Evaluation of Comprehensive Community Initiatives: Progress, Prospect & Problems. In New Approaches to Community Initiative. (II), *Theory, measurements & analysis*. Washington: Aspen Institute.

Denis, J., & Champagne, F. (1997). *Análise da implantação. Avaliação em Saúde: Dos modelos Conceituais à Prática na Análise da Implantação dos Programas*. Rio de Janeiro: ENSP/FIOCRUZ.

Ferreira, J. R., & Buss, P. M. (2002). O que o Desenvolvimento Local tem a ver com a Promoção da Saúde? In L. Zancan, R. Bodstein, & W. B. Marcondes (Eds.), *Promoção da saúde como caminho para o desenvolvimento local: a experiência em Manguinhos-RJ* (pp. 15–37). Rio de Janeiro: ABRASCO/FIOCRUZ.

Fundação Centro de Defesa dos Direitos Humanos Bento Rubião. (2000). *Diagnóstico Rápido Participativo das Comunidades de Manguinhos*. Rio de Janeiro.

Giddens, A. (2002). *Modernidade e Identidade*. Rio de Janeiro: Jorge Zahar.

Hartz, Z. (1999). Pesquisa Avaliativa em Promoção da Saúde. In P. M. Buss (Ed.), *Promoção da Saúde e Saúde Pública: Contribuição para o Debate entre as Escolas de Saúde Pública da América Latina.* (manuscript).

Hartz, Z. M. A., Ramos, C. L., & Marcondes, W. (2002). Lições Aprendidas do Projeto Promoção da Saúde em Ação. In L. Zancan, R. Bodstein, W. B. Marcondes (Ed.), *Promoção da saúde como caminho para o desenvolvimento local: a experiência em Manguinhos-RJ* (pp. 61–78). Rio de Janeiro: ABRASCO/FIOCRUZ.

Health Action Zones/Just do something. (n.d.). Web site: http://www.justdosomething.net

Health Action Zones/ Merseyside. (n.d.). Web site: http://www.mhaz.org.uk

Health Action Zones/Our Healthier Nation. (n.d.). Web site: http://www.ohn.gov.uk

Jackson, S. F., Cleverly, S., Poland, B., Burman, D., Edwards, R., & Robertson, A. (2003). Working with Toronto neighborhoods toward developing indicators of community capacity. *Health Promotion International, 18*(4), 339–350.

Jacobi, P. (2002). Políticas Sociais Locais e os Desafios da Participação Citadina. *Ciência e Saúde Coletiva, 7*(3).

Krutman, H. M. (2004). *Fatores Críticos no Êxito da Gestão de Projetos de Desenvolvimento Local Integrado e Sustentável*. Tese da Universidade Federal do Rio de Janeiro, COPPE. Engenharia de Produção.

Pawson, R. (2002). Evidence-based policy: the promise of "Realist Synthesis". *Evaluation, 8*(3), 340–358.

Pawson, R. (2003). Nothing as practical as a good theory. *Evaluation, 9*(4), 471–490.

Pawson, R., & Tilley, N. (1997). *Realistic evaluation*. London: Sage.

Peres, F., Bodstein, R., Marcondes, W., Ramos, C., & Lazer. (2005) Esporte e Cultura na Agenda Local: a experiência de Promoção da Saúde em Manguinhos. *Ciência e Saúde Coletiva, 10*(3).

Potvin, L., & Richard, L. (2001). Evaluating community health-promotion programmes. In I. G. Rootman et al. (Eds.), *Evaluation in health promotion: Principles & perspective*. WHO Regional Publications, European Series 92.

Potvin, L., Haddad, S., & Frohlich, K. L. (2001). Beyond process & outcome evaluation: A comprehensive approach for evaluating health-promotion programmes. In Rootman et al. (Eds.), *Evaluation in Health Promotion: Principles & Perspective*. WHO Regional Publications, European Series 92.

Putnam, R. (1996). *Comunidade e Democracia: a experiência da Itália Moderna*. Rio de Janeiro: FGV.

Reis, I. N. C., & Vianna, M. B. (2002). Promoção da Saúde e Reorientação do Serviço: a experiência do Centro de Saúde Escola Germano Sinval Faria. In L. Zancan, R. Bodstein, W. B. Marcondes (Eds.), *Promoção da saúde como caminho para o desenvolvimento local: a experiência em Manguinhos-RJ* (pp. 111–157). Rio de Janeiro: ABRASCO/FIOCRUZ.

Rinaldi, A. (1998). Marginais, delinqüentes e vítimas: um estudo sobre a representação da categoria favelado no tribunal do júri da cidade do Rio de Janeiro. In A. Zaluar & M. Alvito (Eds.), *Um século de Favela*. (pp. 299–322). Rio de Janeiro: FGV.

Rootman, I. (2001). *Evaluation in health promotion: Principles and perspective*. WHO Regional Publications, European Series, 92.

Santos, J. L., & Martins, I. (2002). O Fórum Acorda Manguinhos. Um olhar sobre a participação Comunitária e o Desenvolvimento Local. In L. Zancan, R. Bodstein, & W. B. Marcondes

(Eds.), *Promoção da saúde como caminho para o desenvolvimento local: a experiência em Manguinhos-RJ* (pp. 215–224). Rio de Janeiro: ABRASCO/FIOCRUZ.

Senna, M., Mello, A., & Bodstein, R. (2002). A estratégia da saúde da Família no DLIS Manguinhos. In L. Zancan, R. Bodstein, W. B. Marcondes (Eds.), *Promoção da saúde como caminho para o desenvolvimento local: a experiência em Manguinhos-RJ* (pp. 189–214). Rio de Janeiro: ABRASCO/FIOCRUZ.

Shadish, W. R., Jr., Cook, T. D., & Leviton, L. C. (1991). *Foundations of program evaluation: Theories of practice.* Thousands Oaks, California: Sage.

Springett, J. (2005). Geographically-based approaches to the integration of health promotion into health systems: a comparative study of two Health Action Zones in the UK Promotion & Education. *IUPHE/UIPES Supplement,* 39–44.

Sullivan, H., Barnes, M., & Matka, E. (2002). Building collaborative capacity through "Theories of Change" – early lessons from the evaluation of HAZ. *England. Evaluation, 8*(2), 205–226.

Sullivan, H., Judge, K., & Sewell, K. (2004). In the Eye of the Beholder: Perceptions of Local Impact in English Health Action Zones. *Social Science & Medicine,* 59, 1603–1612.

Thurston, W., & Potvin, L. (2003). Evaluability assessment: A tool for incorporating evaluation in social change programmes. *Evaluation, 9*(4), 453–469.

Wacquant L. (2001). *Os condenados da cidade: Estudo sobre marginalidade avançada.* [tradução de João Roberto Martins Filho . . . et al.] Rio de Janeiro: Ed. Revan; FASE, 224pp.

Weiss, C. H. (1972). Utilization of evaluation: toward comparative study. In C. H. Weiss (Ed.), *Evaluating action programs: Readings in social action and education. needham heights.* Mass, Allyn & Bacon.

Weiss, C. H. (1998). Understanding the program. In C. H. Weiss (Ed.), *Evaluation – methods for studying programs and policies* (pp. 46–70). New Jersey: Prentice Hall.

Zaluar, A. (1997). Exclusão e Políticas Públicas: dilemas teóricos e alternativas políticas. *Revista Brasileira de Ciências Sociais, 12*(35), 29–47.

Zancan, L., Bodstein, R., & Marcondes, W. B. (2002). *Promoção da Saúde como Caminho para o Desenvolvimento Local: a experiência em Manguinhos-RJ.* Rio de Janeiro: ABRASCO/IOCRUZ.

Chapter 14
Multi-strategy in the Evaluation of Health Promotion Community Interventions: An Indicator of Quality

Zulmira Hartz, Carmelle Goldberg, Ana Claudia Figueiro, and Louise Potvin

There is a general agreement in the specialized literature on the need to design and conduct multi-strategy evaluation in health promotion and in social sciences. "Many community-based health interventions include a complex mixture of many disciplines, varying degrees of measurement difficulty and dynamically changing settings ... understanding multivariate fields of action may require a mixture of complex methodologies and considerable time to unravel any causal relationship" (McQueen & Anderson, 2001, p. 77). The meaning of the term multi-strategy, however, varies greatly. For some, multi strategy corresponds to the use of multiple methods and information data that allow for the participative evaluation of multiple dimensions, like outcome, process, and social and political context (Carvalho, Bodstein, Hartz, & Matida, 2004; Pan American Health Organisation, 2003). For others, the support for using multiple methods and strategies is rooted in wills to deploy multi-paradigm designs (Goodstadt et al., 2001). More generally, however, the term refers to studies mixing qualitative and quantitative methods of enquiry (Gendron, 2001; Green & Caracelle, 1997). Exceptionally, in the evaluation literature, multi-strategy also refers to the possibility to mix all kinds of evaluation approaches or models from diverse categories, such as advocacy, responsive, and theory-driven evaluation (Yin, 1994; Datta, 1997a,b; Stufflebeam, 2001). In all these references, the use of multi-strategy evaluation is justified as the best approach to minimize validity problems in dealing with the complexity of multi-strategy interventions and in multi-centers evaluation research.

Unfortunately, in examining research synthesis studies it is often impossible to estimate the real utilization and the effective contribution of multi-strategy evaluation, despite the fact that such multi-strategy evaluation is largely recommended to improve knowledge resulting from health promotion intervention evaluations. Meta-analysis and other research synthesis methods are based on a very limited classification system of evaluation study design that consists in whether a Randomized Control Trial (RCT) has been used (Hulscher, Wensing, Grol, Weijden, & Weel, 1999; International Union for Health Promotion and Education, 1999). This impedes the capacity to judge the appropriateness of evaluation approaches, in

Z. Hartz
Department at the National School of Public Health (ENSP/Fiocruz) in Rio de Janeirao, Brazil

L. Potvin, D. McQueen (eds.), *Health Promotion Evaluation Practices in the Americas*,
DOI: 10.1007/978-0-387-79733-5_14, © Springer Science+Business Media, LLC 2008   253

particular for the multi-strategy interventions characterizing complex community-based actions.

Considering the additional difficulties associated with conceptual definitions of health promotion in community settings (Boutilier, Rajkumar, Poland, Tobin, & Badgley, 2001; Potvin & Richard, 2001) and the absence of a standardized typology for multi-strategy evaluations and their implications to research validity and practical utility, this chapter explores the approaches and multi-strategy models implemented by evaluators in health promotion. To do so, we carried out a systematic review of scientific articles reporting on community health promotion evaluation conducted in countries from any of the three Americas, between 2000 and 2005, and available through electronic databases until May 2005. We were further interested in assessing the quality of these evaluation studies using quality indicators derived from international standards of meta-evaluation adequacy and from health promotion principles and values.

Two questions guided our work: (1) What are the characteristics of health promotion intervention evaluation studies? and (2) To what extent do these studies conform to common and specific evaluation standards? The need for using specific standards comes from the fact that, in order to convincingly demonstrate both expected and unintended effects, evaluation must use methodological approaches that are congruent with the principles and values of complex community health promotion interventions.

Methods

The Meta-Evaluation Approach

Meta-evaluation, in an informal sense, has been around for as long as someone has recognized that evaluators are professionals and, like in other professional practices, the quality of their products must be assessed. Cooksy and Caracelli (2005) have underlined that meta-evaluations conducted on a set of studies are useful to identify strengths and weaknesses in evaluation practice. It serves the general goal of capacity development in the field of evaluation.

In short, meta-evaluation is the systematic evaluation of an evaluation study, mainly based on four categories of evaluation standards that have reached consensual agreement from the American Evaluation Associations (AEA) for the evaluation of social programs (Stufflebeam, 2001, 2004; Yarbrough, Shulha, & Caruthers, 2004), public health interventions (Centers for Diseases Control, 1999; Hartz, 2003; Moreira & Natal, 2006), and also for Community Programs (Baker, Davis, Gallerani, Sanchez, & Viadro, 2000). These four categories are defined as follows and the complete list of standards that were used in this study for each category is provided in Appendix 1.

The first category is labelled utility standards. It is composed of criteria concerned with whether the evaluation is useful. Together these criteria answer questions directly relevant to users. Three standards from this category were selected for this study. The second category is composed of feasibility standards that assess whether the evaluation makes sense. The single criterion selected from this category assesses whether interests from various relevant groups were taken into account in evaluation design. The third category is made of propriety standards and concern evaluation's ethic. The three criteria selected assess whether evaluation was conducted in respect of the rights and interests of those involved in the intervention. The fourth category is composed of accuracy standards. The ten criteria selected relate to whether the evaluation conveyed technically adequate information regarding the determining features of merit of the evaluated program.

In addition to those four categories of standards and as an answer to concerns regarding international applications, the notion of open standards is now being developed to face the difficulties associated with transferring standard categories into different cultures and contexts (Love & Russon, 2004). According to Stufflebeam (2001), the main challenge in a meta-evaluation is one of balancing merit and worth in answering how the evaluation studies analyzed meet the requirements for a quality evaluation (merit) while fulfilling the audience's needs for evaluative information (worth). Despite the fact that these standards are recognized by evaluators' professional associations, these associations also recognize that standards are not recipes. They are useful starting points to develop trade-offs and adaptations for specific situations faced by meta-evaluators (Whorthen, Sanders, & Fitzpatrick, 1997).

Another category of open standards was defined for this meta-evaluation study. This category, called specificity standards, assesses whether the evaluation was theorized in accordance with community-based health promotion principles. Indeed, the complex nature of health promotion community interventions requires innovative and complex evaluative approaches, using a variety of methods that are coherent and consistent with initiatives that target changes at various levels. In addition, evaluation studies should be valid and allow the identification of theories and mechanisms by which actions and programs lead to changes in specific social contexts (Fawcett et al., 2001; Goodstadt et al., 2001; Goldberg, 2005). For this exploratory meta-evaluation, we adopted specific standards and criteria of a quality evaluation that follow three fundamental community-based health promotion principles: community capacity-building and accountability; disclosed theory or mechanisms of change; and multi-strategy evaluation. Multi-strategy evaluation was defined as an evaluation which combines quantitative/qualitative analyses and makes appropriate links between theory and methods, and process and outcome measures.

Based on these criteria, we assessed and gave a score to selected articles reporting on evaluation of community-based interventions. This scoring was performed in anonymous meta-evaluation format, in the same spirit than that of professional evaluators societies, i.e., to enhance the quality and credibility of knowledge resulting from evaluation studies (Stufflebeam, 2001).

Data Collection and Analysis

The first step was to select the articles to be included in the meta-evaluation. A systematic review of community-based health promotion program evaluation available in major data bases, such as CINHAL (Cumulative Index to Nursing & Allied Health

Literature) and the Virtual Health Library of the Pan-American Health Organization registry, was undertaken. This registry was chosen for its ability to house English, French, Spanish, and Portuguese studies conducted throughout the Americas by taping into prominent scientific databases in the field of health promotion. These databases include Lilacs (Latin American and Caribbean Health Sciences), SCIELO (Scientific Electronic Library Online), and Medline (International Database for Medical Literature).

Three search terms were used to identify eligible references, namely: health promotion, program evaluation, and community. Our initial search lead to the identification of 58 references from the Lilacs-SCIELO (L&S), and 120 references from Medline and CINHAL (M&C), that moved on to the second round of analyses, where abstracts were reviewed for their adherence to the specified definition of community interventions in health promotion. Differences in Medline's default search settings lead to slight modifications to our search specification, while restriction possibilities lead to fairly large differences to search results. Medline's default search settings required the specification of residence characteristics attributed to community as a search term, and allowed both full text documents and evaluation studies to be used as search restrictions. The former restriction lead to the identification of 53 studies, which excluded systematic reviews of the literature, commentaries, books, and editorials, while the latter lead to the identification of 23 studies that were rated as evaluation studies by authors.

In a second step, 29% (17/58) of the abstracts referenced in L&S and 23% (28/120) of those in M&C were selected according to a broad definition of "community health promotion interventions". The definition we used was based on Potvin & Richard (2001) and on Hills, Carrol, and O'Neill (2004), who restrict the term community interventions to interventions that use complex multiple strategies, focus on various targets of changes (individuals and environment changes), and engage communities with a minimum level of participation. Such interventions are generally characterized as community development, community mobilization, community-based intervention, and community-driven initiatives (Boutilier et al., 2001). The third and final step of article selection was based on the agreement of two reviewers who have read the complete texts. In the case of disagreement, a third reviewer was called. In this final stage, we selected articles that were designed to answer at least one evaluative question regarding the program under study, based on the Potvin, Haddad, and Frolich (2001, p. 51) five-category classification of evaluation questions. These are: (1) Relevance questions: How relevant are the program's objectives to the target of change? (2) Coherence questions: How coherent with the theory of problem is the theory of treatment linking the program's activities? (3) Responsiveness questions: How responsive is the program to changes in implementation and environmental conditions? (4) Achievement questions: What do the program's activities and services achieve? (5) Results: To which changes are the program's activities and services associated?

All 27 articles selected and listed in Appendix 2 (among which 19 are from North America) were read by two independent coders. Four dimensions adapted from Goodstadt et al. (2001, p. 530) were used to describe the program that was evaluated. These were: (1) the intervention goals (improve health and well-being, reduce mortality and morbidity, or both); (2) the level of the targeted changes as stated in the intervention objectives (enhance individual capacity, enhance community capacity, or develop supportive institutional and social environment); (3) the health promotion strategies used (health education, health communication, organizational development, policy development, intersectoral collaboration, or research); and (4) the main reported results. According to Goodstadt et al. (2001), model, health promotion actions should have goals that extend beyond reducing and preventing ill health to include improving health and well-being, focusing on different levels and determinants of health and adopting strategic and operational activities to reach objectives in the areas given priority by the Ottawa Charter.

Three dimensions have been coded to characterize the evaluation approaches used in evaluation studies. The first dimension relates to the question that guided the evaluation study (relevance, coherence, responsiveness, achievements, or results). The second dimension assesses the main focus of the evaluation (process, outcome, or both). The third dimension concerns the methods used (qualitative, quantitative, or mixte).

Finally, each evaluation study was rated using the four American Evaluation Association's standards listed in Appendix 1 and the five criteria of the specificity standards designed for this study. Because many of the information required to assess the criteria of the American Evaluation Association standards were only available in original reports or in evaluability assessment studies, each standard category was assessed globally. Each standard category and each of the five specificity criteria were given a score ranging from 0 to 10 by two independent reviewers, following Stufflebeam's (1999) classification: Poor 0–2; Fair 3–4; Good 5–6; Very Good 7–8; and Excellent 9–10. A correlation coefficient of 0.86 between the reviewer's scores was estimated using three randomly selected articles. All statistical analyses were performed using Epiinfo 3.3.2.

Results

Table 14.1 presents the characteristics of programs evaluated in the selected articles. Two characteristics are in line with health promotion principles. As shown in Table 14.1, only a minority of the programs targeted the reduction of mortality and morbidity as program sole objectives. Another positive result is the fact that, in addition to individual level change objectives, the great majority of programs also target middle and macro level change objectives, this in 70% and 48% of cases respectively. Concerning the health promotion strategies adopted or the activities carried out to ensure that the objectives can be achieved, health education and communication are the two most often implemented and they appear to be always associated in local practices. Interestingly as well, all programs were composed of at least two types of actions meeting the minimal requirement for being labeled multi-strategy interventions. More interestingly, 20 out of 27 programs were made up of three or

Table 14.1 Main characteristics of evaluated interventions ($n=27$)

Characteristics	No.	%
Health Promotion Goals		
Improved health and well-being	9	33.3
Reduced mortality and morbidity	5	18.5
Both	13	48.1
Objectives/Levels*		
Enhanced individual capacity/Micro	20	74.1
Enhanced community capacity/Meso	19	70.4
Supportive institutional and social environments/Macro	13	48.1
Generic Strategies*		
Health education	20	74.1
Health communication	20	74.1
Organizational development	16	59.3
Community development	12	44.4
Policy development	8	29.6
Intersectoral collaboration	11	40.7
Research	13	48.1
Main Results*		
Improved awareness, knowledge, skills, decision-making & behaviors	19	76.0
Enhanced organizational capacity	13	52.0
Increased community capacity & participation	11	44.0
Increased equitable access to health care	7	28.0
Increased focus on prevention and health promotion in health systems	13	52.0
Enhanced coordination of efforts & resources in policies	6	25.0
Enhanced health promotion public policies	7	28.0
Knowledge development and dissemination	12	48.0

* Categories within these dimensions are not mutually exclusive.

more components. The presence of research activities, as part of 13/27 interventions, seems also to indicate an integration of knowledge development as an intervention strategy. Less encouraging however is the fact that only a minority of programs address issues of public policies. As for the evaluation results, not surprisingly the majority of them reported improved awareness, skills, and behaviors. Only a few reported positive effects on public policies and increased equity.

Table 14.2 describes the main characteristics of the evaluation approaches implemented in the articles selected. It is interesting to note that evaluation studies seem to be covering a broad range of evaluation questions, overcoming the traditional dichotomies between process versus result evaluations, or between formative versus summative evaluation. Indeed, our results clearly illustrate the richness of using a typology of questions to characterize the evaluation focus, compared to categorizations based on the traditional dichotomy. Our results also show that the use of multi-strategy approaches to evaluation is still somewhat limited. Only 40% of the reported studies focus on a mixture of process and outcome, and 36% used a mix of quantitative and qualitative analyses. We will come back to the relevance of this dimension as a quality indicator of health promotion evaluative research in the discussion.

Table 14.2 Main characteristics of evaluation designs ($n = 27$)

Characteristics	No.	%
Types/Questions*		
Coherence	6	22.2
Achievements	13	48.1
Relevance	3	11.1
Responsiveness	11	40.7
Results	18	66.7
Focus		
Process	8	29.6
Outcomes	8	29.6
Both	11	40.7
Data analysis		
Mixed	9	36.0
Quantitative	8	32.0
Qualitative	8	32.0

* Categories within this dimension are not mutually exclusive.

The second issue addressed in this chapter has to do with to the extent to which the evaluations meet common and specific evaluation standards. Figure 14.1 presents ratings given to the 27 selected evaluation studies on the five meta-evaluation standard categories and on the 5 criteria that form the specificity standard category. In general, published evaluation studies are of very high quality. Not surprisingly, standards of accuracy are the most commonly met, with almost 80% of studies (21/27) classified as very good or excellent. Conversely, specificity standards, related to whether the evaluation was theorized in accordance with community-based health promotion principles, are the least often met in our sample. Only 52% (14/27) obtained a very good or excellent rating. An examination of the

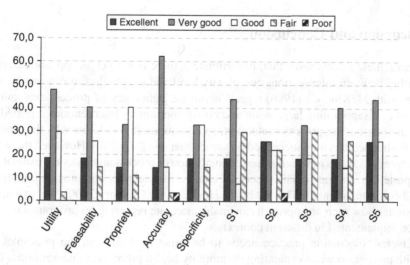

Fig. 14.1 Histogram of ratings on quality standards ($n = 27$)

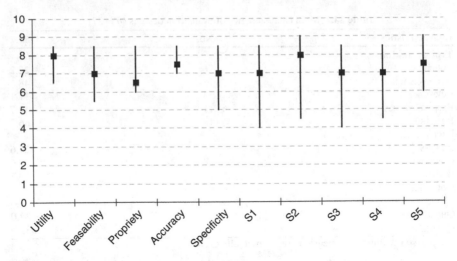

Fig. 14.2 Median, percentiles 25 and 75 of ratings on quality standards ($n = 27$)

various dimensions of the specificity standards show that 30% (8/27) of the reported evaluations had scores lower than 5,0 (fair) related to the appropriate use of theory (S1) and to the use of multi-strategy evaluation (S3).

It is also worth noting that there seems to be greater variation in quality when evaluations are assessed with standards specific to health promotion, rather than with common standards. Figure 14.2 shows that although the medians of the rating distributions are similar across standards, the range of ratings is broader for standards specific to health promotion evaluation.

Discussion and Conclusion

Overall, these results show that, unfortunately, there is not yet an appropriate relationship between interventions complexity level and approaches to evaluation. We agree with McKinlay's (1996) regrets about the deficiency of process evaluation: "Most of disappointing large-scale and costly community interventions reported in recent years had no process evaluation, so it is impossible to know why they failed or whether perhaps they succeeded on some other level" (p. 240). However, there are examples of studies in which some reconciliation of process and outcome evaluation supported by an appropriate theory of change for complex community initiatives has been implemented. The study by Hughes and Traynor (2000), for example, illustrates how such an approach can enable accurate reporting on program's results when implemented in different contexts.

Overall, evaluation practice needs to be better aligned with the principles of health promotion when evaluating community health promotion interventions. The intervention's high degree of complexity is very seldom matched by multi-methods approaches to evaluation. With all the limitations associated with an explanatory meta-evaluation of a limited number of evaluation research reports, we think that three main messages can be drawn from this work.

The first message is that a relatively simple way to improve the usefulness and relevance of evaluation research for health promotion is to examine the quality of health promotion evaluation using both common and specific meta-evaluation standards. The systematic meta-evaluation using a broad range of common criteria and of criteria specific to health promotion allows a much better assessment of the field of health promotion than using the traditional dichotomous category such as process versus outcome evaluation, or experimental versus non-experimental designs. Our broad, inclusive strategy may have biased our sample of studies toward 19/25 showing positive results, in contradiction with Merzel and D'Afflitti's (2003) comments apparently, which state on the modest impact of community-based programs from the past 20 years. But it is also possible that Merzel and D'Afflitti (2003) results were an artefact of them including criteria that limited their analysis to experiment-control study design, thus restricting the expression of intervention effectiveness "precisely because ... the phenomena under study do not lend themselves to an application of that methodology" (De Leeuw & Skovgaard, 2005, p. 1338).

The second message is to plea for a better alignment of health promotion with the evaluation of health promotion. If we are really serious about the principles that health promotion interventions are multi-strategy, then we should require multi-strategy evaluations. This is the condition for us to be able to demonstrate both beneficial and detrimental effects. The development and use of health promotion specific quality criteria for the meta-evaluation of health promotion evaluation have to be encouraged. Our exploratory meta-evaluation shows that there are quality deficiencies on those specific criteria and that the performance of health promotion studies is much less consistent regarding such specific criteria compared to common criteria.

The third message is the reiteration of the hypothesis that the interventions demonstrated that effectiveness is not independent from the evaluation models implemented to study it. Given that among the six evaluation studies that showed negative results, five were multiple strategy interventions evaluated with single data analysis strategy, it would be interesting to conduct a larger meta-evaluation to test the relationship between the use of multi-strategy evaluation and the conclusion of the evaluation. Conversely, it would be critical to analyze the real meaning of positive evaluation results for studies with a low rating on health promotion specificity criteria. A meta-evaluation based in a "realistic synthesis" review (Pawson, 2003), grouping different programs and contexts with a common theoretical framework and mechanisms, could also increase the ability for highlighting the role of multi-strategy evaluation for constructing the case of an effective intervention. As noted, there is "a tendency to underrate and invalidate knowledge derived from a deductive process applied to theoretical knowledge and to overrate the accumulation of empirical observations even if the empirical basis is not sufficient" (Potvin, 2005, p. S97).

These messages, however, are to be taken in the light of the inherent problems of our meta-evaluation study that limit the generalization of our observations. The first has to do with the content validity of the ratings according to the four common standard categories (utility, feasibility, propriety, and accuracy), using an overall impression instead of a series of detailed criteria. The only source of information regarding the programs that were evaluated was the published evaluation result papers, thus limiting our ability to provide nuances to quality assessment substantially. Another problem, particularly important for evaluations carried out in Latin America, was the fact that, given the time and resource restrictions, we were not able to include the grey literature, and half of the selected studies were part of graduate study thesis. The small number of published articles available also limited our possibility to contrast the patterns of evaluation in North America and South America.

We would like to conclude this chapter with some empirical remarks. At this point, we do not have meta-evaluation criteria for the evaluation of complex multi-strategy health promotion interventions. It is therefore quite difficult to assess whether multi-strategy evaluations are most capable to provide valid results while evaluating such interventions.

Acknowledgment We wish to acknowledge Prof. Luis Claudio S. Thuler, for his valuable collaboration in the management of our database.

Appendix 1 – Meta-evaluation Checklist for Health Promotion Programs, Adapted from Centers for Diseases Control (1999), Stufflebeam (2001), Goodstadt et al. (2001), and Goldberg (2005)

Utility standards: the evaluation will serve the information needs of intended users.

   U1 – Stakeholder identification. The individuals involved in or affected by the evaluation should be identified so that their needs can be addressed.
   U4 – Values identification. The perspectives, procedures, and rationale used to interpret the findings should be carefully described so that the bases for value judgments are clear.
   U7 – Evaluation impact. Evaluations should be planned, conducted, and reported in ways that encourage the follow-through by stakeholders to increase the likelihood of the evaluation being used.

Feasibility standards: the evaluation will be realistic, prudent, diplomatic, and frugal.

   F2 – Political viability. During planning and conduct of the evaluation, consideration should be given to the varied positions of interest groups so that their cooperation can be obtained and possible attempts by any group to curtail evaluation operations or to bias or misapply the results can be averted or counteracted.

Propriety standards: the evaluation will be conducted legally, ethically, and with regard to the welfare of those involved in the evaluation, as well as those affected by its results.

P1 – Service orientation. The evaluation should be designed to assist organizations in addressing and serving effectively the needs of the targeted participants.

P5 – Complete and fair assessment. The evaluation should be complete and fair in its examination and recording of strengths and weaknesses of the program so that strengths can be enhanced and problem areas addressed.

P6 – Disclosure of findings. The principal parties to an evaluation should ensure that the full evaluation findings with pertinent limitations are made accessible to the persons affected by the evaluation and any others with expressed legal rights to receive the results.

Accuracy standards: the evaluation will convey technically adequate information regarding the determining features of merit of the program.

A1 – Program documentation. The program being evaluated should be documented clearly and accurately.

A2 – Context analysis. The context in which the program exists should be examined in enough detail to identify probable influences on the program.

A3 – Described purposes and procedures. The purposes and procedures of the evaluation should be monitored and described in enough detail to identify and assess them.

A4 – Defensible information sources. Sources of information used in a program evaluation should be described in enough detail to assess the adequacy of the information.

A5 – Valid information. Information-gathering procedures should be developed and implemented to ensure a valid interpretation for the intended use.

A6 – Reliable information. Information-gathering procedures should be developed and implemented to ensure sufficiently reliable information for the intended use.

A7 – Systematic information. Information collected, processed, and reported in an evaluation should be systematically reviewed and any errors corrected.

A8+A9 – Data analysis. Information should be analyzed appropriately and systematically so that evaluation questions are answered effectively.

A10 – Justified conclusions. Conclusions reached should be explicitly justified for stakeholders' assessment.

Specificity standards: the evaluation was theorized in accordance with community-based health promotion principles.

S1 – Theory or mechanisms of change. The evaluation discloses the theory or mechanisms of change in a clear fashion (logic model of the evaluation).

S2 – Community capacity-building. The evaluation adheres to empowerment and community capacity-building principles ("participatory users").

S3 – Multi-strategy evaluation. The evaluation combined quantitative and qualitative analyses that made appropriate links between theory & methods and process & outcomes measures.

S4 – Accountability. The evaluation provided information regarding community (stakeholder) accountability.

S5 – Effective practices. The evaluation helped spread effective practices.

Appendix 2 List of References for the Meta-evaluation Study

Becker, D., Edmundo, K., Nunes, N. R., Bonatto, D., & Souza, R. (2004). Empowerment e avaliação participativa em um programa de desenvolvimento local e promoção da saúde. *Ciência & Saúde Coletiva, 9*, 655–667.

Bodstein, R., Zancan, L., Ramos, C. L., & Marcondes, W. B. (2004). Avaliação da implantação do programa de desenvolvimento integrado em Manguinhos: Impasses na formulação de uma agenda local. *Ciência & Saúde Coletiva, 9*, 593–604.

Cabrera-Pivaral, C. E., Mayari, C. L. N., Trueba, J. M. A., Perez, G. J. G., Lopez, M. G. V, Figueroa, I. V., et al. (2002). Evaluación de dos estrategias de educación nutricional vía radio en Guadalajara, México. *Cadernos de Saúde Pública, 18*, 1289–1294.

Carrasquilla, G. (2001). An ecosystem approach to malaria control in an urban setting. *Caernos de. Saúde Pública, 17(Suppl)*, 171–179.

Cheadle, A, Beery, W. L., Greenwald, H. P, Nelson, G. D., Pearson, D., & Senter, S. (2003). Evaluating the California Wellness Foundation's health improvement initiative: A logic model approach. *Health Promotion Practice, 4*, 146–156.

Chiaravalloti, V. B., Morais, M. S., Chiaravalloti Neto, F., Conversani, D. T., Fiorin, A. M., Barbosa, A. A. C., et al. (2002). Avaliação sobre a adesão às práticas preventivas do dengue: O caso de Catanduva, São Paulo, Brasil. *Cadernos de Saúde Pública, 18*, 1321–1329.

Chrisman, N. J., Senturia, K., Tang, G., & Gheisar, B. (2002). Qualitative process evaluation of urban community work: A preliminary view. *Health Education & Behavior, 29*, 232–248.

Conrey, E. J., Frongillo, E. A., Dollahite, J. S., & Griffin, M. R. (2003). Integrated program enhancements increased utilization of farmers' market nutrition program. *Journal of Nutrition, 133*, 1841–1844.

D'Onofrio, C. N., Moskowitz, J. M., & Braverman, M. T. (2002). Curtailing tobacco use among youth: Evaluation of Project 4-Health. *Health Education & Behavior, 29*, 656–682.

Figueiredo, R., & Ayres, J. R. C. M. (2002). Intervenção comunitária e redução da vulnerabilidade de mulheres às DST/Aids em São Paulo, SP. *Revista de Saúde Pública, 36(4 Suppl)*, 96–107.

Figueroa, I.V., Alfaro, N. A., Guerra, J. F., Rodriguez, G. A., & Roaf, P. M. (2000). Una experiencia de educación popular en salud nutricional en dos comunidades del Estado de Jalisco, México. *Cadernos de Saúde Pública, 16*, 823–829.

Hawe, P., Shiell, A., Riley, T., & Gold, L. (2004). Methods for exploring implementation variation and local context within a cluster randomized community intervention trial. *Journal of Epidemiology and Community Health, 58*, 788–793.

Kelly, C. M., Baker, E. A., Williams, D., Nanney, M. S., & Haire-Joshu, D. (2004). Organizational capacity's effects on the delivery and outcomes of health education programs. *Journal of Public Health Management Practice, 10*, 164–170.

Kim, S., Koniak-Griffin, D., Flaskerud, J. H., & Guarnero, P. A. (2004). The impact of lay health advisors on cardiovascular health promotion using a community-based participatory approach. *Journal of Cardiovascular Nursing, 19*, 192–199.

Lantz, P. M., Viruell-Fuentes, E., Israel, B. A., Softley, D., & Guzman, R. (2001). Can communities and academia work together on public health research? Evaluation results from a community-based participatory research partnership in Detroit. *Journal of Urban Health, 78*, 495–507.

Lima-Costa, M. F., Guerra, H. L., Firmo, J. O. A., Pimenta, F., Jr., & Uchoa, E. (2002). Um estudo epidemiológico da efetividade de um programa educativo para o controle da esquistossomose em Minas Gerais. *Revista Brasileira de Epidemiologia, 5*, 116–128.

MacLean, D., Farquharson, J., Heath, S., Barkhouse, K., Latter, C. & Joffres, C. (2003). Building capacity for heart health promotion: Results of a 5-year experience in Nova Scotia, Canada. *American Journal of Health Promotion, 17*, 202–212.

Markens, S., Fox, S. A., Taub, B., & Gilbert, M. L. (2002). Role of black churches in health promotion programs: Lessons from the Los Angeles mammography promotion in churches program. *American Journal of Public Health, 92*, 805–810.

McElmurry, B. J., Park, C. G., & Busch, A. G. (2003). The nurse-community health advocate team for urban immigrant primary health care. *Journal of Nursing Scholarship, 35*, 275–281.

Moody, K. A., Janis, C. C., & Sepples, S. B. (2003). Intervening with at-risk youth: Evaluation of the Youth Empowerment and Support Program. *Pediatric Nursing, 29*, 263–270.

Naylor, P-J., Wharf-Higgin, J., Blair, L., Green, L. W., & O'Connor, B. (2002). Evaluating the participatory process in a community-based heart health project. *Social Science & Medicine, 55*, 1173–1187.

Nuñez, D. E., Armbruster, C., Phillips, W. T., & Gale, B. J. (2003). Community-based senior health promotion program using a collaborative practice model: The escalante health partnerships. *Public Health Nursing, 20*, 25–32.

Quinn, M. T., & McNabb, W. L. (2001). Training lay health educators to conduct a church-based weight loss program for African American women. *The Diabetes Educator, 27*, 231–238.

Reininger, B. M., Vincent, M., Griffin, S. F., Valois, R. F., Taylor, D., Parra-Medina, D., et al. (2003). Evaluation of statewide teen pregnancy prevention initiatives: challenges, methods, and lessons learned. *Health Promotion Practice, 4*, 323–335.

Schulz, A. J., Zenk. S., Odoms-Young, A., Hollis-Neely, T., Nwankwo, R., Lockett, M., et al. (2005). Healthy eating and exercising to reduce diabetes: exploring the potential of social determinants of health frameworks within the context of community-based participatory diabetes prevention. *American Journal of Public Health, 95*, 645–651.

Stewart, A. L., Verboncoeur, C. J., McLellan, B. Y., Gillis, D. E., Rush, S., Mills, K. M., et al. (2001). Physical activity outcomes of CHAMPS II: A physical activity promotion program for older adults. *Journal of Gerontology: Medical Sciences, 56A*, 465–470.

Williams, J. H., Belle, G. A., Houston, C., Haire-Joshu, D., & Auslander, W. F. (2001). Process evaluation methods of a peer-delivered health promotion program for African American women. *Health Promotion Practice, 2*, 135–142.

References

Baker, Q. E., Davis, D. A., Gallerani, R., Sanchez, V., & Viadro, C. (2000). *An evaluation framework of community health programs*. Durham NC: The Center for Advancement of Community-Based Public Health. Downloaded in November 2007 from: www.cdc.gov/eval/evalcbph.pdf

Boutilier, M. A., Rajkumar, E., Poland, B. D., Tobin, S., & Badgley, R. F. (2001). Community action success in public health: Are we using a ruler to measure a sphere? *Canadian Journal of Public Health, 92*, 90–94.

Carvalho, A. I., Bodstein, R. C., Hartz, Z. M. A., & Matida, A. H. (2004). Concepts and approaches in the evaluation of health promotion. *Ciência & Saúde Coletiva*, 9, 521–544.

Cooksy, L. J., & Caracelli, V. J. (2005). Quality, context and use. Issues in achieving the goals of metaevaluation. *American Journal of Evaluation*, 26, 31–42.

Centers for Diseases Control. (1999). Framework for program evaluation in public health. *MMWR, 48 (RR-11)*.

De Leeuw, E., & Skovgaard, T. (2005). Utility-driven evidence for health cities: Problems with evidence generation and application. *Social Science & Medicine, 61*, 1331–1341.

Datta, L. E. (1997a). A pragmatic basis for mixed-method designs. *New Directions for Program Evaluations, 74*, 33–46.

Datta, L. (1997b). Multimethod evaluations: Using case studies together with other methods. In E. Chelimsky, & W. Shadish (Eds.), *Evaluation for the 21st century* (pp. 344–359). Thousand Oaks: Sage.

Fawcett, S. B., Paine-Andrews, A., Francisco, V. T., Schultz, J., Richter, K. P., Berkley-Patton, J., et al. (2001). Evaluating community initiatives for health and development. In I. Rootman, M. Goodstadt, B. Hyndman, D.V. McQueen, L. Potvin, J. Springett, & E. Ziglio (Eds.), *Evaluation in health promotion. Principles and perspectives* (pp. 241–270). Copenhague: WHO regional publications. European series; No. 92.

Gendron, S. (2001). Transformative alliance between qualitative and quantitative approaches in health promotion research. In I. Rootman, M. Goodstadt, B. Hyndman, D.V. McQueen, L. Potvin, J. Springett, & E. Ziglio (Eds.), *Evaluation in health promotion. Principles and perspectives* (pp. 107–122). Copenhague: WHO regional publications. European series; No. 92.

Goldberg, C. (2005). The effectiveness conundrum in health promotion (work in progress).

Goodstadt, M., Hyndman, B., McQueen, D. V., Potvin, L., Rootman, I., & Springett, J. (2001). Evaluation in health promotion: synthesis and recommendations. In I. Rootman, M. Goodstadt, B. Hyndman, D.V. McQueen, L. Potvin, J. Springett, & E. Ziglio (Eds.), *Evaluation in health promotion. Principles and perspectives* (pp. 517–533). Copenhague: WHO regional publications. European series; No. 92.

Green, J. C., & Caracelle, V. J. (Eds.). (1997). Advances in mixed-method evaluation: The challenges and benefits for integrating diverse paradigms. *New Directions for Program Evaluations, 74*.

Hartz, Z. (2003). *Significado, validade e limites do estudo de avaliação da descentralização da saúde na Bahia: uma meta-avaliação*. Anais Congresso da Abrasco.

Hills, M. D., Carrol, S., & O'Neill, M. (2004). Vers un modèle d'évaluation de l'efficacité des interventions communautaires en promotion de la santé: compte-rendu de quelques développements Nord-américains récents. *Promotion & Education, suppl. 1*, 17–21.

Hughes, M., & Traynor, T. (2000). Reconciling process and outcome in evaluating community initiatives. *Evaluation, 6*, 37–49.

Hulscher, M. E. J. L, Wensing, M., Grol, R. P. T. M., Weijden, T. van der & Weel, C. van (1999). Interventions to improve the delivery of preventive services in primary care. *American Journal of Public Health, 89*, 737–746.

International Union for Health Promotion and Education (1999). *The evidence of health promotion effectiveness. Sahping public health in a new Europe*. Bruxelles: ECSC-EC-EAEC.

Love, A., & Russon, C. (2004). Evaluation standards in an international context. *New Directions for Evaluation, 104(winter)*, 5–14.

McQueen, D. V., & Anderson, L. M. (2001). What counts as evidence: issues and debates. In I. Rootman, M. Goodstadt, B. Hyndman, D.V. McQueen, L. Potvin, J. Springett, & E. Ziglio (Eds.), *Evaluation in health promotion. Principles and perspectives* (pp. 63–81). Copenhague: WHO regional publications. European series; No. 92.

McKinlay, J. B. (1996). More appropriate methods for community-level health interventions. *Evaluation Review, 20*, 237–243.

Merzel, C., & D'Afflitti, J. (2003). Reconsidering community-based health promotion. Promise, performance and potential. *American Journal of Public Health, 93*, 557–574.

Moreira, E., & Natal, S. (Eds.). (2006) . *Ensinando avaliação, vol.4*. Brasil: Ministério da Saúde, CDC, ENSP/FIOTEC.

Pan American Health Organisation. (2003). Recomendações para formuladores de políticas nas Américas (GT municípios e Comunidades Saudáveis). Mimeo.

Pawson, R. (2003). Nothing as practical as a good theory. *Evaluation, 9*, 471–490.

Potvin, L., & Richard, L. (2001). The evaluation of community health promotion programmes. In I. Rootman, M. Goodstadt, B. Hyndman, D.V. McQueen, L. Potvin, J. Springett, & E. Ziglio (Eds.), *Evaluation in health promotion. Principles and perspectives* (pp. 213–240). Copenhague: WHO regional publications. European series; No. 92.

Potvin, L., Haddad, S., & Frolich, K.L. (2001). Beyond process and outcome evaluation: a comprehensive approach for evaluating health promotion programmes. In I. Rootman, M. Goodstadt, B. Hyndman, D.V. McQueen, L. Potvin, J. Springett, & E. Ziglio (Eds.), *Evaluation in health promotion. Principles and perspectives* (pp. 45–62). Copenhague: WHO regional publications. European series, No. 92.

Potvin, L. (2005). Why we should be worried about evidence-based practice in health promotion. *Revista Brasileira de Saúde Maternal Infantil, Suppl.1*, 2–8.

Stufflebeam, D. (1999). *Program evaluations metavaluation checklist*. Downloaded in November 2007 from: www.wmich.edu/evalctr/checklists/program_metaeval.htm

Stufflebeam, D. L. (2001). The metaevaluation imperative. *American Journal of Evaluation, 2*, 183–209.

Stufflebeam, D. L. (Ed.). (2001). Evaluation models. *New Directions for Program Evaluation, 89, Spring*.

Stufflebeam, D. L. (2004). A note on purposes, development and applicability of the Joint Committee Evaluation Standards. *The American Journal of Evaluation, 25*, 99–102.

Whorthen, B. R., Jr., Sanders, J. R., & Fitzpatrick, J. L. (1997). *Evaluation: Alternative approaches and practical guidelines*. New York: Longman.

Yarbrough, D. B., Shulha, L. M., & Caruthers, F. (2004). Background and history of the Joint Committee's Program Evaluation Standards. *New Direction for Evaluation, 104(winter)*, 15–30.

Yin, R. K. (1994). Discovering the future of the case study method in evaluation research. *Evaluation Practice, 15*, 283–290.

Chapter 15
The Contribution of A Systematization Evaluative Approach to Implement A Health Promotion Project in Capela do Socorro, Sao Paulo, Brazil

Marcia Faria Westphal and Juan Carlos Aneiros Fernandez

The Capela do Socorro is one of the 31 Regional City Halls of the city of Sao Paulo (Fig. 15.1). It is the most heavily populated and has a high rate of urbanization and population growth (Table 15.1). However, with its $134.2 \, km^2$ of area, it does not have the highest population density in the city.

The industrial development of the 1970s had a significant impact on Capela do Socorro. Because it had a large rural area and was relatively close to the Jurubatuba industrial center, and because of the dynamic trade and services center located at the southern and south-western parts of the metropolitan area, the region has been absorbing a portion of the city's urban growth. A large working class population flocked to Capela in search of areas where urban land was affordable and had not yet any urban infrastructure in place, such as public transportation, water supply, public lighting, and social facilities.

The Headwaters Protection Act[1], enacted in 1976, covering 82% of the territory of Capela do Socorro, defined density limits for occupation of the land and hindered the development in the area. As a result, the land was virtually excluded from the formal real estate market and consequently land prices dropped significantly. Instead of protecting the natural water reserves as expected, this depreciation of land value led to the quick expansion of clandestine land division and to the setting up of slums around the region's water reserves. The end result was a highly concentrated low-income population living in poor housing in Capela do Socorro (Tables 15.2 and 15.3), neighboring a smaller portion of the territory (18%) with better infrastructure, where a higher average income population lived.

The Healthy Cities strategy was adopted in 2003 to provide a structure to actions undertaken by the Deputy-mayor and his advisory group. An earlier initiative had

---

[1]Law Number 1172/76, State of São Paulo, on the protection of natural reservoirs for drinking water.

M.F. Westphal
University of Sao Paulo, Sao Paulo, Brazil

L. Potvin, D. McQueen (eds.), *Health Promotion Evaluation Practices in the Americas*,
DOI: 10.1007/978-0-387-79733-5_15, © Springer Science+Business Media, LLC 2008   269

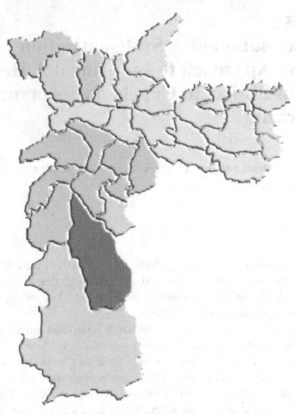

Fig. 15.1 Capela do Socorro Regional city hall area in the São Paulo city

been the Inter-Department Nucleus (*Núcleo Intersecretarial da Capela do Socorro –* NICS), set up in 2001 to plan intersectoral actions within the purview of what was then the Regional Administration for Capela do Socorro. Over a two-year period, the multi-professional group that was developing this earlier initiative, put into practice an integrated and participatory management model that later was formalized and expanded to the municipal administration as a whole with the creation of the Decentralization Law for the City of Sao Paulo. In March 2002, based on the experience

Table 15.1 Demographic indicators

Total population	563,922
Demographic density (Hab/Km^2)	4,202.1
Growth rate 1991–2000 (%)	3.72
Urbanization rate (%)	93.57
Working age population	381,267

Source: Brazilian Institute of Geography and Statistics (IBGE) Demographic Census 1991 and 2000; Municipal Law 10932 enacted 15 January 1991

Table 15.2 Income, heads of family

(1 Minimum Salary = US$ 133)	% Capela do Socorro	% Sao Paulo
No income	16.09	10.43
Up to 5 times Minimum Salaries	57.01	47.55
Over 5 and up to 20 times Minimum Salaries	24.53	32.58
Over 20 times Minimum Salaries	2.36	9.44
Average income of heads of family (US$ 1 = R$ 2.26)	US$ 306.45	US$ 586.47

Source: Brazilian Institute for Geography and Statistics (IBGE) – Demographic Census 2000

Table 15.3 Sub-standard housing and annual growth rate

Sub-standard housing	Capela do Socorro	Sao Paulo
Number of Slums	221	2018
Slum Population	132,177	1,160,590
Percentage of the Population living in Slums (%)	23.44	11.12
Annual growth rate, slum-dwelling population (%)	4.67	2.97

Source: Secretariat of Housing and Urban Development/PMSP and City of Sao Paulo Data Processing Company (PRODAM) Digital Map Basis for Slums in the Municipality of Sao Paulo 2000.

of this Nucleus, the City Administration of Sao Paulo decreed the creation of Local Administrations that would pave the way for the partition of the city into Regional city halls. The Decentralization Law was at that time going through the Municipal Legislative Branch.

From March to June 2002, the Local Government of Capela do Socorro carried out an intergovernmental strategic planning process that led to the following mission statement of the local administration: *To construct an environmentally healthy Capela do Socorro through sustainable and joint development, encouraging and enabling the participation of the population and the exercise of their citizenship.* (Local Government Capela do Socorro, 2002a).

The Healthy Capela pilot plan, which later became a framework for the pursuit of institutional partnerships and the engagement of the communities and the population as a whole, was also drafted at this time. Among the Healthy Capela Program's goals, of interest to this paper is that of carrying out integrated intersectoral actions between the public and private spheres. Associated with this goal is the following strategy: linkage of the various forums and participation channels in the region, comprising Health Management Councils (unit-level and district-level), School Boards, Forum of Delegates to the Participatory Budget, Neighborhood Civil Defense Nuclei, among others, regarding health promotion.

In May 2003, the Healthy Capela do Socorro Seminar officially launched the Healthy Capela Program. It was proposed at this seminar to set up four local Healthy Capela commissions. Following the recommendation of the regional office of the Pan American Health Organization (PAHO) in Brazil, the management group of Capela do Socorro County, the Center for Studies, Research and Documentation on Healthy Cities – CEPEDOC and the School of Public Health of the University of Sao Paulo began to work closely together. A partnership was set up and extended to other key stakeholders, including the business community, social movements, non-governmental organizations, and universities in the region. This partnership developed several joint actions, involving four planning workshops, which were attended by representatives of the four commissions initially set up by the project, an international seminar and the assessment of the management model based on the principles of Healthy Cities.

This chapter will examine part of the Healthy Capela Program assessment project, focusing on the systematization of the experience lived in the period from 2001 to 2004 (Jara, 1996, 2001).

Choosing a Method to Systematize Experiences

The Healthy Capela Program assessment research project was designed to analyze the development of the experience and its results, aiming to enhance the management model. It was submitted and approved by the State of Sao Paulo Research Foundation – FAPESP (Fundação de Amparo a Pesquisa do Estado de Sao Paulo) Public Policy program, to be performed in two phases. The first phase involved the preparation of researchers, to identify the issues to be investigated – problems and potentialities of the Healthy Capela Program – and the creation of possible categories and indicators to be used in the assessment project. The second phase aimed at assessing the effectiveness of an integrated and participatory management model to improve the quality of life and decrease the inequalities of a population that shares a territory.

In order to achieve the objectives of the first phase, the method chosen was Systematization of Experiences. This enabled the group of researchers to discuss and assess, with local managers, strategies that would be suitable to ensure the involvement of all sectors of the government and all stakeholders in the process of reflection upon integrated and participatory management, and its advances and limitations. The actors involved in the program and in the evaluation clearly valued these aspects, and were concerned about implementing them despite regular setbacks in doing so. The adoption of this method also catered to the concerns raised by the Deputy-mayor, who faced some difficulty in linking and organizing the management processes in an integrated and participatory perspective. This method also suited the objectives of the first phase, which were to develop a formative process, and detail the following phases of the project. Thus, the context of that phase made it easy for the University and CEPEDOC researchers to involve the group of managers – Deputy-mayor, coordinators, and several other professionals in the systematization of lived-through experience as a means of enabling the group to carry out critical reflection on the Healthy Capela initiative.

The systematization of experiences method, which aims to review, analyze, interpret and communicate lived-through experience, may help to explain the factors that negatively and positively affect the proposed management process. It is, thus, a suitable method for working with dynamic, complex states of affairs which have the social setting as their source of data, and for attaining the general objective of the project: to enhance the management of public policies in an integrated participatory perspective so as to improve quality of life in the region of the Capela do Socorro Regional City Hall.

Hence, throughout the process experienced by the systematizing group, there was an ongoing concern to overcome the gap that usually exists between the subject and the object of the research, and the ownership of the results by all those involved in the study, enabling this group of people to produce together a body of knowledge concerning the management of local integrated public policies. The participation of the Deputy-mayor and professionals from a range of coordination offices of the Regional City Hall, as well as the group of researchers of both institutions, assured this collective process throughout the first phase of the study.

We adopted Oscar Jara's experience with the systematization method, through which "the experiences [are understood] as historical processes, complex processes, in which different players intervene and that are carried out within a given socio-economic context and institutional moment in which they take part" (Jara, 2001, p. 2). According to the author, systematization "is that critical interpretation of one or several experiences that, from their ordering and reconstruction, discovers or makes explicit the logic of the process experienced, the factors that intervened in the process, how they related to each other, and why they did so." (Jara, 1996, p. 29).

Originally developed out of popular education experiences in Latin America, this method has also proved suitable for the assessment of management and health promotion experiences, particularly more complex ones, owing to the multiplicity of settings and players and also to the long period required for its development. Application of this method can be suitable in early stages of program development, when important issues for the implementation of intersectoral actions are dealt with. The examination of, and reflection upon, the conditions necessary for setting up the process of systematization help create a context in which joint production of knowledge is valued. Furthermore, the constitution of a "systematization group" is also an opportunity to assert subjects that are plural and diverse, with starting and finishing points in real life experiences.

Systematization begins with the discussion and definition of the object – what experience we want to systematize ; objective – what we want to systematize for; and axis of systematization – what core aspects of this experience we want to systematize. This is followed by the stages of the "recovery of the lived", which is performed through the indication of objective, subjective, and contextual elements related to such experience: "particular situations are faced; actions directed to get to a certain end; perceptions, interpretations, and intentions of different subjects that take part in the program; and, the relations and reactions of these participants" (Jara, 1996, p.25). In short, to recover things which were experienced means "to reconstruct history and order and classify information" (Jara, 1996, p. 85). Added to that is an effort to understand the meaning of experiences through critical interpretation – making a deep reflection requiring the group to analyze, synthesize, and interpret facts and situations that were experienced, that is, to understand the reasons why the experience took place and how the experience occurred. Finally, the group works out its conclusions and communicates the results, in order to give feedback to the participants about the experience. All this process was developed in the Healthy Capela project first phase of assessment, and will be reported further on.

Challenges to and Queries Concerning the Healthy Capela Project

The Healthy Capela project, referenced in the proposal for Healthy Cities of the World Health Organization (OPS, 1997), was set up as a framework for local actions' management. It should therefore be governed by an intersectoral team in order to develop work plans and promote social participation. The first actions carried out already showed that changing the logic of management would not be an easy task. An experimental area was chosen to test the methodology, and local actions planned in a participatory manner were successful. However, since the beginning of the project, coordinators of different sectors of the local administration found it difficult to work along the principles of Healthy Cities, whether planning actions, including always sharing and analyzing the results of the actions conducted with the participation of the local population. There was dissatisfaction among the agents responsible for local actions toward their superiors and with regard to the program itself. Concomitantly, other actions were performed, such as the design of the local rector plan and creation of the Regional Planning and Sustainable Development Council, without establishing relations with the framework selected – the Healthy Capela project.

The planning of workshops began, outlining an integrated participatory management model that was included to strengthen intersectoral actions in the territory as a whole. Unfortunately, the steering committee of the Regional City Hall interrupted the planning process before the international seminar could be held. The ending of the workshops ushered in a period of loosening relations among the partners, only to be strengthened six months later when the research project was approved by the State of Sao Paulo Research Foundation. It seems that the management model under construction was – in a period of six months – replaced by a self-absorbed management style that was distant from partnerships.

The apparent uncertainty or doubt of the Deputy-mayor with regard to the maintenance of the intersectoral and participatory model that would at one moment mobilize players, and the next move away from them, was the major motivation for the conduct of systematization, the object of this chapter. The questions that guided the process were: "What could have led the group, which had been building a successful experiment from the point of view of intersectoral action and social participation, to abruptly change the direction of the process? What information and contexts could have caused this?"

Answering these questions was the aim of a research project developed in response to the State of São Paulo Research Foundation's special program in public policy, in its first phase. Thanks to this support, a discussion was reinitiated between local managers and researchers from the University and the Center of Research and

Documentation on Healthy Cities concerning the project entitled "Healthy Capela and the integrated and participatory management of public policies."

We believe that this illustrates the key enabling role that funding agencies such as the State of São Paulo Research Foundation can play in setting up innovations in the field of health promotion. The production of knowledge, the possibility of evaluating the introduction of an innovative practice in the field of healthy public policies and the increased prestige and visibility that they could generate sensitized managers and provided incentives for the latter to welcome research projects. In the Capela case this would appear to have played a decisive role. It is a fact that no other element or event was cited or acknowledged as a reason to resume discussions on the project.

Assessment of Healthy Capela Process by Systematization

We decided to take, as object, the Healthy Capela Project during the period from February 2003 to July 2004, with the objective of constructing new integrated and participatory work strategies for improvements in quality of life. We chose as the axis of analysis, the influence of other agendas (projects, programs, other commitments going on in the community) in the Healthy Capela Project.

In the phase of recovering what was experienced, participants are invited to verbalize the elements they consider relevant. When presented to the group, the element is transformed by a facilitator, with the support of the group, into a term or expression, recorded on a paper plate and is finally posted on a place visible to all those present. The participants may indicate as many elements as they believe necessary. In this stage of development of the method, it is important that people respect the diversity and plurality of opinions, assessments, and emotions in relation to the declared experience. Once the group finishes indicating elements, it is invited to define categories that can group these elements. As the following example suggests, the definition of categories and the starting point used to interpret the experience is already part of the re-signification the group produces with the help of the method. Their choices, throughout the entire systematization process, evidence what is most significant in the experience lived.

During recovery of the live-through process, 75 significant elements of experience were listed, and grouped into six themes, as shown in Fig. 15.2. These were decentralization, the Capela/city relation; participation; city management; local management; and local projects. Figure 15.2 orders and classifies information, reconstructing the "different aspects of the experience, already seen as a process" (Jara, 1996, p. 104).

The whole work was then guided to unveil the reasons for what happened. The process focused on locating the tensions or contradictions that marked the experience and, with these elements, going back to the whole processes, that is, making a summary that enabled conceptualizing the systematized practice (Jara, 1996).

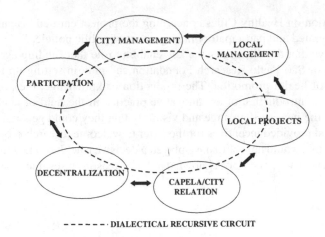

Fig. 15.2 Aspects of healthy capela project

Under the decentralization heading, only budget issues and those concerning the lack of human resources were not addressed directly during the process of reflection. On the other hand, none of the elements under the local projects heading were addressed throughout the systematization of experience.

Under the Capela-city relation heading, the group dwelt on the outstanding position enjoyed by this local city hall in relation to other regional city halls, examining mainly the situations when relations proved more difficult. The result thus acquires a certain self-critical nature and all the elements listed were present in later discussions.

With regard to participation, the group focused on examples of the setting up of participatory spaces such as the Regional Planning and Sustainable Development Council, the carrying out of the Integrated Participatory Rector Plan encompassing all regions of the city, the setting up of the Local Committees of the Healthy Capela Project, and forming the General Committee, which included Districts, Regional Committees, and other partners. The group referred to other actions taken where participation was one of the elements present and also stated that popular participation fell below expectations and those partners, even the Regional Committees, distanced themselves.

Under the heading city management, three out of the seven listed elements were discussed by the group throughout the systematization process. These were: (1) the existence of a vertical relation between Departments and Counties, felt particularly strongly in the education and social work sectors, which tended to maintain centralized control and sectoral practice; (2) changes in command within the Municipal Department of the Regional City Halls, which significantly reduced the influence of Capela within the municipal scope; and (3) the strong influence of the ongoing electoral dispute on decisive City Administration actions and decisions.

Under the heading local management and this despite reference having been made to positive aspects, accounts of perceived difficulties, flaws, and shortcomings predominated, especially with regard to intersectoral action, integrated planning, and the link between actions and objectives.

As laid down by the adopted method, the systematization group was required to define the way in which it would approach the critical interpretation phase of the experience, in which participants would ask themselves: why did things happen in the way they did? Grouping the significant elements of the experiment under themes was merely a way of approaching the problem, though the themes may or may not be used.

The systematization group decided to open the interpretation based upon the nostalgia for the Inter-Department Nucleus—NICS element, which had been added to the issue of decentralization. Later examination of the minutes of meetings enabled us to see that more than half of the elements initially listed were addressed at the time of the discussion of a chosen element. One might suppose that if any other element had been chosen, we would have discussed the same issues anyway, since what is at stake in the systematization process is the attempt to link issues and relate them in order to understand the overall experience, as we intend to show in Fig. 15.2.

Nonetheless, the choice made by the group is believed significant and some points revealed during the reflection helped understand the choice. The tension created by the political and administrative decentralization process in the city of Sao Paulo was apparently felt more intensely in the Capela do Socorro region due to the large investment that had been made there in constructing a new benchmark for local management and due to the high degree of visibility and exposure resulting from this. One example of this investment was the setting up of the Inter-Department Nucleus of Capela do Socorro (NICS). It is worth pointing out that the NICS became a model for decentralized, intersectoral, and participatory management and was a benchmark for the creation of local governments throughout the city approximately one year later. When referring to the process and principles of the NICS, the group particularly focuses on a series of positive aspects: involvement/identity, a context of euphoria, regularity, group, exchange, participation, production of synergy and clarity; it aimed at integration, public policy, idealism, leadership, and motivation.

Some accounts of the workshops[2] reinforce these aspects:

> ...whoever took part felt that it had been an enriching process; it was the richest period of intersectorality...it was a disorganized form with a great deal of participation and the feeling of participation...

> ...we brought together all those working in the Capela territory, which was the great step taken.

Additionally, when the NICS was placed on a timeline – as it was to become first the Local Government of Capela do Socorro and then a Regional City Hall – this reflection showed its ability to reflect and record important moments in the political and administrative decentralization process in the city of Sao Paulo.

Another factor that seems to have influenced the choice of this element stems from a certain internal conflict within the group about the importance placed on the

---

[2] All sentences originally selected from another text - (Fernandez, Bógus & Mendes 2006).

nostalgia issue, given that part of the group had not lived through the experience, but took it further when the Regional City Hall was set up and people were appointed to their positions in the sector's coordination offices. Even the wording of the item – nostalgia for the Inter-Department Nucleus – NICS – expressed a certain irony on the part of the systematization group. This also led people, during the process of interpretation of the experience, to demystify the NICS, accepting what had been said and adding what appeared to be present but remained unspoken in meetings.

Along these lines, a text written during the interpretation of the experience phase (Fernandez, 2004b) states that:

> The NICS is, for the County as a whole, an on/off-type cleavage. It is the switch that turns on or off the attentions and the lighting. It is the NICS that prescribed the axes of operations and the goals that the group that was formed when the County was set up is to accept and pursue. It is the NICS that armed with undeniable legitimacy and rules out possible alternatives. It is the NICS that confers skills, knowledge, and experience to some people. The NICS is, in a nutshell, also and therefore, a statement of what Marilena Chauí calls 'competent discourse'(Chauí, 1969), that is to say, it is a statement that it is not simply anyone and any place that is able to and allowed to say what it wants. Thus, it is only those who are entrusted and hold a place in a bureaucratic organization that are legitimated and have the competence defined so as to be able to say-utter a likewise defined discourse to which institutionalized authority is ascribed.

The NICS is thus the message of integrated and participatory management and its own shadow. Moreover, it is at the same time the promise of change and the affirmation of the status quo. With such expressivity, the work of the NICS and its meanings for the group would have to be investigated and debated if the NICS is actually to understand the experience and review its practices.

Focus on Decentralization

It should be stressed that the processes of decentralization must not be understood only from the standpoint of the institutional or legal apparatus, mainly serving decentralization through legislation, normalization, and workflow definitions. Subjective, contextual, and situational issues that explain behaviors of groups and that depart from a merely positive and organizational logic, such as those revealed during the experience systematization process, must also be considered. There is a recent bibliography (Arretche, 1999; Santos & Barreta, 2004; Capucci & Garibe Filho, 2004; FINATEC, 2004) containing analyses grounded on the first point of view, and the Capela do Socorro experience can help broaden such analyses.

This is attributable above all to the particularity it presents in relation to the other Regional City Halls of the city of Sao Paulo – virtually all of them derived from the former Regional Administrations – in that it foreshadowed an integrated participatory management model corresponding to the promised setting up of the Regional City Hall. As early as February 2001, Capela do Socorro set up the NICS, preparing itself to function as a County, although this would only be created legally as of August 2002 (Governo Local da Capela do Socorro, 2002a,b).

What was the reason, or what were the reasons behind this particularity?

One reason that is important to highlight is its profile as a local manager that triggered, through its strong leadership and powers of creativity and innovation, synergy in the process centered on Capela do Socorro. This was possible due to the fact that it had delegated the bulk of its characteristic caretaker[3] powers as the then Regional Administration, - which might have demanded the manager's full-time energies and probably kept the remaining regional administrations of the city busy – to other members of its team, engaging itself in a liaison between other local managers for other departments, associations, universities and other partners centering on projects for the region. The participants of the systematization process expressed feelings of enthusiasm reflecting the manager's idealism and trust in change.

> (The manager) presented an innovative idea, as he said: – I have not come to be the regional administrator. There was idealism, a goal in life, it was excellent, and there was trust in the change. It gave us a strychnine injection and we had to prepare ourselves for that. It brought an impetus.

The concrete manifestation of this way of working was the NICS, which brought together as many as 40 people in its fortnightly meetings, where information was exchanged, and shared actions were planned. This corroborates what Junqueira lays down when stating that decentralization and intersectoral action are processes "that complete each other and together determine a new way of managing a city's public policies" (Junqueira, 1998, p. 15).

There was also a unique situation of positive mutual influence between Capela do Socorro and the Department of the Regional City Halls, from 2001 to December 2002, which allowed Capela to intervene substantively in central administration decisions affecting decentralization. Examples of this are the drafting of the documents to set up the local governments (Decree 41813 enacted 15 March 2002)[4] – along the lines of the working of the NICS – and organizational structuring of the Regional City Halls (Interdepartment Administrative Act 6/SMSP/SGM/ SGP/ 2002)[5] – largely based on the local government of Capela do Socorro. The members of the systematization process related the decree of the Sao Paulo mayor that changed substantially the way to manage the city, with their local experience with NICS.

> Based on experience with the NICS, we proposed the Administrative Act to set up the Local Governments. Many administrators did not know what was happening, the Regional Administrations were in a state of panic, and did not know what to do.

> It (the Administrative Act) came out virtually exactly as we had proposed, except for the CASD (Coordinating Office for Social Action and Development). It is like winning a prize.

---

[3] "Caretaker" means the conservation and upkeep of the roadways and public spaces, the clearing up of brooks and drains, etc.

[4] See. http://www3.prefeitura.sp.Gov.BR/cadlem/secretarias/negocios_juridico/cadlem/pesqfonetica. Asp?p=Governo+local&var=o&t=D&A.

[5] See. http://www3.prefeitura.sp.Gov.BR/cadlem/secretarias/negocios_juridico/cadlem/pesqfonetica. Asp?p=subturas&var=o&t=PI&A=2002.

The accounts of the participants support the conclusion that the local manager was willing to interfere in the process, and enjoyed political space to do so.

The technical and political profile of the professionals involved in the NICS project must also be underlined. They were people with experience in public management, who had worked in social projects and in decentralization and participation actions in their respective fields. We have highlighted all these aspects here as examples that go beyond the scope of central technical and administrative decisions, and, did in fact interfere in the process and were reported throughout the systematization workshops, as discussed above.

With the setting up of the subprefectures and the definition of their organizational structure – landmarks in the city's decentralization process – changes occurred that significantly marked the Capela do Socorro experience: there was less proximity to central power and discussions of local policies became the exclusive task of the recently-appointed group of coordinators. The focus of the project ceased to be regional and intersectoral and became centered on organizational issues for the region. The following quote expresses feelings of the members of the systematization workshop showing that, the fact of achieving their objectives, was not always an incentive to keep going.

> We threw our energy into building the coordinating bodies and modeling the internal, losing this for the whole: building something new. Before, it was a process of making. Today one does less together. Why? Because we have to set up the coordinating body.

These changes produced a strong repercussion in the group, which reacted to them by departing from the discussion about decentralization in the city, thus beginning another type of relationship with the municipal power. These changes were considered a defeat by the group, who saw them as half-hearted in regard to the decentralization project they had been constructing.

The group may have carried out a partial evaluation of the meaning of the process and, for this reason, understood it as a clear indication that changes would occur much more slowly than hoped for, failing to take into consideration other aspects of the complex process of decentralization in a city of 10 million inhabitants. This means that in general they related the issue to the government political will or lack thereof to conclude the process, and ignored the political, physical, and financial capacity of the government to make the investments that the decentralization process demanded. Toward the end of the term, shortage of investment had made too difficult the task of organizing the Regional City Hall that it diverted the attentions of the management group from innovative intersectoral actions.

The same assessment process reveals that the management group ignored an even more important point: the educational aspect of the decentralization experience. By withdrawing from the discussion, it abandoned the involvement that had characterized the group – not without repercussions as the systematization process demonstrated – and failed to contribute to the advancement of decentralization in the city as well as in the Regional City Hall itself.

The following phrases express the discouraged feelings of the members of systematization group, when they perceived their management proposal for the city of Sao Paulo was not considered in its essence:

I gave up the decentralization debate. . . I abandoned the debate in the city.

This proposal (administrative reform of secretariats) is defeated in the government. . .We lost, that was the context. Here is where we make our decision (to give up the debate).

We had this dream of building something new, and we were building it, when this happened, from top to bottom. Reality hit us. The tool that we had in the District to build the dream was not enough.

Another element that interfered in the city decentralization process was the maintenance of the local management as a means of exchange in negotiation, aiming to have projects and laws of interest to the City Administration approved by the legislative branch. This weakened the Deputy-mayors as interlocutors of the decentralization process, therefore bringing the worker to question and divert the process, as we would be able to perceive in those expression of the members of the systematization group.

Decentralize and hand over power to the 70% who don't believe in it? Is that why I should decentralize?

What I am going to give the guy, I said. . .

. . .if power goes to our enemies we shouldn't decentralize? If it is for society then it doesn't make any difference regarding parties.

What comes through clearly from the experience is how these decentralization processes need to remain alert to local potential and to the strengthening of their own autonomy. One may suppose that these processes will be stronger insofar as they are open to dialogue with the multiple actors that have been investing in building decentralized public policies, and more permeable to civic practices. These same processes, depending on how they are managed, may neutralize advances achieved at local level.

The study of the decentralization experience that occurred within the City Administration of Sao Paulo and particularly in the process experienced in the Capela do Socorro Regional City Hall, shows the tension that exists between the founder and its discovery (Castoriadis, 1982; Lourau, 1975; Maffesoli, 1997), or rather, between the setting up of a project for change and a project for power and maintenance of the status quo; between a project that is mediated by participatory decisions, concerned with the complexity of urban problems, in other words, mediated by intersectorality, guided by a communicative reason (Habermas, 1989), rather than one that is produced by the excessively technical view of isolated managers, unable to liaise with and negotiate so as to involve the several social players present in the political arena (Junqueira, 1998). In short, the study illustrates a process that oscillates between innovation and bureaucratization in building the management processes.

Conclusion

As pointed out by Jara (1996, p.108), "all interpretative reflection conducted in a systematization process should result in the formulation – as clear as possible – of both theoretical and practical conclusions." The conclusion presented herein stems directly from what was reflected from the experience of the systematization method in relation to the Healthy Capela experience.

What quality of life improvement outcomes for the population of Capela do Socorro might one attain by identifying key elements for the assessment of the Healthy Cities experiment by systematizing the experience? Without wishing to shun the challenge of evidencing the effectiveness of actions in the field of health promotion, into which the 'healthy cities' initiatives fit, we feel that outcomes can only be detected with the continuity of the process that, as we said, began with the setting up of the NICS, which was fed by the Healthy Capela project and was to be threatened eventually by the alternating changes in municipal political power.

Several lessons can be drawn from this systematization experience. First, the de-mobilization of the management group regarding integrated and participatory management can be explained by the same factors that, to a different extent, accounted for initial mobilization. What we see is that the best and the worst moments experienced by the Healthy Capela group are closely linked to the true and false paths followed during the decentralization process by the municipality of Sao Paulo, from 2001 to 2004. Second, certain conditions enable concretization of intersectoral action and social participation, the pursuit to integrate both as guiding principles and not as ends in themselves, and the concrete possibility of mobilizing resources to attain specific desired goals. What the experience underlined was the understanding that intersectoral action, participation and the outcomes promoted in actions guided by them, are the tributaries of their association to other equally important issues – in this case, political and administrative decentralization. Third, it is only apparently paradoxical that the best and worst of the Capela do Socorro experience should be closely linked to the political process of administrative decentralization. The experience is above all about the dynamics between the founder and the founded, and relates a process in which intersectoral action – motivated by decentralization and driven by autonomy – as a project for change, gives way to (or should one say, is defeated by?) bureaucracy, in the control of decentralization and given up to its own dynamics, as a project of power. Fourth, the policies guiding innovation processes in Third World countries like Brazil, based on relations of subordination and domination, founded on "clientelism" and paternalistic hand-out, an element of resistance to changes while simultaneously driving them. Any manager committing to a type of integrated and participatory management jeopardizes this relation of inferiority, counter to this training and action of citizens, who might set in motion a process of changing relations within society. No other methodology would enable one to reveal these elements that hinder the implementation of a real integrated participatory management.

Stakeholders Challenge the Systematization Process

Participants reported that in one NICS meeting, a representative of the central authority, expressing his admiration for the advances achieved by the group, said: "I don't know if this is good for you or bad for you." The episode remained in the group's memory and, was expressed by one metaphor, written by one of the members of the systematization workshop that we thought it will be interesting to reproduce to the readers:

> this episode represents the first or the most meaningful meeting of our characters with the dialectical field of conflicting relations between the founder and the founded, between bound social energy and subject groups, and between free social energy and subject groups, as Paula Carvalho well wrote. It was the moment where that innovative energy with freedom to build the vehicle of its dreams met the transport 'system', with its regulatory and norm-defining agencies, in short, with the institution, already founded and which struggles above all for its own preservation (...) It was the fortune or the misfortune of our characters to discover themselves in the midst of a counter-institutional act, with whatever this means when you want to be 'with', when you want to be 'inside' and not knocking at the door demanding that the institution speak – and speak differently. (Fernandez, 2004a).

The equation encountered between creative energy and the strength of the already-founded, where autonomy gives way to heteronomy – and perceived in the priority given to the organization of sector coordinating agencies, in the departure from the discussion that was taking place in the city, in the distancing from spaces where there was interlocution with the other partners, in short, in the dissolution of the energy that mobilized the group – is only a fragment or a single frame from a feature film dealing with the processes of decentralization. However, it is at the same time a unique opportunity to think about participation and intersectoral action and the conditions in which it might be better developed.

References

Arretche, M. T. S. (1999). Políticas sociais no Brasil: Descentralização em um Estado federativo [*Social policies in Brazil: decentralization in a federative State*]. *Revista Brasileira de Ciências Sociais, 14*(40), 111–141.

Capucci, P. F., & Garibe Filho, R. N. (2004) Gestão local nos territórios da cidade: ciclo de atividades com as subprefeituras. [*Local management in the city's territories: the cycle of activities with the subprefectures*] São Paulo: Mídia Alternativa/Secretaria Municipal das Subprefeituras.

Carvalho, M. C. B. (2001). Avaliação de Projetos Sociais. [*Evaluation of Social Projects*] In A. M. Ávila (org). Gestão de Projetos Sociais. 3a edição, São Paulo, AAPCS – Associação de Apoio ao Programa Capacitação Solidária, 61–91.

Castoriadis, C. (1982). A instituição imaginária da sociedade. [*The imaginary institution of society*] 3. ed. Rio de Janeiro: Paz e Terra.

Chaui, M. S. (1969). O discurso competente e outras falas. [*The competent discourse and other utterances*] São Paulo: Moderna.

Fernandez, J. C. A. (2004a) Senhores passageiros do "Capela para...". [*Passengers on board the "Capela to..."*] Retrieved January 28, 2008, from http://www.cidadessaudaveis.org.br/noticias.asp

Fernandez, J. C. A. (2004b). Sistematização de experiência: Capela do Socorro, fase: interpretação. [The systematization of experience: Capela do Socorro, interpretation phase]. Retrieved January 28, 2008, from http://www.cidadessaudaveis.org.br/noticias.asp

Fernandez, J. C. A., Bogus, C. M., & Mendes, R. (2006) O método da sistematização: uma leitura crítica do processo. [The method of systematization: a critical reading of the process] In (orgs.) WESTPHAL, M.F. & PAIS, T.J.A.D. Capela saudável: gestão de políticas públicas integradas e participativas. [A healthy Capela: an integrated and participatory management of public policies] São Paulo: Editora EDUSP.

FINATEC, Fundacão de Empreendimentos Científicos e Tecnológicos. (2004). Descentralização e poder local: a experiência das subprefeituras no município de São Paulo. [Decentralization and local power: the experience of the sub-prefectures of São Paulo] São Paulo: HUCITEC/FINATEC.

Governo Local da Capela do Socorro. (2002a). Planejamento estratégico. [strategic planning]. São Paulo: PMSP.

Governo Local da Capela do Socorro. (2002b). Plano de ação local. [local planning] São Paulo: PMSP.

Habermas, J. (1989). Consciência moral e agir comunicativo. [Moral awareness and communicative action] Rio de Janeiro: Tempo Brasileiro.

Jara, O. (1996). Para sistematizar experiências. [To systematize experiences] Translated Maria V.V. Rezende. UFPB – Editora Universitária EQUIP.

Jara, O. (2001). Dilemas y desafios de la sistematización de experiências. [Dilemmas and challenges of the systematization of experiences] Seminário ASOCAM, Cochabamba.

Junqueira, L. A. P. (1998) Descentralização e intersetorialidade: a construção de um modelo de gestão municipal. [Decentralization and intersectorality: the construction of a model for municipal management] RAP, 32(2), 11–22.

Lourau, R. (1975). El análisis institucional [Institutional analysis] – Buenos Aires: Amorrortu editores.

Maffesoli, M. (1997). A transfiguração do político: a tribalização do mundo. [The transfiguration of the political: the tribalization of the world] Translated Juremir Machado da Silva. Porto Alegre: Editora Sulina.

OPS. (1997). Municípios saludables. [Healthy Cities] Washington, DC. OPS.

Paula Carvalho, J.C. de. (1990). Antropologia das organizações e educação: um ensaio holonômico. [The anthropology of organizations and education: a holonomic essay] Rio de Janeiro: Imago Editora.

Santos, U. P., & Barreta, D. (orgs.). (2004). Subprefeituras de São Paulo: descentralização e participação popular em São Paulo. [Sub-prefectures of São Paulo: decentralization and popular participation in São Paulo] São Paulo: HUCITEC/ Prefeitura do Município de São Paulo.

Chapter 16
Issues in Evaluating Equity

Mita Giacomini and Jeremiah Hurley

Equity entails the fair distribution of resources, whether these are health services, nutrients, education, or something else. When evaluating a health program, it is often important to understand the program's impact not only in terms of the total benefits it has achieved (effectiveness), or its cost relative to these benefits (efficiency), but also how its benefits have been distributed amongst individuals or groups within the target community (equity). To evaluate equity, we must formulate what an ideal distribution of resources would look like. For example, we may want a program to narrow gaps in health between rural and urban communities, or to simply improve the health of the sickest children whatever its effects on others. Evaluation then assesses how well the program achieves the equity ideal. Another important role of equity evaluation is to investigate whether inequities were unintentionally created or exacerbated by the program.

Equity evaluation is appropriate when either (1) the aim of the program is to improve equity or (2) the program has other aims but there are concerns about its incidental effects on equity. As an evaluative criterion, equity is widely embraced by many decision-makers and jurisdictions, and could apply in principle to any type of health program. Despite its nearly universal ethical appeal, however, there is less consensus in the health policy community over how best to operationalize, measure, and judge equity. In this chapter, we discuss some options and approaches for applying the equity concept in the context of health program evaluation. We address the equity evaluation of a program that is already implemented, whether it was originally aimed directly at the problem of inequity or at some other goal.

Defining Equity

The contemporary concept of equity stems from Aristotle's original imperative to treat those who are alike the same, and those who are not alike differently in proportion to their relevant differences (Aristotle, 350 B.C., 2000). The term horizontal equity is sometimes used to refer to the equal treatment of equals, whereas vertical

M. Giacomini
McMaster University, Hamilton, Canada

L. Potvin, D. McQueen (eds.), *Health Promotion Evaluation Practices in the Americas*,
DOI: 10.1007/978-0-387-79733-5_16, © Springer Science+Business Media, LLC 2008
285

equity refers to appropriately differential treatment of those who are different. Each is important in the evaluation of the fairness of a program's distributive impacts.

When policy makers raise concerns about equity, they are usually referring to how intervention outcomes are distributed: who ends up with what, and whether this pattern looks fair. This is sometimes referred to as end-state or distributional equity. For example, we may want to see all community members have equal access to preventive care. Sometimes, policy interest may turn instead to procedural equity, which specifies fair distributive processes without judging further where the resources actually end up. Some might argue, for example, that a fair process for an immunization clinic is to treat individuals on a first-come, first-served basis. Procedural equity is often pursued when fairness matters but fair end-states are difficult to prescribe or to measure. Most of our attention here will be on determining the equity of end-state distributions, but we will also briefly discuss implications of procedural equity for program evaluation.

The World Health Organization defines equity as follows: "Equity is the absence of avoidable or remediable differences among populations or groups defined socially, economically, demographically, or geographically; thus, health inequities involve more than inequality—whether in health determinants or outcomes, or in access to the resources needed to improve and maintain health—but also a failure to avoid or overcome such inequality that infringes human rights norms or is otherwise unfair." (World Health Organization, 2005)

A major challenge for the evaluation of equity in the health sector is identifying which differences are avoidable or remediable, and thus all under the purview of public health, health care, or social programs. Fundamental policy goals and questions for the evaluation of equity are summarized in Box 16.1.

Box 16.1 Examples of Basic Policy Goals and Questions for Equity Evaluation

Horizontal equity: Treating likes alike
Policy goals:

> *All enjoy an equal level of health, equal access to services when they need them or equal protection from health risks*

Evaluation question:
Do some identifiable groups – and specifically, which – receive less, or benefit less?

Vertical equity: Treating unlikes differently
Policy goals:

> *Sicker people receive proportionately more health services or health improvement from services given; at-risk people receive proportionately more health protection*

Evaluation question:
Do those who need more receive, or benefit, proportionately more?

Equity must also be understood in relation to equality and social justice. Equality simply refers to giving everyone an equal amount of a resource. This is an appropriate approach to basic human rights, such as equality under the law, and it applies in an idealistic way to good health, although realistically it is also understood that a fully equal distribution of health is not achievable. However, equality is often not appropriate when applied to health care, health programs, and many other determinants of health because not everyone needs the same amount of these resources to achieve good health. To be fair and equitable, we must assign such goods not strictly equally, but in proportion to meaningful and relevant differences among individuals. Social justice is a broader ethical imperative that entails the fair distribution of resources, but may also entail obligations outside this realm, such as equal citizen rights, equality under the law, or health as a fundamental human right. The United Nations clearly links health with social justice: "Health is a fundamental human right indispensable for the exercise of other human rights. Every human being is entitled to the enjoyment of the highest attainable standard of health conducive to living a life in dignity" (United Nations Economic and Social Council & Committee on Economic Social and Cultural Rights, 2000).

As argued by Nobel Laureate Amartya Sen (2002), equity in health plays a central role in achieving social justice more broadly. Health is not like any other good: it is an essential feature of human existence, and determines our capability and freedom to achieve basic life goals (Sen, 1987, 1992, 2002). Broader social justice, then, is conditional in part on equity in health and the resources that generate health.

Three Analytical Tasks for Evaluating Distributive Equity

The key evaluative question for distributive equity is: To what degree does the actual distribution of resources conform to an ideally equitable distribution? For program evaluation in particular, we ask: Has the program brought us any closer to the ideally equitable distribution of resources? These questions are both descriptive and normative, because they require a clear vision of the good and of what constitutes fairness.

Returning to Aristotle's maxim: those alike should receive equal amounts of the resource, and those unalike should receive different amounts in proportion to their relevant differences. This lays out three analytic tasks necessary to evaluating equity: (1) identify the resource to be distributed equitably, (2) in relation to this resource, identify differences amongst potential recipients that are relevant to their need of, or claim upon, the resource; and (3) specify in quantifiable terms how the differences among recipients should determine their equitable proportion of the resource.

Consider, for example, the resource of prenatal education classes distributed among rural villages, with the policy objective of lowering the maternal-infant mortality rate of an entire region. Equity-relevant differences among these communities might include fertility rates, morbidity and mortality among women and infants, etc. Differences less relevant to equity may include proximity to paved roads, predominant ethnicities or religions, and so forth. To be fair, villages with higher fertility rates perhaps should receive a greater number of classes; however, this depends on the nature of the classes and may not be necessary if one class could accommodate any number of participants. After the region-wide program was implemented, evaluation of its equity impacts would proceed in a similar order: identify the resource (classes), identify differences relevant to an equitable distribution (fertility, health), identify irrelevant differences that should not matter beyond their coincidence with relevant differences (geography, ethnicity) and measure how well the actual distribution of classes meets the equitable ideal. Evaluators should also be interested in differences in ultimate health outcomes across the villages, and whether the program leveled these. Equity-oriented evaluation may be separate from broader effectiveness-oriented evaluation, which would determine whether and how the program lowered maternal-infant mortality rates for the region. It is possible for a program to be effective overall because it lowers regional mortality while being inequitable because it preserves or exacerbates a mortality gradient between villages.

To develop a program aimed specifically at inequity, the three analytic tasks may be approached in a different order: identifying and measuring relevant differences first, and selecting the most appropriate resources next. For example, the equity problem might be identified as differences in maternal-infant mortality rates across villages. Prenatal classes may help level these, but depending on the nature of the problem, other interventions focused on nutrition or women's general education might do a better job of both lowering and equalizing mortality. The final policy task becomes determining how best to match the level of need with specific levels of the various programs (prenatal, nutritional, educational) at hand. Evaluation would focus more squarely on health outcomes, with attention to both levels and differences across villages.

Identifying the Resources

The fundamental resource of concern in health policy and health promotion is health itself: health is what we would like to see distributed more equitably. Analysis of health equity, however, is complicated by two facts. First, health itself cannot be directly distributed, only some of its determinants may be. Second, health is both determined by, and determines, resources beyond health programs and health care. Equity oriented evaluation may be interested in the fairness of the distribution of both resources that determine health, and ultimate health outcomes. Evaluators must also take into account initial health problems and disparities to understand how well the program succeeded in alleviating them.

Many factors determine health status. Contributors to health include broad social determinants such as wealth disparities, working conditions, environmental conditions, and the status of women; public health services and programs; the availability, accessibility, and quality of healthcare services; genetics; congenital conditions; the existence and nature of pathogens; individual behaviors and choices;

and collective behaviors and choices. Often for the purposes of policy and politics, those interested in equity try to distinguish between health problems caused by society, nobody, or individual themselves, with the implication that the former two merit collective intervention in a way that the last may not, or that disparities in the last are more tolerable from a social justice perspective. In practice, however, these distinctions are nearly impossible because health determinants interact with each other in nested relationships such that each cause also has its causes to consider (Krieger, 1994). For example, a genetic feature such as lactose intolerance may or may not be a health problem depending on the prevailing culture (Gannett, 1999); a personal choice not to exercise regularly may be determined in part by poverty that offers little time and opportunity for this kind of activity (Krieger, 1994). A disease such as diabetes may be explained by nearly all of these determinants. Whether inequalities in rates of diabetes among income, ethnic, gender, geographic, or age groups should be considered inequitable is a further value judgment.

Health affects access to other resources. Its relationship to basic freedoms, opportunities and privileges in life is in part why people value health, both for themselves and for others (Sen, 1992). The World Health Organization explains: "Reducing health inequities is important because health is a fundamental human right and its progressive realization will eliminate those inequalities in the opportunity to enjoy life and pursue one's life plans that result from differences in health status (i.e., diseases, disabilities, etc.) and that in turn exacerbate these differences" (World Health Organization, 2005).

Researchers operationalize health in a variety of ways. There is typically a gap between what ought to be measured in principle and what most evaluators are able to measure in practice. Sophisticated models and measures of health and well-being typically require data such as population surveys or detailed administrative data, which are unavailable or expensive in many contexts. For these reasons, the most common empirical indicators of health are life expectancy, mortality rates, selected mortality causes (e.g., accidents, infectious disease, violence, chronic disease, etc.), and morbidity rates. Broad health system level monitoring of equity tends to rely on data such as birth and death records, census data, and population health or standard of living surveys (Braveman, 1998).

Equity evaluation in the health sector often focuses on equity in the distribution of resources necessary to produce health rather than health outcomes per se. There is widespread interest in equitable distribution of good quality and adequate quantity of necessities for generating, maintaining, and restoring health. Such health-determining inputs can be measured in the physical units, such as providers, technologies, services, service quality, capital; funding levels (adjusted for price differences across regions or groups) or the barriers and opportunities for access, or rates of actual access and utilization. A full evaluation of the equity of a health system must also consider sources of funding: for example, how progressively is the health system financed (Mills, 1998)? All of these aspects of a health system have the appeal of being relatively easy to measure, compared to actual health outcomes. They often relate directly to the concrete activities and traceable data of health programs. All share the common drawback, however, of representing efforts rather than successes.

Identifying the Relevant Differences

Having established the resource being allocated, the next question is to whom it goes. Returning to Aristotle, the task for equity analysis is to identify the relevant differences between people (or groups) in relation to the resource. For health resources, health status is obviously a potentially relevant difference, as is the ability to benefit from the health resources. However, other categories are often applied in equity analyses of health systems and programs, for example gender, poverty, or geographic location. Several considerations underlie the construction of relevant subgroups for an equity evaluation.

For the determination of horizontal equity, we must start by asking: who should get equal shares of health resources? The immediate answer in most jurisdictions is: those with an equal level of need. The question may then be posed in a slightly different way: given equal needs, who should not get unequal shares of resources? This leads the evaluator to consider the categories used in the community to assign equal rights or to identify people at risk for discrimination in general, including but not restricted to, discrimination in health programs. Such groups may be encoded in antidiscrimination law or they may represent popular understandings of socially or economically vulnerable or disadvantaged groups. Typical constructs include for example race, ethnicity, gender, age, disability, poverty, and so forth. An illustrative list appears in Table 16.1. Many of these variables are also correlated with health status, and this is addressed in the following discussion of vertical equity. The important point regarding horizontal equity is that these categories do not derive their

Table 16.1 Examples of potentially relevant group characteristics for equity evaluation of health programs

Justice variables[a]		Health need variables
Poverty	Education	Health status
Social status	Employment	Health risk
Discrimination history	Occupation	Ability to benefit
Age	Insurance status	
Developmental stage	Geography	
Gender	Culture	
Ethnicity	Language	
National origin	Stigmatization	
Aboriginal status	Etc.	
Sexuality		
Disability		

[a] Note: some of these justice oriented variables are hybrid variables that could also correspond to health needs, but they are characterized here as justice variables because they may be of analytic interest even when not correlated with health status. This is most often true when assessing the horizontal equity of resources for producing health (inputs).

entire value for health program evaluation from their relationship to health status or ability to benefit from health programs. They are interesting in their own right because of broader concerns about justice, rights and discrimination.

The evaluation of vertical equity examines whether disparities in resources are fair. For this, we turn primarily to the characteristic of need and ask whether those who need more get more, and whether the increment is proportionate with their greater need. There are many ways of characterizing need (Culyer & Simpson, 1980; Culyer, 1998; Robertson, 1998), and of course not all needs are relevant to all resources. As noted above, some equity evaluations begin with a given resource, and ask whether it is distributed according to need. While in other cases, the evaluation begins with a given need, then determine which resources are required and whether they are provided in proportion to needs. Both approaches share a central concern with equity, although the latter is more clearly directed at leveling health differences as well. Returning to the example above, equity motivated policy may ask either, "Which villages should get these prenatal classes to lower maternal-infant mortality?" or "What shall we do to level differences in maternal-infant mortality between villages?"

The various formulations of need may be divided into two major types. The first type represents how badly off people are and may be expressed in terms of health or risk status. The second type relates to how much better off a given resource would make people and is linked to people's ability to benefit. Many economists argue that ability to benefit should be the fundamental attribute of need and that health status is at best an imperfect proxy for ability to benefit. However, health status can be relevant in its own right because it is associated with ethical imperatives such as a duty to care or the rule of rescue, especially in clinical contexts. In practice, health status and ability to benefit both have salience for assessing equity, and measurements of need will be constructed from available – and often less than ideal – proxy variables that may represent a mix of health status, ability to benefit, and social justice claims.

If need is equated with health status, or with health risk in the case of preventive or protective programs, evaluators would measure whether people who are sicker or more vulnerable get more resources. Many measures are available. Some rely on subjective report, others on externally measured indicators of risk, disability, quality of life, diagnosis, disease severity, and so forth. If need is equated with ability to benefit from the resource in question, an evaluator must measure whether those with greater ability to benefit get more resources. Notions of need based on ability to benefit flow from a consequentialist position, which judges ethicality by consequences rather than acts or intentions. Such position, for example, would hold that it is not equitable to give disadvantaged people extra resources if they cannot make productive use of them. This is easier to justify when the evaluation question is framed as, "Who should receive these resources?" than when it is framed as, "Which resources do the disadvantaged need, and are they getting them?" This latter question opens up the possibility not only that different groups have different levels of need, but also that qualitatively distinct resources or technologies may be appropriate for meeting those needs. Although these formulations rest on the same concepts, they may have different implications for practice and intervention. Policy makers may address the latter problem either by allocating different things to different target populations, or by allocating a resource that recipients can exchange for the exact technologies they need (e.g., funds rather than services).

In practice, actual resource allocations are not made directly to needs in the abstract, but to groups of people targeted through available institutions. This distinction between the reason for the allocation and the institutions and groups who actually receive the resource is crucial for two reasons. First, real groups must serve as appropriate proxies for differing levels of need. For example, resources are often apportioned to local governments or providers rather than to the sick or the healthy, men or women. Most of these real groups contain individuals with heterogeneous needs, even if average needs vary between the groups. Second, because resources are allocated by institutions and within social, political, and economic contexts, these target groups must be regarded and treated as something more than empty buckets of health needed to be filled with equitable amounts of health resources. As the World Health Organization explains:

> A characteristic common to groups that experience health inequities (e.g., poor or marginalized persons, racial and ethnic minorities, and women) is lack of power in political, social, and/or economic terms. Thus, to be effective and sustainable, interventions that aim to redress inequities must typically go beyond remedying a particular health inequality and also help empower the group in question through systemic changes, such as law reform, changes in economic or social relationships, or the like. (World Health Organization, 2005)

One might ask whether justice based characteristics such as gender, age, or ethnicity matter at all if health differences are fully accounted for, that is, if any apparent inequality of health-generating resources such as health promotion programs, insurance coverage, care, between groups could be explained and justified by differences in their health status, or needs. Equity analyses based on demographic and justice-related variables remain particularly salient when: (1) health need is difficult to measure and control for, (2) the resource corresponds imperfectly or uncertainly to actual benefit, and, (3) when the resource in question represents investments or efforts rather than an outcome.

Distributing Resources by Relevant Differences

Once the evaluator has characterized the resource and intended recipients or beneficiaries, there remains the final matter of determining the equitable correspondence between resources and recipients. This depends on the moral underpinnings of the community's particular commitment to equity. It is a value judgment. We illustrate some basic models assuming that health is the resource ultimately being allocated by the program and measured by evaluators. Other variations on this sort of typology and elaborations of specific models can be found elsewhere (Beauchamp & Childress, 2001; Williams & Cookson, 2000).

A utilitarian view of equity looks to allocations that produce greatest good for the greatest number. The distribution of the resource across individuals or groups within the population does not matter. This subordinates the equity question to efficiency, a criterion likewise concerned with producing the greatest amount of benefit possible with limited resources. For the utilitarian, inequalities are tolerable and even desirable if they have the effect of making the population as a whole better off. In the extreme, a utilitarian view would even condone the sacrifice of individuals' health or lives for the net benefit of the group. Strict utilitarianism is broadly rejected in health policy. In most legal and ethical systems it would violate human rights to require some individuals to sacrifice for the benefit of others.

An equality of health view aims not to maximize net population health, but to equalize the distribution of health in the population, that is, to decrease the differences between the least and most healthy. The maximin criterion focuses only on the degree to which an allocation improves the lot of those worst off, without regard to net benefit for the population as a whole. A more utilitarian variant maximizes overall population health conditional on a minimum standard of health for all. It establishes a floor beneath which nobody can fall, while it raises the overall average health for the group as a whole. These models are consistent with a contractarian approach to social justice, which asks policy makers to allocate goods as if they themselves could be in any of the receiving positions, but do not know which (Rawls, 1971). Ignorance of one's own position and interests is particularly conducive to establishing a floor of minimum entitlement.

Three more models focus on improving the positions of those worst off, but differ in their interpretation of what worst off means and how resources are supposed to help. The models invoke respectively the two different constructs of need summarized in Table 16.1. First, resources may be allocated according to health status, with those in worst health receiving the most. It is based on the assumption that the resources are helpful, and proportionately more so when health is worse. Allocation by health status also has the symbolic virtue of making greatest efforts in areas of greatest distress.

Another approach allocates resources more discriminatingly according to ability to benefit, with those who have the most to gain also receiving the most. These recipients are not necessarily the sickest. It is based on principles of triage, which view futile or unsuccessful efforts as wasted.

A final model pursues equality of opportunity (Rawls, 1971). In health policy, this means, recognizing that some health differences are inevitable and beyond policy remedy, while others are capricious or artifacts of broader injustices such as discrimination by gender or race, and for this reason deserve especially energetic intervention. Resources are aimed to equalize individuals' opportunities to gain health (Daniels, 1985).

Which of the foregoing models is most appropriate for envisioning an ideally equitable distribution? The stock answer to this question is that it is a value judgment. This is particularly true where there are tensions between improving overall population health versus helping those who are worst off. The choice between the specific allocation criteria of health status versus ability to benefit, however, is determined in part by technical features of the program. Those technical features are (1) the policy level at which resources are allocated, and (2) the specificity of both resources (in terms of technologies) and needs (in terms of qualitative categories in addition to degree). If the resource is not particularly specialized (e.g. money, personnel, clinics that could address many health challenges) and recipient groups are determined by broad characteristics such as justice variables (see Table 16.1) or by administrative features (e.g., local jurisdictions), then it makes more sense to use broad health indicators as proxies for need, and to allocate according to health status. However, if the resource is more specific (e.g., programs for a specific disease, medical specialists) and if the population can be segmented and targeted by health-relevant features (e.g., people at risk for a specific disease or requiring a particular specialist), ability-to-benefit might be considered.

Assuming that a health program is targeted to needs, we return to the two distinct ways to pose an equity question. Recall that the first is: "We have resources, how should we allocate them according to need?" This is the presumption underlying many models. However, in some situations the second will be more relevant: "We have people in need, which resources should we give them to equalize or fulfill their needs?" For the first question, ability to benefit depends not only on the recipients' condition, but also on technological capacity. If the type of technology or program is not negotiable, and it does not address the most severe and inequitably distributed health problems, then it can be regarded less as a resource and more as a barrier to equity when the second question is asked. Whether either question can be asked productively, and whether anything can be done to tailor technologies, programs, or resources to specific needs, will vary with the policy and institutional context. Braveman's proposed cycle for monitoring equity in health, for example, is initiated by the identification of disadvantaged groups and their needs, describes a variety of implications for measurement, intervention, and evaluation (Braveman, 1998).

Procedural Justice and Equity

The models we have described so far are often referred to as end state formulations of equity. In contrast to end-state models, procedural justice models do not prescribe equitable distributions. Rather, they prescribe processes for deciding distributions in specific cases. Examples of popular procedural features include for example the participation of the public in priority setting, rules of engagement around the table where decisions are made, or mechanisms for transparency and appeal.

There may be philosophical reasons for choosing to focus on procedural means rather than end distributions for defining what is just and equitable. In the context of health policy and program planning, certain conditions may make procedural justice particularly appealing. First, allocation procedures become more important where needs vary greatly and are difficult for policy makers or service providers to measure, and thus are best assessed from the ground up rather than the top down. Second, when a resource is scarce and not easily divisible, a fair process may be necessary to allocate between equally deserving recipients, as in the case for example where there is only one organ available for two equally sick and promising transplant candidates. Third, communities with inadequate consensus on a broad vision of end-state equity may aim to suit various local values, and the procedure for making allocation decisions may be of more immediate ethical interest than the decisions themselves. Procedural dimensions are important to protect certain rights or enforce obligations such as the right of citizens to appeal decisions that affect them, or the accountability of policy makers to the public. Finally, particular procedural models are popular wherever there is a prevailing libertarian ideology that rejects the distribution of resources by governments or programs in favor of allocation through free exchange. A great deal has been written on fair processes in health resource allocation, and there are various proposed models (Daniels & Sabin, 2002; Gutmann & Thompson, 2002). Most extreme procedural justice theories hold that fair processes necessarily lead to equitable outcomes, or that outcomes are by definition equitable only if they result from fair process. This is the libertarian standard articulated by Nozick (1974). However, in health policy, most recognize that fair processes may be valuable in themselves and necessary, but not always sufficient, for achieving equity.

Even where there is a primary commitment to procedural equity, it may be desirable to evaluate impacts on distributional equity. For program evaluation, process models of equity may be relevant especially for programs that devolve resource allocation decisions. It may also be important in some formative evaluations for understanding how specific resource allocation decisions are developed, justified, and revised. Summative evaluations of the equity of the material impacts of a program, however, require an end-state model of equity.

Equity and Efficiency

It is often believed that equity and efficiency inevitably conflict with each other as evaluation criteria: a maximally efficient program will be inequitable to some degree, and a maximally equitable program will be inefficient. This is not necessarily true. It depends upon how efficiency and equity are defined, and the particular situation at hand.

Efficiency is often praised as a policy goal. Yet, efficiency is not a goal in itself but rather a means for achieving goals. We can ask whether objectives are reached efficiently, but we cannot ask whether efficiency has been achieved without knowing first what the policy objective was. Economists speak of three types of efficiency: technical, cost-effectiveness, and allocative. Technical efficiency refers to producing maximal outputs with a given mix of inputs, for example, immunizing the greatest number of children possible with a given number of health workers. If health workers are not engaged to their full capacity given their skills, the program becomes relatively less technically efficient. Cost-effective efficiency requires considering the inputs in terms of their costs. For example, we might ask not only whether we have used the minimum number of health workers required, but whether we have used the lowest-cost combination of health workers. If a physician provides a service that a nurse or trained layperson could provide just as well, this is relatively less cost-effective. Allocative efficiency adds the question of whether the final product ends up in the hands of the people who value it the most. A clinic that immunizes many children and employs appropriate clinicians may seem technically efficient and cost-effective, but it would be allocatively inefficient if it missed many high risk children, favoured one gender, or targeted those not at risk.

Efficiency and equity need not conflict. For instance, allocation according to need may be both efficient if those most in need benefit the most from care (i.e., the health gain is greatest) and equitable if need is judged to be the key variable for judging equity. They may conflict, however, if those with relatively lesser needs actually derive greater health benefit from a given resource than those with greater need. Many health systems are not operating at full efficiency or equity and it is possible to identify programs and reforms that could improve both efficiency and equity. The precise nature of any potential conflict between efficiency and equity depends critically on the definitions of efficiency and equity adopted and the empirical relationship between benefit and the receipt of health resources. It is possible to ask whether the goal of equity is achieved as efficiently as possible, or whether efficiency in relation to some other goal (cost-effectiveness or technical productivity) comes at a gain or loss in equity.

Conclusion

Equity means treating similarly situated people equally and treating differently situated people in a manner appropriate to their differences. This concept challenges evaluators to identify the relevant difference as well as the appropriate rule for portioning resources in relation to differences. In evaluation, then, actual achievements can be measured against equity ideals. Equity must be operationalized specifically for the context in which it will be applied and measured. There are many possible formulations and no universally right way to do it, either ethically or technically. Some of the variations in defining equity depend on differences across value systems. However, variation is also necessitated by the diverse nature of the social institutions, groups, and technologies involved in resource distribution. Resources vary in their divisibility and generalizable value; needs differ in their qualities as well as degree.

To evaluate whether equity has been achieved, or inequities have been exacerbated, the evaluator must envision what an ideal distribution of resources would look like, then compare the actual distribution against this ideal. These idealized models take various forms based on different underlying ethics. Utilitarian models focus solely on the total amount of benefit, ignoring the distribution of benefit across members of society; others put more weight on benefits to relatively disadvantaged groups within the population; still others attempt to consider the full distribution across all members of society. Dilemmas include whether to aim for more equal levels of health or to raise the level of those in poorest health, and how to consider severity of health problems versus ability to benefit from intervention. It is important to recognize that the variables prescribed by ideal models do not always map well onto the realities of actual resources, recipients, or the intervening institutions that do the allocating. The use of proxy variables for need, such as gender, age and geographic location, is the norm in equity research in health fields. These variables are often correlated or conflated with other justice imperatives, claims on resources, political or social interests, and so forth.

Finally, the presumed tradeoff between equity and efficiency is often overstated. Efficiency is a feature of means, and as such can only be evaluated in relation to an end. If the end is a particular vision of equity, then it may be reasonable to ask whether equity is achieved efficiently, or effectively, safely, at affordable cost, or some other criterion. In some cases, the utilitarian goal of maximizing health may conflict with the goal of equity, meaning that gains in equity come at a cost to overall productivity. Choosing which outcome to favor in these cases is a moral task, not a technical one.

References

Aristotle. (350 B.C., 2000). *Nicomachean ethics, book 5, chapter 3* (W.D. Ross, Trans., Vol. 2007). Adelaide: Adelaide Library eBooks @ Adelaide.

Beauchamp, T. L., & Childress, J. F. (2001). Justice. In *Principles of biomedical ethics* (5th ed., pp. 225–282). Oxford: Oxford University Press.

Braveman, P. (1998). *Monitoring equity in health: A policy-oriented approach in low- and middle-income countries. Equity initiative paper No. 3* (No. WHO/CHS/HSS/98.1). Geneva: World Health Organization Department of Health Systems.

Culyer, A., & Simpson, H. (1980). Externality models and health: a Rückblick over the last twenty years. *Economic Record, 56*, 220–230.

Culyer, A. J. (1998). Need: is a consensus possible? *Journal of Medical Ethics, 24*, 77–80.

Daniels, N. (1985). *Just health care*. New York: Cambridge University Press.

Daniels, N., & Sabin, J. E. (2002). Accountability for reasonableness. In *Setting limits fairly; Can we learn to share medical resources?* (pp. 43–66). New York: Oxford University Press.

Gannett, L. (1999). What's in a cause? The pragmatic dimensions of genetic explanations. *Biology and Philosophy, 14*, 349–374.

Gutmann, A., & Thompson, D. (2002). Just deliberation about health care. In M. Danis, C. Clancy, & L. R. Churchill (Eds.), *Ethical dimensions of health policy* (pp. 77–96). New York: Oxford University Press.

Krieger, N. (1994). Epidemiology and the web of causation: has anyone seen the spider? Social Science and Medicine, *39*, 887–903.

Mills, C. (1998). *Equity and health: Key issues and WHO's role. Equity initiative paper No. 5* (No. WHO/CHS/HSS/98.3). Geneva: World Health Organization.

Nozick, R. (1974). *Anarchy, state, and utopia*. New York: Basic Books.

Rawls, J. (1971). *A theory of justice*. Cambridge, Massachusetts: Harvard University Press.

Robertson, A. (1998). Critical reflections on the politics of need: Implications for public health. *Social Science and Medicine, 47*, 1419–1430.

Sen, A. (1987). *The standard of living*. Cambridge: Cambridge University Press.

Sen, A. (1992). *Inequality reexamined*. Cambridge, Massachusetts: Harvard University Press.

Sen, A. (2002). Why health equity? *Health Economics, 11*, 659–666.

United Nations Economic and Social Council, & Committee on Economic Social and Cultural Rights (CESCR). (2000). *General comment No. 14: The right to the highest attainable*

standard of health (Available at: http://www.unhchr.ch/tbs/doc.nsf/(symbol)/E.C.12.2000.4.
En?OpenDocument).

Williams, A., & Cookson, R. (2000). Equity in health. In A. J. Culyer & J. P. Newhouse (Eds.),
Handbook of health economics (pp. 1863–1910). New York: Elsevier Science.

World Health Organization. (2005). *Glossary of globalization, trade, and health terms: Equity*.
(http://www.who.int/trade/glossary/en): World Health Organization.

Chapter 17
Context as a Fundamental Dimension of Health Promotion Program Evaluation

Blake Poland, Katherine L. Frohlich, and Margaret Cargo

Context can be broadly defined as "the circumstances or events that form the environment within which something exists or takes place" (Encarta, 1999). That 'something' can be health behavior, another health determinant, an intervention, or an evaluation. Each of these events unfolds, not in a vacuum, but in a complex social context which necessarily shapes how the phenomena are manifest, as well as how they may be taken up, resisted or modified. In this chapter we unpack the nature and significance of social context for health promotion practice and evaluation. Drawing on critical realism, we develop a framework for understanding key dimensions of social context that impact on three key levels: the target phenomena (what health promotion practice is seeking to change or enhance), the intervention (how it is received and plays out, its impact), and efforts to evaluate health promotion interventions (we propose that evaluation practice is also embedded in social context).

That social context matters is widely recognized and nothing particularly new. Context is identified as a fundamental dimension of program evaluation (Suchman, 1967; Weiss, 1972), and person-environment and program- environment interactions can be traced back to the human ecology work of Broffenbrenner (1977, 1979). Applications of these concepts and ecological systems theory, in various guises, are found in the health promotion literature (see Best et al., 2003; Chu and Simpson, 1994; Green and Kreuter, 2005; Green, Richard and Potvin, 1996; Stokols, 1992, 2000). Although context receives attention in many health promotion texts (Bartholomew, Parcel, Kok, & Gottlieb, 2000; Green & Kreuter, 2005), it is not routinely integrated into or adequately accounted for in most program evaluations. The complexities involved in mapping contextual factors in evaluation pose significant evaluation challenges. Some interventionists and evaluators may lack the necessary theoretical breadth and methodological skills to adequately unpack, theoretically and empirically, how context matters. Nor may they feel they have the 'luxury' of time or breadth of mandate to tackle what may be seen as more challenging conceptual and methodological issues associated with doing so. This

B. Poland
Department of Public Health Sciences, University of Toronto, Toronto, Canada

L. Potvin, D. McQueen (eds.), *Health Promotion Evaluation Practices in the Americas*,
DOI: 10.1007/978-0-387-79733-5_17, © Springer Science+Business Media, LLC 2008   299

chapter identifies some of these challenging issues and proposes a critical realist framework for addressing these lacunae.

The overwhelming emphasis within the dominant post-positivist paradigm in health promotion evaluation research has been to treat context as a source of potential confounders that need to be either 'factored in' (as variables that apply across cases) or 'factored out' ('controlled for' statistically or through study design such as randomization). Identification of 'best practices' that can be disseminated across space and time with predictable outcomes following the results of promising pilot research, also treats context as something of a nuisance to be addressed only insofar as it threatens to seriously compromise implementation fidelity or program outcomes. Further, following Malpas (2003), we believe that increasingly dominant managerial regimes that privilege efficiency and tight fiscal and legal accountability in health and social service delivery seek to tighten administrative control through the standardization of practice. Standardization accords only grudging acknowledgement to the difference that context makes. The inherent 'messiness', unpredictability, and uniqueness of context is difficult to reconcile with an administrative rationality intent on procedural standardization. In short, epistemological, political, and administrative factors have conspired to either obscure the relative importance of social context to program design, implementation, and evaluation or, at the very least, leave largely unexamined or unexplained the ways in which context matters.

From studies of small area variations in healthcare practice (Wennberg & Gittelsohn, 1973), to studies of community-based health promotion interventions (Bracht, 1990; Minkler, 1990, 1997), the evidence that context matters is increasingly difficult to ignore. In some fields, such as tobacco control, there is growing awareness that the failure to sufficiently understand the social context of smoking has compromised the field's success record (Flay & Clayton, 2003; Poland et al., 2006). The social distribution of smoking has changed, and thus the social distance between target populations and interventionists, whose assumptions and world view are reflected in programming (Poland et al., 2006). The popularity of a settings approach in health promotion reflects, in part, an understanding of the importance of aligning program design and intervention activities with the realities of the setting for which they're intended (Chu & Simpson, 1994; Dooris et al., 2007; Mullen et al., 1995; Poland, Green, & Rootman, 2000, Poland, Lehoux, Holmes, & Andrews, 2005; Whitelaw et al., 2001). For example, considerable expertise has emerged in school-based health promotion with respect to the essential features of schools, as well as variability in their expression (e.g., inner city versus rural), that impact on program delivery and outcomes. The identification of aspects of context that impact on practice has also been undertaken with respect to community-based programming, workplace health promotion, and interventions tailored for other settings such as hospitals, Aboriginal communities, and prisons, among others.

Context is fundamental to understanding the adequacy of program conceptualization and design: do interventions adequately address the social context within which target phenomena, such as health behaviors, are created, sustained and socially distributed in time and space? Context is also fundamental to program implementation and outcomes: are interventions optimized to take advantage of the unique confluence of opportunities available in each local context and which intervention components produce which results under what conditions? Finally, context shapes the production and utilization of evaluation findings: the influence of key assumptions and stakeholders on the design and implementation of the evaluation, as well as the impact of timing and other factors on research uptake. The organization of this chapter reflects the ways in which social context is implicated at three overlapping levels: (a) the nature of the phenomena that are the object of health promotion intervention (the social context of target phenomena); (b) interventions themselves (the social context of health promotion practice); and (c) knowledge development and utilization (the social context of evaluation research).

At this juncture it is worth clarifying what we mean by evaluation. We adopt the definition proposed by Rossi and Freeman (1985, p. 19): "the systematic application of social research procedures in assessing the conceptualization and design, implementation, and utility of social intervention programs". We prefer this over less comprehensive definitions because it explicitly makes room for a critique of the adequacy of program conceptualization and design, whereas many evaluation definitions do not and are restricted to determining the extent to which intended outcomes are achieved.

The premise of this chapter is that although context is of inescapable importance in health promotion program evaluation, better conceptual, theoretical, and methodological tools are needed to reposition it at the centre of evaluation efforts. Following a review of each of the three layers of context identified above, we draw on diverse disciplinary perspectives to assemble some of the conceptual, theoretical, and methodological tools necessary for a deeper and more satisfying treatment of context in health promotion program evaluation. In particular, we draw on critical social theory and critical realist perspectives to fashion an understanding of how social relations (at the heart of any social intervention) function in different social contexts, for these are critical to understanding how context matters.

Three Layers of Context

The Social Context of Target Phenomena

The determinants of the status quo are an obvious starting point for thinking about what interventions are needed and how should be structured to shift those determinants most critical for health enhancement. Understanding what created and sustained the phenomena that interventionists wish to change, be it specific lifestyle behaviors, organizational practices, or policies, is fundamental.

Health promotion seeks to influence human behaviors as a key target of intervention (either as a means or as an end in itself). The focus may be risk behaviors linked to particular disease outcomes (e.g., diet, exercise, smoking), organizational behaviors (organizational policies and practices), or the decisions of policy makers.

For Agnew, "in order to explain human behavior one must deal with the 'micro-episodes' of everyday life and their embeddedness in concrete milieux or contexts" (1993, p. 264). Interventions need to address not only the cognitive or psychosocial elements of behavior change, be that lifestyle behavior, organizational behavior, or the behavior of policy-makers, but also the social environments in which these behaviors are shaped or maintained. For example, in school-based health promotion, there is an attempt to integrate curriculum components with school level changes (e.g., removal of soft drink vending machines; changes in cafeteria menu), extra-curricular activities, parental involvement, community programming, peer-to-peer, and other initiatives in comprehensive, multi-component (and multi-modal) approaches. These have been shown to be more effective at bringing about and sustaining healthier behaviors than more narrowly cast interventions (Soubhi & Potvin, 2000).

When it comes to health behavior modification (which remains a central focus in health promotion practice), it is still the case that for the most part social context is understood primarily in terms of 'social influences' (peers, parents, media personalities), 'social norms' (as a focus for 'denormalization' efforts in tobacco control, for example), or as 'social environment' (in, for example, ecological and systems theory models that specify the inclusion of variables from a variety of interacting contextual levels). Health promotion and health education efforts aimed at smoking is an instructive example of how social context matters and how it has been addressed. Attention has traditionally focused on genetics, parental influence, peer influences, pricing and availability of cigarettes (including retailer compliance regarding sales to minors), restrictions on smoking in public places, visibility and impact of public education campaigns, local pro-smoking or non-smoking community norms and social sanctions (see Chaloupka, 2003; Flay & Clayton, 2003). However, more recently researchers have drawn on anthropology and sociology, and on qualitative, feminist and cultural studies traditions, that focus attention on the role smoking plays in adolescent cultures (Amos, Gray, Currie, & Elton, 1997; Ioannou, 2003; McCracken, 1992; Plumridge, Fitzgerald, & Abel, 2002), the role of gender (Elkind, 1985; Greaves, 1996; Graham, 1987; 1993), and other dimensions of social context.

The concept of "collective lifestyle practice" (Frohlich, Corin, & Potvin, 2001) captures many of these dimensions of social context. Drawing on Giddens and Bourdieu, the heuristic, "collective lifestyles", is a framework for understanding behaviors like smoking, as social practices, that is, routinized and socialized behaviors common to groups (Frohlich et al., 2001; see also Cockerham, Rutten, & Abel, 1997). Collective lifestyles comprise interacting patterns of behaviors, orientations and resources adapted by groups of individuals in response to their social, cultural and economic environment (Abel, Cockerham, & Niemann, 2000, p. 63). These practices are generated at the intersection of social structure (norms, resources, policy and the institutional practices that organize society), and agency (individual action, volition and sense of identity). This is expressed recursively, with social structure influencing agency and agency, in turn, influencing the structure. Conceptualising health behaviors in terms of collective lifestyles has the potential to offer more to an understanding of the social context of target phenomena than serving as a synonym for patterns of individual risk behaviors. A theory-driven collective lifestyles approach helps not only to prevent a reductionist and individual centered perspective, but also takes into account both behaviors and social circumstances (Abel et al., 2000).

The collective lifestyles was extended by Frohlich, Poland and colleagues (Poland et al. 2006), who propose a model for understanding the social context of smoking and other 'behavioral risk factors'. Highlighting the centrality of power relations in shaping the uneven socio-spatial distribution of smoking, their model identifies the following dimensions of the social as key to our understanding of smoking: the sociology of the body as it relates to smoking, collective patterns of consumption, the construction and maintenance of social identity, the ways in which desire and pleasure are implicated in these latter two dimensions in particular, and smoking as a social activity rooted in place.

Sometimes the 'social context' is the primary target of intervention. In a settings approach to health promotion, there has been growing recognition of the need to move beyond simply seeing setting as a way of targeting 'captive' audiences, but instead to act on the setting itself (Poland, Green, & Rootman, 2000). For example, workplace health promotion can include not just educational and stress reduction seminars for employees, but also changes to the workplace to reduce injuries and exposures to noxious substances, improvements in cafeteria menu, installation of a breastfeeding room, family-friendly workplace policies, and efforts to address labour-management relations, workload issues and decision latitude (democratization of the workplace) (Polanyi, et al., 2000).

The Social Context of Health Promotion Interventions

As previously noted, context impacts both program delivery and program outcomes (Potvin, Haddad, & Frohlich, 2001). A key issue is the fit and responsiveness of interventions to situational context. Intervention success reflects the ability to embed programs in context over time (community ownership, routinization). Responsiveness to environment (adaptiveness) is key. Several attempts have been made to systematize evidence regarding the effectiveness of interventions in different settings (e.g. school-based health promotion, community development). But few attempts have been made to systematically 'unpack' those aspects of settings that most impact health promotion practice, and how interventions are experienced by program participants, in a way that could directly impact policy, practice, and research. Context is of great interest when a program 'fails', but its contribution to program success is rarely examined.

Poland, Krupa & McCall (2008) propose a framework that can be utilized by practitioners to systematically analyze features of settings that impact intervention design and delivery, in the form of a nested series of questions to guide analysis. The analytic framework addresses how settings are commonly understood (unpacking assumptions, variability within and between types of settings, etc), localized determinants of health (including local manifestations of broader economic, socio-political and cultural trends), making explicit stakeholder interests, and understanding power relations. With respect to context, specifically, we address the history of health promotion efforts in the category of setting (e.g. schools vs. workplaces), then the specific setting itself. What efforts have been aimed at changing behaviors within the setting or changing the setting itself? How have approaches changed over time, and how might we explain these changes? We ask what the health promoter brings to this particular setting: the skills, capacities, resources, and relevant sensitivities. This includes similarities or differences with key stakeholder groups (e.g., race, class, gender, physical ability, sexual orientation) that may act as points of friction or affinity. An analysis of the context for change efforts must also grapple with what supports must be in place (or barriers removed) outside the setting in the broader socio-political, community, and/or economic context. This may necessitate advocacy, coalition building, strategic partnerships or deepening and widening community participation.

The Social Context of Health Promotion Evaluation

Having briefly reviewed the first layer of social context in which determinants of health are created and sustained, and the second layer of social context within which interventions are inserted and unfold, a third layer of context must be addressed: that in which the evaluation itself is conducted.

Evaluations do not take place in a vacuum: they are deeply shaped by context. Context shapes the many assumptions that animate the evaluation, including what is considered knowable and worth knowing, how it can be known, and what is seen as doable within given time and resource constraints. It also shapes the agendas of key stakeholders, including funders, intervention staff, and those targeted or impacted by the intervention. There is always potential for stakeholders to hold different perspectives on what is important and what is doable. And there are ways in which stakeholders can intentionally or unintentionally selectively share or withhold information, seek to discredit, derail, downplay or ignore the evaluation, or steer it in directions more favourable to their perceived interests (e.g. Brousselle, 2004). Evaluations often require the consent, cooperation, and permission of gatekeepers who control access to certain settings and populations. This influences the evaluation through subtle pressure to frame the evaluator's stance in 'gatekeeper-friendly' terms or through effects on respondents to appear aligned with the gatekeeper (e.g. employee candour when workplace health promotion evaluation requires implicit endorsement of the workplace manager).

Evaluation research is inherently political (Shadish, Cook, & Leviton, 1991) because programs are embedded within dynamic organisational, interorganisational and community systems which may relegate evaluation research as secondary to program delivery interests (Weiss, 1972). In the evaluation of health promotion programs, researchers develop relationships with a variety of health professionals, practitioners, bureaucrats, politicians, and members of special interest groups (e.g., teachers, nonprofit organisations, recreation workers, health and social policy makers, Aboriginal representatives, community members, parents). The nature of relationships developed between evaluation researchers and program professionals or advocates can range the spectrum from friendly to hostile.

Evaluation research is differentiated from other forms of research because it takes place in an action setting, marked by competing agendas and power relations that can become extremely asymmetrical depending on the issue at hand. Most service organisations see the first order of priority as implementing the program; evaluating the program often is considered secondary to program delivery (Weiss, 1972). Weiss argues that researchers may try to change the order of priority and for good reason. The mandate of the evaluation researcher is to determine whether the program works, under what conditions and for whom (see earlier discussion of Rossi's definition of evaluation). Differences in perspective on the primacy of program delivery versus program evaluation from different stakeholders can lead to tensions. The evaluator must be sensitive to the political landscape within which their program is embedded when making evaluation decisions, otherwise their evaluation efforts can be undermined. Where multiple stakeholders and agendas are implicated in complex interventions, evaluability assessment may be warranted (Smith, 1989; see also Poland, 1996, for an application in health promotion evaluation).

The uptake of research findings needs to be considered in any discussion of the social context of program evaluation. Here too, contextual factors weigh heavily on the possibilities for successful knowledge translation and uptake. The *Ottawa Model of Health Care Research Use* is one example of a framework that explicitly addresses the nature of the practice environment and the need for an adequate diagnosis prior to knowledge translation intervention (Logan & Graham, 1998; Santesso & Tugwell, 2006).

While these and other issues have been raised in the evaluation literature, the dimension of context that we address here is the politics of evaluation associated with understanding and navigating competing stakeholder interests. These can be seen as 'extrinsic' to the evaluation (something to be avoided, skillfully managed, or factored in) or as 'intrinsic' to more participatory forms of evaluation research. We have argued that all three layers of context – the context of the target phenomena, the context of intervention, and the context of evaluation – can be essential to solid program planning and evaluation. What is missing is a framework for identifying which elements of context are most critical in each layer. This is discussed in the next section.

A Framework for Understanding Key Dimensions of Social Context

Interventions in health promotion are essentially complex, *social* interventions: they are intentional change efforts inserted into pre-existing social relations. To quote Pawson and Tilley (1997), "it is not programs that make things change, it is people, embedded in their context who, when exposed to programs, do something to activate given mechanisms, and change" (cited in Stame, 2004, p. 62) Further, following Pawson, Greenhalgh, Harvey, and Walshe (2004), we can assert that in many cases in health promotion the interventions themselves are people. It is therefore necessary to take into account how programs, as complex social interventions, manage to embed themselves in these social contexts by aligning with existing incentive structures and mobilizing key opinion leaders. Or, alternatively, how they fail to take hold by generating unanticipated resistance, and attempts to discredit, resist, reframe or ignore change efforts. One promising, and as yet underutilized approach to unpacking how interventions work or fail in particular contexts (viz., which elements of context matter, and why), is critical realist evaluation.

A Critical Realist Approach

Critical realism is a logic of inquiry, drawing on the foundational work of Roy Bhaskar (1979) whose central premise is that constant conjunction (empirical co-occurrence) is an insufficient basis for inferring causality, and that what is required is the identification of generative mechanisms whose causal properties may or may not be activated, depending on the circumstances (Connelly, 2001; Julnes, Mark, & Henry, 1998; Stame, 2004; Williams, 2003). It is a theory-driven approach whose point of departure is in the distinctions made between the *empirical* (what is observed), the *actual* (events and experiences that may or may not be observed/ observable), and the *real* (the domain of underlying causal mechanisms) (Williams, 2003). Further, mechanisms can coincide under real world conditions to produce *emergent properties* that are contingent in time and space (Sayer, 2000).

From a critical realist perspective, context is not an undifferentiated social ether in which programs and phenomena float, but rather it is a series of generative mechanisms in constant interaction with complex and contingent combinations of events and actors. The notion of contingency stands in contrast to positivist notions of universal logical necessity (natural laws, generalisable truths) by calling attention to the uncertain nature of phenomena (viz., that propositions may hold true under some circumstances but not others). The 'ideal-typical' positivist view is that the causal relationship can be said to exist when A is always or very nearly always followed by B. Such stance is consistent with relatively 'closed' systems, where external factors can be 'controlled for'. Yet we know factors which have 'causal powers' often manifest only under particular conditions – hence the importance of the total 'situation' or context.

Since underlying generative mechanisms may only be discernable on account of the effects they generate and since such effects are contingent in space-time, critical realist program evaluations must be grounded in theories that specify what generative mechanisms are triggered, or suppressed, by which intervention elements, under which conditions. Generative mechanisms refer to program mediators that interventions seek to modify. Weiss (1995, 1997) makes a strong case for developing sound program theory during the conceptualization and design phase of the evaluation so that program mediators can be prospectively assessed and understood through multiple methods. Program theory can be made explicit through specifying the inter-related sequence of events that are expected to occur and how they relate to each other in space and time. Thus program theory is based on a series of micro-steps that aims to make transparent the underlying logic and assumptions of a given intervention.

Critical realism can be distinguished from two other meta-paradigms of social research that are often found in program evaluation: post-positivism which is associated with most controlled designs and quantitative evaluation methods, and hermeneutics which is most closely associated with qualitative methods and designs. Table 17.1 illustrates, in broad terms, how each of these differ in terms of key assumptions about what is knowable (ontology) and how it can come to be known (epistemology), the role of theory, and preferred choice of methods.

Critical realism is a logic of inquiry that privileges neither 'objective' facts nor subjective lived experience or narrative accounts, but rather seeks to situate both in relation to a theoretical understanding of the generative mechanisms that link them together, as a basis for interpreting the empirical or observable world. It follows that the questions posed in critical realist evaluation are of a different order from those derived from other evaluation approaches. As in other areas of social research, how the question is framed has fundamentally important consequences for what is found and consequent funding and intervention decision-making. In much conventional evaluation research, the central animating question that drives the study is either "which interventions work best?" (the best practice option), or "what are the vital ingredients of success?" (generalizable recipe for success). The question of context is largely ignored, except to specify what needs to be factored

Table 17.1 Three contrasting paradigms within which evaluations can be situated

Dimension	Post-positivist	Hermeneutic	Critical realist
Ontology (the nature of reality)	Verifiable evidence	What people perceive to exist	Appearances differ from underlying mechanisms (but mechanisms leave observable traces)
Epistemology (what is knowable)	Knowledge objectively acquired through rigorous application of method	Knowledge socially constructed, subjective	Knowledge actively constructed from facts, events & experience
Theory	Formal, predictive	Understanding people in their environments	Explain underlying structures
Methodology	Verification	Interpretation of meaning	Explanation based on theory + observation
Methods	Survey research Modelling, Manipulation	Depth interviews Observation	Mixed methods Case studies

in or factored out of the model. From a critical realist perspective, the central evaluative question is not so much *whether* certain programs, or parts of, work, what Stame (2004) refers to as 'black box' evaluation, but "to unpack the mechanism[s] of *how* complex programs work, or *why* they fail, in particular contexts and settings" (Pawson et al., 2004). It is precisely these how and why questions which are critical to decision-making regarding which programmatic components are worth replicating in which other contexts and settings.

A key author in critical realist evaluation is Ray Pawson. Pawson and colleagues have articulated a theory of interventions that they argue is essential to critical realist evaluation (Pawson & Tilley, 1997; Pawson, 2006). It is the underlying intervention theory which drives the purposive, theoretical sampling of a wide variety of types and forms of evidence to shed light on the different generative mechanisms thought to be at play, and the conditions under which their causal properties are activated (or not), as well as how these combine to form emergent properties which in turn impact upon and become absorbed into the social context. As a point of departure, Pawson et al. (2004) identify a number of basic assumptions concerning the nature of interventions that inform a critical realist approach to program evaluation. First, they maintain that *interventions are theories*, which is to say that they are constellations of hypotheses about what will happen, which are resourced (funded, equipped, supplied with personnel) and inserted into existing social systems. Second, *interventions are active*: they work through stakeholder reasoning and intentionality, and understanding these is key to understanding how outcomes are achieved or thwarted. Third, *intevention chains are long and thickly populated*. A series of stakeholders and social processes are implicated over time (and space), and the chain of events can misfire or break down at any time, with unintended (and sometimes unpredictable) results. When multiple stakeholder groups with different power bases vie for influence, *interventions can sometimes follow a very non-linear path or even be thrown into reverse*. This is the fourth tenet. The relative influence of these actors to affect and direct implementation must therefore be considered as part of any evaluation exercise. Fifth, *interventions are embedded in multiple social systems*. Individuals, interpersonal relations, organizations, and broader infrastructural and policy elements are implicated, and the influence of factors at all these levels need to be considered. Sixth, Pawson et al. (2004) characterize interventions as *"leaky and prone to be borrowed"*. As actors struggle to achieve their interests and optimize interventions in the face of sometimes unique local obstacles and setbacks, processes of lateral communication and active agency cause programs to be copied (in part or *in toto*), refined, reinvented, adapted from one context to the next. These processes of informal adaptive learning are also underscored in the literature on 'communities of practice' (e.g., Brown and Duguid, 1991; Wenger, 1998; Wenger, McDermott, & Snyder, 2002). These dynamic aspects can be difficult, but no less important, to capture. Last, but not least, *interventions are open systems that feed back on themselves*: in changing the conditions in which they operate, they also act on themselves in ways that call for new adaptations, which in turn alter the conditions of practice, in infinitum. Both intended and unintended consequences must be considered.

One of the advantages of a critical realist approach is that it requires us to be explicit about our assumptions. Assumptions are often embedded and implicit (Eakin et al., 1996). This also fits well with, but also extends in several important ways, the use of logic models in health promotion program evaluation (Julian, 1997).

Drawing on the work of Sayer, Pawson, and others, we can thus (re)define context as: the local mix of conditions and events, social agents, objects and interactions which characterize open systems, and whose unique confluence in time and space selectively activates, triggers, blocks or modifies causal powers and mechanisms in a chain of reactions that may result in very different outcomes depending on the dynamic interplay of conditions and mechanisms over time and space.

Pawson and colleagues concern themselves primarily with the social context of intervention implementation, and secondarily with some of the politics of evaluation itself. What we add here is a third dimension critical to the adequacy of program design: the social context of the phenomena that are the target of change efforts. Here, it is incumbent upon us to more fully address what we see as some of the key enduring features of social context that evaluators need to pay closer attention to.

Key, Enduring Features of Social Context

In the same way that Pawson and colleagues offer a general conceptual schema regarding the key characteristics of interventions that they believe have important consequences for program evaluation, so too it's incumbent upon us to identify a few of the most salient features of the social to frame our general understanding of the generative mechanisms at work in most social contexts. In doing so, we wish to underscore that these take different forms in different contexts.

The Dialectic of Agency and Structure

Our first basic assumption is that phenomena are neither the result of unencumbered agency nor purely of structural constraints and opportunities, but rather result of the relationship between the two. Proponents of structural explanations emphasize the power of structural conditions in shaping individual behavior (Cockerham, 2005). Advocates of agency, on the other hand, accentuate the capacity of individual actors to choose and influence their behavior regardless of structural influences. Rather than view this as a dichotomy, we posit that health outcomes, behaviors, and social relations are the result of both of these spheres in a dialectical relationship with each other; each informing, producing and reproducing the other (Giddens, 1984). This has been termed recursivity by Giddens (ibid).

Our earlier discussion of 'collective lifestyle practices' (Cockerham et al., 1997; Frohlich et al., 2001) exemplifies how an understanding of the dialectical nature of agency and structure translates into an understanding of the social context of human behavior. As previously noted, practices are generated at the intersection of social structure (norms, resources, policy and the institutional practices that organize society), and agency (individual action, volition and sense of identity). This is expressed recursively, with the social structure influencing agency and agency, in turn, influencing the structure.

We have noted that evaluation research is subject to the same contextual influences outlined in our earlier section on critical realist theory of interventions: evaluations are theories, active, long chains, non-linear, embedded in multiple social systems, leaky, open systems with feedback loops. The blurred boundaries between program and context identified by Potvin (2007) are relevant here, insofar as the problematic they address (and to which, they argue, only critical realism has an adequate response) reflects the inherently recursive and dialectical relationship between intervention and conditions, program and context.

Power Relations

With few exceptions (e.g., Kuyek & Labonte, 1995; Eakin et al., 1996), power relations are frequently acknowledged but rarely adequately unpacked in health promotion. This is the more surprising given the emphasis that health promotion places on empowerment (Rissel, 1994), and the relative sophistication with which issues of power have been addressed in the sociological literature (Grabb, 2002; Jones, 2003). Indeed, according to Jones (2003, p. 130), "a key to understanding experiences of health and illness in late modern society is the operation of power at different interacting levels". Poland, Coburn, Robertson, & Eakin with members of the Critical Social Science in Health Group (1998) argue that such analyses are largely missing in contemporary debates in social inequalities in health which focus more on identifying the bio-psychosocial pathways through which social hierarchies impact on health than they do on explaining how social inequalities are produced and maintained in the first place.

Drawing on the work of Michael Mann, Jones (2003) argues that power is exercised by individuals and groups in a manner that is simultaneously *diffuse* (unconscious, decentred) and *authoritarian* (commanding obedience), *intensive* (actors are heavily invested in the exercise of power) and *extensive* (far-reaching in space and time). He argues that issues of exploitation and adaptation are keys to understanding how power is exercised.

In his review of sociological theories of inequality, from Marx and Weber to Giddens, Edward Grabb (2002) goes further, proposing a framework that acknowledges how power and exploitation operate via three key mechanisms, each of which are further stratified in their effects by race, class, gender and other social cleavages: control of material resources in the form of means of production, natural resources, capital; control over human resources and labour power; and control over ideas (ideology, hegemony, cultural dominance, control of media, ability to impact representation and social meaning).

An analysis of power and how power relations come into play in the field invites the practitioner to adopt a reflexive stance regarding her own role in reproducing or resisting existing asymmetrical power relations. Kuyek and Labonte (1995),

Poland (1992) and Boutilier, Cleverly, and Labonte (2000), address how health promotion practitioners can transform their inherent 'power-over' marginalized groups with whom they may be working into 'power-with'.

Emplacement

"Every action is situated in space and time, and for its immediate outcome [is] dependent on what is present or absent as help or hindrance where the events take place" (Hagerstrand, 1984). In other words, social relations are contingent in time and space. For contextualists, space or place becomes both 'condition' and 'consequence' of human activity (Gregory, 1994, p. 92). Deriving from the work of Hagerstrand (1984), and Giddens (1984), contextual theory is an approach which helps us identify "relations of coexistence, connection or 'togetherness', rather than the relations of 'similarity' that characterize compositional theory" (Gregory, 1994, p. 90) that "remove different classes of being from their habitats and place them in a classification system" (Hagerstrand, 1984 in Gregory, 1994). One of the protagonists of contextual theory, Simonsen (1991) has sought to codify the contextuality of social life in terms of the trajectories of social actors across time and space, emphasizing how different kinds and units of time and space thread together to constitute the social. He writes about the importance of situated life stories or biographies of human agents bounded in time and space, as a methodology for accessing these aspects of reality.

If contextual theory helps us understand how place matters for health promotion, then the concept of *culture of place* helps us understand how these factors come together in particular places to imbue them with a distinctive 'feel'. Jary and Jary (1995) note that culture of place encompasses the symbols, artifacts, manners, customs, language, norms and systems of belief that make up 'culture' as the 'way of life' of any society, setting or social grouping. A distinctive culture of place emerges from the pragmatic and routinised interactions between engaged participants and social processes (Poland et al., 2005). These are shaped by the ways in which material objects (artifacts), social relations (socio-facts) and ideas (mentifacts) come together in ways that are contingent in time and space (Gesler & Kearns, 2002). This understanding of 'culture of place' as infused with technologically-mediated power relations (Poland et al., 2005), allows us to represent in Fig. 17.1 the relationship of culture of place, technology, and power to health promotion practice.

There are, understandably, many other generative mechanisms identified by various authors as being central to understanding the production, consumption and social geography of health: neoliberalism (Coburn, 2000), capitalism (Navarro, 2000, 2004; Navarro & Muntaner, 2004), racism (Porter, 1993), class (Bourdieu, 1990), to mention only a few. A detailed examination of each of these is beyond the scope of this chapter, but the reader is referred to Grabb (2002) for a useful overview in the context of explaining social inequality.

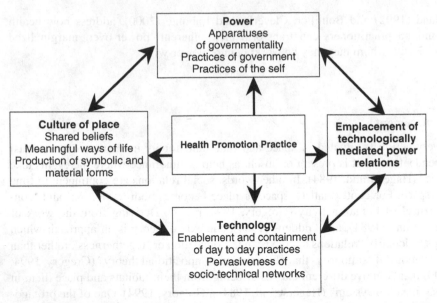

Fig. 17.1 Technologically mediated power relations, culture of place, and the constitution of health promotion practice in space-time
Source: Adapted from Poland et al., 2005

Conclusion

In this chapter, we have tackled the thorny issue of context as it applies to the evaluation of health promotion initiatives. We have argued that understanding context is fundamental to understanding how interventions thrust into such contexts (and seeking to be absorbed and routinised into these practice environments) are received, modified, resisted, and reinvented from place to place. Furthermore, we extend conventional discussions of context considerably by showing that context needs to be considered at three nested and overlapping levels: (a) the context of the target phenomena (what interventionists are seeking to change) as a basis for assessing the adequacy of program conceptualization and design (does it address the salient determinants and levers of change?), (b) the contexts in which interventions are mobilized and (c) the contexts in which program evaluations are conducted, and their results disseminated and taken up by others (or not). We have described critical realism and core tenets of critical realist evaluation, as proposed by Pawson and others. Our thesis is that critical realism allows a more sophisticated assessment of the relationship between context and program, and it offers a third alternative to the sometimes polarized debate about the relative merits of quantitative or experimental versus qualitative approaches.

Furthermore, we have sought to identify several enduring features of social relations as possible 'generative mechanisms' that can be said to act in each context, albeit somewhat differently from site to site. Those mechanisms are the dialectical relationship between agency and structure, power relations, and processes of emplacement. We show, drawing on some of our earlier work, how power relations can be shown to be technologically mediated and constituted in, by and through, and constitutive of, particular places, as embodied in 'cultures of place'.

The complex and expansive nature of the social, together with the diversity of disciplinary and epistemological perspectives that can be brought to bear on it, mean that any chapter seeking to unpack social context will necessarily leave out as much as it includes. We have not, for example, addressed participatory approaches (Green et al., 1995; Israel et al., 2003; Macaulay et al., 1998, 1999) to evaluation, nor initiatives for the development of reflexive practice (McCormack, Manley, Kitson, Titchen, & Harvey, 1999; Schon, 1991), although we consider both highly relevant to this discussion. Nevertheless, we believe that the way we have brought together critical realism with an understanding of the overlapping levels of context implicated in health promotion practice has the potential to contribute to the field.

Acknowledgment We would like to acknowledge Louise Potvin and John Garcia for helpful comments on an earlier draft, as well as participants of the 2006 Annual Symposium in *Healthcare Technology and Place* (Toronto, May, 2006) for their provocative and challenging questions.

References

Abel, T., Cockerham, W. C., & Niemann, S. (2000). A critical approach to lifestyle and health. In J. Watson & S. Platt, (Eds.), *Researching Health Promotion* (pp. 54–77). London: Routledge.

Agnew, J. (1993). Representing space: Space, scale and culture in social science. In J. Duncan & D. Ley (Eds.), *Place/culture/representation*. London: Routledge.

Amos, A., Gray, D., Currie, C., & Elton, R. (1997). Healthy or druggy? Self-image, ideal image and smoking behavior among young people. *Social Science and Medicine 45*, 847–858.

Bartholomew, L. K., Parcel, G. S., Kok, G., & Gottlieb, N. H. (2000). *Intervention mapping: Designing theory – and evidence – based programs*. New York: McGraw-Hill Higher Education.

Best, A., Moor, G., Holmes, B., Clark, P. I., Bruce, T., Leischow, S., et al. (2003). Health promotion dissemination and systems thinking: Toward an integrative model. *American Journal of Health Behaviour, 27*, s206–s216.

Bhaskar, R. (1979). *The possibility of naturalism*. Atlantic Heights, NJ: Humanities Press.

Bourdieu, P. (1990). *The logic of practice*. Stanford, CA: Stanford University Press.

Boutilier, M., Cleverly, S., & Labonte, R. (2000). Community as a setting for health promotion. In B. Poland, L. W. Green, & I. Rootman (Eds.), *Settings for health promotion: Linking theory and practice*. Thousand Oaks, CA: Sage Publications.

Bracht, N. (1990) *Health promotion at the community level*. Thousand Oaks, CA: Sage Publications.

Broffenbrenner, U. (1977). Ecological systems theory. In R. Vasta (Ed.), *Annals of child development* (Vol .6). Greenwich, CT: JAI Press.

Broffenbrenner, U. (1979) *The ecology of human development*. Cambridge, MA: Harvard University Press.

Brousselle, A. (2004). What counts is not falling… but landing. Strategic analysis: An adapted model for implementation evaluation. *Evaluation, 10*, 155–173.

Brown, J. S., & Duguid, P. (1991). Organisational learning and communities of practice: Toward a unified view of working, learning, and innovation. *Organization Science, 2*, 40–57.

Chaloupka, F. J. (2003). Contextual factors and youth tobacco use: policy linkages. *Addiction*, 98, 147–150.

Chu, C., & Simpson, R. (1994) *Ecological public health: From vision to practice*. Nathan: Institute of Applied Environmental Research, Griffith University, Queensland, Australia and Centre for Health Promotion, University of Toronto, Canada.

Coburn, D. (2000). Income inequality, social cohesion and the health status of populations: the role of neo-liberalism. *Social Science and Medicine, 51*, 135–146.

Cockerham, W. (2005). Health lifestyle theory and the convergence of agency and structure. *Journal of Health and Social Behavior, 46*, 51–67.

Cockerham, W. C., Rutten, A., & Abel, T. (1997). Conceptualising contemporary health lifestyles: moving beyond Weber. *The Sociological Quarterly, 38*, 321–342.

Connelly, J. (2001). Critical realism and health promotion: effective practice needs an effective theory. *Health Education Research, 16*, 115–120.

Dooris, M., Poland, B., Kolbe, L., De Leeuw, E., McCall, D., & Wharf-Higgins, J. (2007). Healthy settings: Building evidence for the effectiveness of whole system health promotion. In D. V. McQueen & C. M. Jones (Eds.), *Global prespectives on health promotion effectiveness* (pp. 327–352). New York: Springer.

Eakin, J., Robertson, A., Poland, B., Coburn, D., & Edwards, R. (1996). Toward a critical social science perspective on health promotion research. *Health Promotion International, 11*, 157–165.

Elkind A. (1985). The social definition of women's smoking behavior. *Social Science and Medicine, 20*, 1269–1278.

Encarta. (1999). *Encarta world English dictionary*. Microsoft: Bloomsbury Publishing.

Flay, B., & Clayton, R. R. (2003). Contexts and adolescent tobacco use trajectories. *Addiction, 98*, S1.

Frohlich, K. L., Corin, E., & Potvin, L. (2001). A theoretical proposal for the relationship between context and disease. *Sociology of Health & Illness, 23*, 776–797.

Gesler, W., & Kearns, R. (2002) *Culture/place/health*. London, UK: Routledge.

Giddens, A. (1984). *The constitution of society: Outline of the theory of structuration*. Berkeley, CA: University of California Press.

Grabb, E. G. (2002). *Theories of social inequality: Classical and contemporary perspectives* (4th ed). Toronto, ON: Thomson/Nelson.

Graham, H. (1987). Womens' smoking and family health. *Social Science and Medicine, 25*, 47–56.

Graham, H. (1993). *When life's a drag: Women, smoking and disadvantage*. London, UK: HMSO.

Greaves, L. (1996) *Smoke screen: Womens' smoking and social control*. London, UK: Scarlet University Press.

Green, L. W., George, M. A., Daniel, M., Frankish, C. J., Herbert, C. J., Bowie, W. R., et al. (1995). *Participatory research in health promotion*. Ottawa, ON: Royal Society of Canada.

Green, L. W., & Kreuter, M. W. (2005). *Health promotion planning: An educational and ecological approach* (4th Ed). New York, NY: McGraw-Hill.

Green, L. W., Richard, L., & Potvin, L. (1996) Ecological foundations of health promotion. *American Journal of Health Promotion, 10*, 270–281.

Gregory, D. (1994). Geogrophical imagination. Cambridge Mass: Blackwell.

Hagerstrand, T. (1984). Presences and absences: A look at conceptual choices and bodily necessities. *Regional Studies, 18*, 373–380.

Ioannou, S. (2003). Young people's accounts of smoking, exercising, eating and drinking alcohol: being cool or being unhealthy? *Critical Public Health, 13*, 357–371.

Israel, B. A., Schulz, A.J., Parker, E.A., Becker, A.B., Allen, A.J., III, & Guzman, R. (2003). Critical issues in developing and following community based participatory research principles. In M. Minkler & N. Wallerstein (Eds.), *Community-based participatory research for health* (pp. 53–76). San Francisco, CA: Jossey-Bass.

Jary, D., & Jary, J. (1995) *Collins dictionary of sociology* (2nd ed.). Glasgow, UK: Harper Collins.

Jones, I. R. (2003) Power, present and past: for a historical sociology of health and illness. *Social Theory & Health, 1*, 130–148.

Julian, D. A. (1997). The utilization of the logic model as a system level planning and evaluation device. *Evaluation and Programme Planning, 20,* 251–257.

Julnes, G., Mark, M. M., & Henry, G. T. (1998) Promoting realism in evaluation: Realistic evaluation and the broader context. *Evaluation, 4,* 483–504.

Kuyek, J., & Labonte, R. (1995). *Power: Transforming its practices.* Saskatoon, SA: Prarie Region Health Promotion Research Centre.

Logan, J., & Graham, J. (1998). "Toward a comprehensive interdisciplinary model of health care research use". *Science Communication, 20,* 227–246.

Macaulay, A., Delormier, T., Cross, E. J., Potvin, L., Paradis, G., Kirby, R., et al. (1998). Participatory research with the Native Community of Kahnawake creates innovative Code of Research Ethics. *Canadian Journal of Public Health, 89,* 105–108.

Macaulay, A., Gibson, N., Freeman, W., Commanda, L., McCabe, M., Robbins, C., et al. (1999). Participatory research maximises community and lay involvement. *British Medical Journal, 319,* 774–778.

Malpas, J. (2003). Bio-medical Topoi – the dominance of space, the recalcitrance of place, and the making of persons. *Social Science & Medicine, 56,* 2343–2351.

McCormack, B., Manley, K., Kitson, A., Titchen, A., & Harvey, G. (1999). Toward practice development: a vision in reality or a reality without vision? *Journal of Nursing Management, 7,* 255–264.

McCracken, G. (1992). *'Got a smoke?': A cultural account of tobacco in the lives of contemporary teens. Research report for the Ontario ministry of health tobacco strategy.* Toronto, ON: Ontario Ministry of Health.

Minkler, M. (1990). Improving health through community organisation. In K. Glanz, F. M. Lewis, & B. Rimer (Eds.), *Health behavior and health education: Theory, research, and practice.* Oxford, UK: Jossey-Bass.

Minkler, M. (Ed.). (1997). *Community organising and community building for health.* New Brunswick, NJ: Routledge.

Mullen, P. D., Evans, D., Forster, J., Gottlieb, N. H., Kreuter, M., Moon, R., et al. (1995). Settings as an important dimension in health education/promotion policy, programs, and research. *Health Education Quarterly, 22,* 329–345.

Navarro, V. (2000). *The political economy of social inequalities: Consequences for health and quality of life.* Baywood.

Navarro, V. (2004). *The political and social contexts of health.* Baywood.

Navarro, V., & Muntaner, C. (Eds.). (2004). *Political and economic determinants of population health and well-being: Controversies and developments.* Baywood.

Pawson, R. (2006) *Evidence-based policy: A realist perspective.* London, UK: Sage Publications.

Pawson, R., & Tilley, N. (1997). *Realistic evaluation.* London, UK: Sage Publications.

Pawson, R., Greenhalgh, T., Harvey, G., & Walshe, K. (2004) *Realist synthesis: An introduction. RMP Methods Paper 2/2004.* University of Manchester, UK: ESRC Research Methods Programme.

Plumridge, E. W., Fitzgerald, L. J., & Abel, G. M. (2002). Performing coolness: smoking refusal and adolescent identities. *Health Education Research, 17,* 167–179.

Poland, B. (1992). Learning to 'walk our talk': the implications of sociological theory for research methodologies in health promotion. *Canadian Journal of Public Health, 83,* S31–S46.

Poland, B., Coburn, D., Robertson, A., & Eakin, J. with members of the Critical Social Science in Health Group. (1998). Wealth, equity and health care: a critique of a 'population health' perspective on the determinants of health. *Social Science and Medicine, 46,* 785–798.

Poland, B. D., Green, L. W., & Rootman, I. (Eds.). (2000). *Settings for health promotion: Linking theory and practice.* Thousand Oaks, CA: Sage Publications.

Poland, B. D., Krupa, E. & McCall (2007). Settings for health promotion: An analytic framework to guide intervention design and implementation. Manuscript submitted for publication.

Poland, B., Lehoux, P., Holmes, D., & Andrews, G. (2005). How place matters: unpacking technology and power in health and social care. *Health and Social Care in the Community, 13,* 170–180.

Poland, B., Frohlich, K. L., Haines, R., Mykhalovskiy, E., Rock, M., & Sparks, R. (2006). The social context of smoking: the next frontier in tobacco control? *Tobacco Control, 15*, 59–63.

Poland, B. (1996). Knowledge development and evaluation in, of, and for healthy community initiatives. Part I: Guiding principles. *Health Promotion International, 11*, 237–247.

Porter, S. (1993). Critical realist ethnography: the case of racism and professionalism in a medical setting. *Sociology, 27*, 591–665.

Polanyi, M., Frank, J., Shannon, H., Sullivan, T., & Lavis, J. (2000). The workplace as a setting for health promotion. In B. Poland, L. W. Green, & I. Rootman (Eds.), *Settings for health promotion: Linking theory and practice*. Thousand Oaks, CA: Sage Publications.

Potvin, L. (2007). Managing uncertainty through participation. In D. V. McQueen, I. Kickbusch, L. Potvin, J. Pelikan, L. Balbo, & T. Abel (Eds.), *Health & modernity. The role of theory in health promotion* (pp. 103–128). New York: Springer.

Potvin, L., Haddad, S., & Frohlich, K. L. (2001). Beyond process and outcome evaluation: A comprehensive approach for evaluating health promotion programs. In I. Rootman, M. Goodstadt, B. Hyndman, D.V. McQueen, L. Potvin, J. Springett, & E. Ziglio (Eds.), *Evaluation in health promotion: Principles and perspectives* (pp. 45–62). Copenhagen: WHO Regional Publications. European Series, No. 92.

Rissel, C. (1994). Empowerment: the holy grail of health promotion? *Health Promotion International, 9*, 39.

Rossi, P., & Freeman, H. (1985). *Evaluation: A systematic approach* (3rd ed). Thousand Oaks, CA: Sage Publications.

Santesso, N., & Tugwell, P. (2006) Knowledge translation in developing countries. *Journal of Continuing Education in the Health Professions, 26*, 87–96.

Sayer, A. (2000). *Realism and social science*. Thousand Oaks, CA: Sage Publications.

Schon, D. A. (1991). *The reflective practitioner: How professionals think in action*. Aldershot, UK: Arena Books.

Shadish, W. R., Cook, T. D., & Leviton, L. C. (1991). *Foundations of program evaluation: Theories of practice*. Newbury Park, CA: Sage Publications.

Simonsen, K. (1991). Toward an understanding of the contextuality of social life. *Environment and planning D: Society and space, 9*, 417–432.

Smith, M. F. (1989). *Evaluability assessment: A practical approach*. Boston, MA: Kluwer Academic Publishers.

Soubhi, H., & Potvin, L. (2000). Homes and families as health promotion settings. In B. Poland, L. W. Green, & I. Rootman (Eds.), *Settings for health promotion: Linking theory and practice* (pp. 44–67). Thousand Oaks, CA: Sage Publications.

Stame, N. (2004). Theory-based evaluation and varieties of complexes. *Evaluation, 10*, 58–76.

Stokols, D. (1992). Establishing and maintaining healthy environments: Toward a social ecology of health promotion. *American Psychologist, 47*, 6–22.

Stokols, D. (2000). The social ecological paradigm of wellness promotion. In M. Schneider Jamner & D. Stokols (Eds.), *Promoting human wellness: New frontiers for research, practice and policy* (pp. 21–37). Berkeley, CA: University of California Press.

Suchman, E. A. (1967). *Evaluative research: Principles and practice in public service action programs*. New York, NY: Russell Sage Foundation.

Weijer, C. (1999). Protecting communities in research: Philosophical and pragmatic challenges. *Cambridge Quarterly of Healthcare Ethics, 8*, 501–513.

Weiss, C. H. (1972). *Evaluation research: Methods of assessing program effectiveness*. Englewood Cliffs, NJ: Prentice-Hall.

Weiss, C. (1995). Nothing as practical as a good theory: Exploring theory based evaluation for comprehensive community initiatives for children and families. In J. P. Connell, A. C. Kubish, L. B. Schorr, & C. H. Weiss (Eds.), *New approaches to evaluating community initiatives: Concepts, methods and contexts* (pp. 65–92). Washington, DC: The Aspen Institute.

Weiss, C. H. (1997). Theory-based evaluation: past, present, and future. *New Directions for Evaluation, 76*, 41–56.

Wenger, E., McDermott, R., & Snyder, W. (2002) *Cultivating communities of practice: A guide to managing knowledge*. Boston, MA: Harvard Business School Press.

Wenger, E. (1998) *Communities of practice: Learning, meaning and identity*. Cambridge, MA: Cambridge University Press.

Wennberg, J. E., & Gittelsohn, A. (1973) Small area variation in health care delivery. *Science, 182*, 1102–1108.

Whitelaw, S., Braxendale, A., Bryce, C., MacHardy, L., Young, L., & Whitney, E. (2001). Settings based health promotion: A review. *Health Promotion International, 16*, 339–353.

Williams, G. H. (2003). The determinants of health: structure, context and agency. *Sociology of Health & Illness, 25*, 131–154.

Chapter 18
Conclusion

David V. McQueen and Louise Potvin

In this book we have first and foremost attempted to demonstrate and illustrate that health promotion poses unique problems for evaluation and that health promotion evaluators have acquired a great deal of maturity in dealing with the challenges of health promotion evaluation. Founded on an explicit set of humanist values, health promotion cannot be evaluated in ignorance of those values without undermining its potential to produce the desired effects. The contributors we solicited have convincingly demonstrated that it is possible to take health promotion values into account when designing and implementing evaluation research projects. Furthermore, the reflexive exercise that we asked them to perform, and report on, about their evaluation practice proved to be quite challenging. Indeed, beyond the application of methods to collect, analyze and report on data, authors have shown that conducting health promotion evaluation requires an in-depth knowledge of methods in order to operate the adaptations made necessary by the nature of the interventions evaluated. At the end of our project three issues seem worth exploring further—the richness of health promotion practice across the Americas, the omnipresence of preoccupation with participation in health promotion evaluation, and the emerging theme of equity.

Health Promotion Practice Across the Americas

At the outset of producing this book we sought to explore and understand, by both analysis and example, the unique character of health promotion evaluation in the Americas. We had two major assumptions: first, that health promotion in the Americas differed in many ways from that practiced on other continents and second, that there would be significant difference in the practice and evaluation of health promotion between the Anglophone North America and the non-Anglophone Americas. These assumptions were based on the premise that health promotion and health promotion evaluation are ultimately context-based practices.

D.V. McQueen
CDC, Atlanta, Georgia

L. Potvin, D. McQueen (eds.), *Health Promotion Evaluation Practices in the Americas*,
DOI: 10.1007/978-0-387-79733-5_18, © Springer Science+Business Media, LLC 2008   319

We were also cognizant from our experience in the Americas that the academic influences in the region were varied. In the United States there was a strong and well-developed health education base to health promotion. This base emphasized evaluation methods arising from social psychology and behavioral sciences; it also heavily emphasized experimental and quasi-experimental designs in evaluation. The literature that is most often cited originates from the United States with little import from other scientific traditions. Indeed, the U.S. literature is rich in evaluations of health promotion projects that aim at testing hypotheses originating from academia. In the United States, Schools of Public Health and more than 30 CDC funded academically-based Prevention Centers have an established tradition to carry out public health research and programs that are otherwise mostly unavailable through public organizations.

Because of the leading role and early involvement of Canadian scholars and civil servants in the development of the Ottawa Charter, Canadian-based health promotion had been much more influenced by concepts and principles stemming from the European continent. Several Canadian scholars and practitioners became early leaders and worldwide advocates of the Healthy City program and network (see for example Hancock, 1993; Hancock & Duhl, 1986). Original attempts at evaluating these projects raised many issues about the appropriateness and feasibility of the experimentalist tradition. Given the complexity and diversity of the social processes that needed to be implemented in the pursuit of healthy city objectives, it was felt that evaluation should answer questions related to how those projects were working and not be confined solely to attempting to isolate impact (O'Neill, 1993). Also, evaluation research budgets in Canada were never comparable with those available through U.S. research funding agencies. Canadian researchers who wanted to develop a knowledge base about health promotion intervention had to rely heavily on partnerships with public health organizations and negotiate with them how evaluation would improve their program. The Canadian Health Initiative provides an interesting example on how such model was implemented (Stachenko, 2001). In addition, the francophone part of Canada developed partnerships and projects with other francophone countries creating networks and health promotion practices that meet the specific circumstances of those populations. The "Reseau francophone international pour la promotion de la santé" is an example of such intiatives (http://www.refips.org/accueil.php). The absence of language barriers also facilitated access to the French literature not only related to health but also to social scientists such as Michel Foucault, Pierre Bourdieu or Bruno Latour whose impact on Western current conceptions of society and science has been significant.

Further south, in the Spanish and Portuguese speaking areas, very different literatures were influencing health promotion practice. Notably among these literatures were the educational theories of Paulo Freire in Brazil, and the long tradition of using critical theory (among which Marxism) to develop the social dimension in social epidemiology. This literature emphasized knowledge as a social construct and the resulting approaches to assessing interactions stemmed from a different epistemology from that commonly used in North America.

Contributors to this book borrowed heavily from all those literatures as can be observed by examining reference lists at the end of each chapter. Methods developed by South American colleagues such as Program Systematization (Westphal & Fernandez, 2008) had never been referenced in the Anglo-Saxon health promotion evaluation literature until now. Also, the sociology of translation developed by the French anthropologist of science Bruno relevant Latour (2001) proved to provide a powerful and theoretically framework for problematizing and understanding the use of evaluation research results. Thus it is not surprising that the chapters in this book illustrate a much broader perspective on evaluation in health promotion than is generally observed in the limited Anglophone literature. We have in fact several "literatures" on evaluation. We hope that this incursion into those rich literatures will trigger the curiosity of health promotion practitioners and evaluators and lead to much more frequent and systematic imports of those ideas to highlight and debunk health promotion evaluation dilemmas.

Distinguishing Community-Based Participatory Research from Evaluation Based on Participation

The contrast between the various literatures mobilized by health promotion evaluators across the Americas raises challenging questions for many of the fundamental concepts in present day health promotion research and evaluation. One of the key tenants of contemporary health promotion is the idea of participation. This is seen in the large literature on so-called participatory research. It is not the point to review this literature here, but, in summary, a fundamental ethos of health promotion is participation (Potvin, 2007) and this ethos is tied to another guiding principle of action. Fundamentally, in participatory action research (PAR), the idea is that, a group or community in which research is occurring is an active participant in the research process itself. By extension, evaluation research which is participatory must involve the group or community that is being evaluated. This assertion implies that, much of the health promotion evaluation traditionally practiced in North America violates the emerged epistemological basis of health promotion. This is particularly the case because the general experimental approach used requires that there be an objective distance between the evaluator and the group being evaluated. As the underlying epistemology moves from a basis in logical positivism to one involving reflective theory, the meaning of the evaluation experience, and its practice, changes drastically (McQueen, 2007). In brief, PAR is an ill fit to the epistemology stemming from logical positivism, but a better fit to alternative epistemologies. Perhaps this is why the level of comfort for the health promotion practitioner increases as they move away from the standard practice of evaluation based in logical positivism.

While the participatory action-based health promotion practitioners may become more comfortable as they move to an alternative epistemology such as that presented by Freire (1967), the world of public health research outside of health promotion is discomforted. Because most in health promotion work within a setting where evaluation is largely based on experimental method and a more traditional Western-based positivist approach, there is the tendency to retreat to the comfort of models that are understood by those providing the resources for evaluation.

Funding for evaluation is not a minor point. Earlier, the editors of the book *Evaluation in Health Promotion* (Rootman et al., 2001), following a careful discussion and extensive review of the state of evaluation in health promotion, in a report of the WHO European Working Group on Health Promotion Evaluation, supported by WHO(EURO), Health Canada and CDC, called explicitly for 10% of resources devoted to health promotion research and intervention to be set aside for evaluation (WHO European Working Group on Health Promotion Evaluation, 1999). Without specifying the type and character of evaluation it was recognized that evaluation was rarely a part of health promotion practice and would be unlikely to become such without it being specifically mandated by funding agencies. The exact words were: "Analysis of previous experience supports the Working Group's view that the allocation of 10% of total programme resources is a reasonable standard to ensure the development and implementation of appropriate evaluations in health promotion. This does not, however, preclude the allocation of additional resources when necessary"(WHO European Working Group on Health Promotion Evaluation, 1999, p. 10). Almost ten years since this call, the provision of resources for evaluation has rarely reached this level and funding remains a problem and a challenge. In particular this is a problem for those in the South American context where resources for evaluation are very scarce and one reason why this book presented such a formidable challenge to the authors.

However, there is another critical component of PAR in the Americas. The question arises: "Is the evaluation component inherent in PAR an American phenomenon?" More particularly is it a phenomenon that basically arises from the American epistemology in the South? Certainly the evaluation of PAR, as noted and illustrated in several chapters in this book (see for example Allard, Bilodeau, & Gendron, 2008; MacDonald & Mullet, 2008), cannot mesh easily with a traditional epistemology based in logical positivism. There is no well-defined and ontologically clear object of evaluation; there is no tight experimental design; knowledge is contextual. It is clear that the weak theoretical base for health promotion has needed re-examination (McQueen et al., 2007).

Equity and Evaluation

Participation is not the only shibboleth characterizing modern health promotion practice. Equity as a concept is fundamental. The argument is simply that the pursuit of health promotion must be the engagement of research, projects and actions that at a minimum do not reduce equity in a population and in best practice will increase equity. If evaluation is an integral component of health promotion practice it follows, ipso facto, that evaluation must also not disturb the equity balance in a negative way. For example, the finding of an evaluation that such and such a practice is not supported by sufficient evidence to support further funding of such practice may lead to withdrawal of resources from an intervention that is maintaining or increasing equity in a population although there is no evidence that the direct object of evaluation was improved. The methodology based in a positivistic epistemology could easily lead to this outcome.

Also disturbing is the dearth of evaluation research conducted and reported on with values of equity at the forefront. Evaluating equity in health promotion is complex and technical (Giacomini & Hurley, 2008; Potvin, Mantoura, & Ridde, 2007). It requires both a series of valid indicators to quantify inequalities and a normative basis to qualify the degree of fairness of observed inequalities. Unfortunately there is very little public discussion about what would represent a fair distribution of health and its determinants across the various social strata that form a society. This lack of public discourse would leave the evaluator interested in developing equity evaluations in some sort of vacuum. Maybe leading this public debate in a way that would lead to more clarity about what is acceptable or not in terms of health disparities is one task that health promotion practitioners and thinkers should undertake. Potvin et al. (2007) have already underlined that equity has remained a rhetoric in official documents with very little translation into action.

Finally the technical difficulties of evaluating health promotion in terms of equity are also a significant barrier. Technically, evaluating equity requires very large samples in order to estimate the interaction terms with sufficient statistical power. Such samples are not often available or possible given the general lack of funding for health promotion evaluation.

What Do We Have to Tell the Health Promotion and Evaluation Communities?

Based on the chapters in this book, what recommendations do we have for those in health promotion practice and for those concerned with the evaluation of that practice? When we asked contributors to this book to reflect on their experience as health promotion evaluators, many encountered a difficulty in the lack of relevant tools available to describe and critically appraise evaluation practice. The diversity of strategies used by our colleagues range from meta-evaluation (Hartz, Goldberg, Figueiro, & Potvin, 2008), to systematic case-studies (MacDonald & Mullet, 2008), to the presentation of practical tools that supported their practice (Allard et al., 2008) to a more anecdotal report of their practical strategies to illustrate difficulties. Therefore, it seems to us that one message for the overall evaluation community that stems from our project is that outside of realm of the scientific method, evaluators have very few tools to guide them to evaluate the quality of their practice. Indeed, there exist evaluation quality assessment criteria but these are usually designed to be applied when conducting meta evaluation (Stufffflebeam, 2001), and there is very little methodological guidance when it comes to using those criteria on specific projects. In addition, as illustrated by Hartz et al. (2008), many of those criteria are difficult to apply to health promotion and in order to appraise health promotion evaluations one needs also to design more specific criteria.

Another message that this project conveys to the broader evaluation community is that there is a lively and very active community of evaluators in the field of health promotion. These evaluators work from the north to the south of the American continents and the range of interventions that are subject to evaluation is broad and encompassing. Taken together, the practices that are discussed in this book testify to the dynamism of the field. Health promotion evaluators are aware of facing very specific difficulties in their work and they make significant efforts to develop and implement innovative practices. We believe that those practices are a testimony that it is possible to produce rigorous and useful knowledge while taking into account the values and principles promoted in a field of intervention such as health promotion. We hope that the examples developed in this book will be inspirational for evaluators in other fields who are also struggling with the issue of conducting relevant evaluations for social change programs that explicitly promote humanist values.

Finally, we believe that addressing head on the challenges that health promotion, because of its nature, represents for evaluation is also relevant for many other domains of evaluation. Health promotion is not the only intervention domain in which programs are often chaotic and messy, and in which the knowledge base calls for intersectoral work and partnership. In fact, the more open the system in which various types of programs are operating, and the more explicitly value-oriented they are, the more likely they are to present evaluation challenges that are akin to those posed by health promotion and discussed in this book. We do not pretend to have provided the final answer on how to conceive of the evaluation practice in order to better meet those challenges. We believe however, that in the continuity of the work of evaluators such as Schwandt (2005), Mark, Henry, and Julnes (2000), or Pawson and Tilley (1997), our mapping of those challenges and the possible directions in which one can look for guidance is further broadening the debate in a relevant manner.

Finally, we think that our project is important for the health promotion community. In view of the various projects conducted by a diversity of organizations to evaluate health promotion, the practitioners in the field might be under the impression that science, with its striving for rigor and pretension of objectivity represents a threat to what they want to achieve in the field. We hope that this project has opened up a window of opportunity for an increased dialog between researchers and practitioners. We believe that this book is an empirical demonstration that some scientists and evaluators made genuine efforts in order to develop an evaluation practice that aims at increasing the relevance of the knowledge produced by evaluation for their practice, because that knowledge is produced with the intervention principles and values in mind and in conditions that would not automatically undermine those values and principles.

There is still a long way to go for that dialog to be really fruitful. Our own practices as scientists have often promoted a greater divide between the messy world of politics, actions and interventions and the pure world of ideas, scientific rigor and theoretical elegance (Latour, 2005). And even when attempts are made to create that dialog, it seems that, as Latour (2001) tells us, the hierarchical conception of knowledge in which we operate often leads to situations in which scientists systematically undermine the arguments brought forward from a different perspective. There is a need for many more books similar to this one that would give practitioners an opportunity to discuss and expose their own perspectives and answers to the dilemmas associated with increasing the relevance of health promotion evaluation in the pursuit of the health promotion vision and project.

References

Allard, D., Bilodeau, A., Gendron, S. (2008). Figurative thinking and models: Tools for participatory evaluation. In L. Potvin & D. V. McQueen (Eds.), *Health promotion evaluation practices in the Americas: Values and research*. New York: Springer.

Freire, P. (1967). *Educação como prática de liberdade* Rio de Janeiro: Jorge Zahar.

Giacomini, M., & Hurley, J. (2008). Issues in evaluating equity. In L. Potvin & D. V. McQueen (Eds.), *Health promotion evaluation practices in the Americas: Values and research*. New York: Springer.

Hancock, T. (1993). The Healthy City from concept to application. Implications for research. In J. K. Davies & M. P. Kelly (Eds.), *Healthy Cities. Research & Practice* (pp. 14–24). London UK: Routledge.

Hancock, T., & Duhl, L. (1986). (WHO Healthy Cities Paper 1). *Healthy Cities: Promoting health in the urban context*. Copenhagen: FADL.

Hartz, Z., Goldberg, C., Figueiro, A. C., & Potvin, L. (2008). Multistrategy in the evaluation of health promotion community interventions: An indicator of quality. In L. Potvin & D. V. McQueen (eds.), *Health promotion evaluation practices in the Americas: Values and research*. New York: Springer.

Latour, B. (2001). *L'espoir de Pandore. Pour une vision réaliste de l'activité scientifique*. Paris: La découverte.

Latour, B. (2005). *Nous n'avons jamais été modernes. Essais d'anthropologie symétrique*. Paris: La découvcerte.

MacDonald, M., & Mullet, J. (2008). Dilemmas in health promotion evaluation: Participation and empowerment. In L. Potvin & D. V. McQueen (Eds.), *Health promotion evaluation practices in the Americas: Values and research*. New York: Springer.

McQueen, D. V. (2007). Critical issues in theory for health promotion. In D. V. McQueen, I. Kickbusch, L. Potvin, J. Pelikan, L. Balbo, & T. Abel (Eds.), *Health & modernity. The role of theory in health promotion* (pp. 21–42). New York: Springer.

McQueen, D. V., Kickbusch, I., Potvin, P., Pelikan, J., Balbo, L., Abel, T. (Eds.) (2007). *Health & modernity. The role of theory in health promotion*. New York: Springer.

Mark, M. M., Henry, G. T., & Julnes, G. (2000). Evaluation: An integrated framework for understanding, guiding, and improving policies and programs. San Francisco: Jossey Bass.

O'Neill, M. (1993). Building bridges between knowledge and action: the Canadian process of Health Community indicators. In J. K. Davies & M. P. Kelly (Eds.), *Healthy Cities. Research & Practice* (pp. 127–147). London UK: Routledge.

Pawson, R., & Tilley, N. (1997). *Realistic evaluation*. London UK: Sage.

Potvin, L. (2007). Managing uncertainty through participation. In D. V. McQueen, I. Kickbusch, L. Potvin, J. Pelikan, L. Balbo, & T. Abel (Eds.), *Health & modernity. The role of theory in health promotion* (pp. 103–128). New York: Springer.

Potvin, L., Mantoura, P., & Ridde, V. (2007). Evaluating equity in health promotion. In D. V. McQueen & C. M. Jones (Eds.), *Global perspectives on health promotion effectiveness* (pp. 367–384). New York: Springer.

Rootman, I., Goodstadt, M., Hyndman, B., McQueen, D. V., Potvin, L., Springett, J., et al. (Eds.) (2001). *Evaluation in health promotion. Principles and perspectives*. Conpenhagen: WHO Regional Publications, European Series, No 92.

Schwandt, T. A. (2005). The centrality of practice to evaluation. *American Journal of Evaluation, 26*, 95–105.

Stachenko, S. (2001). Case study: The Canadian heart health initiative. In I. Rootman, M. Goodstadt, B. Hyndman, D. V. McQueen, L. Potvin, J. Springett, & E. Ziglio (Eds.), *Evaluation in health promotion. Principles and perspectives* (pp. 463–473). Conpenhagen: WHO Regional Publications, European Series, No 92.

Stufflebeam, D. L. (2001). The metaevaluation imperative. *American Journal of Evaluation, 2*, 183–209.

Westphal, M. F., & Fernandez, J. C. A. (2008). The contribution of a systematization evaluative approach to implement a health promotion project in Capelo Socorro, Sao Paulo, Brazil. In L. Potvin & D. V. McQueen, (Eds.), *Health promotion evaluation practices in the Americas: Values and research*. New York: Springer.

WHO European Working Group on Health Promotion Evaluation. (1999). *Health promotion evaluation: Recommendations to policymakers*. Retrieved in March 2008 from: www.euro.who.int/document/e60706.pdf.

Index